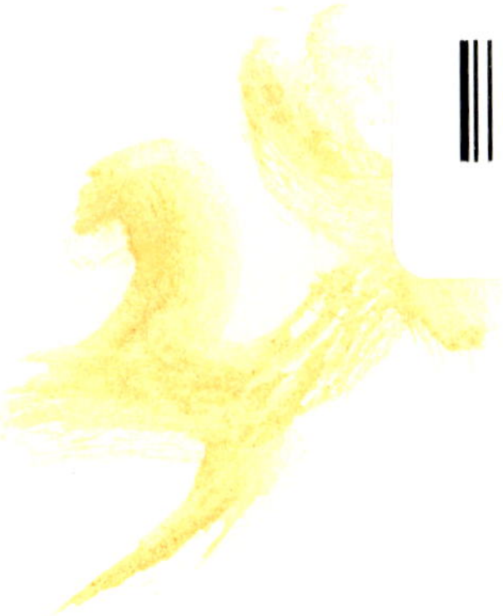

Chronicles from Central India : An Atlas of Rural Health

Jan Swasthya Sahyog, Chhattisgarh

Chronicles from Central India : An Atlas of Rural Health

Edition : 2016

ISBN: 978-93-5098-145-0 (Hb)

ISBN: 978-93-5098-146-7 (Pb)

Publisher :

Jan Swasthya Sahyog

Village and Post Ganiyari,

District Bilaspur,

Chhattisgarh, 495112

Facebook.com/jssbilaspur

Twitter.com/jssbilaspur

www.jssbilaspur.org

Print :

INDIGO

9313852068

Jan Swasthya Sahyog (JSS) is a not for profit organization of health workers and professionals who work in Chhattisgarh. While service is the main objective of the work, we use the force multipliers of training, observational research and advocacy to improve the health status of the marginalized rural communities.

Copies of the book may be obtained from Jan Swasthya Sahyog, by writing to:
janswasthya@gmail.com

“Medicine is a social science, and politics is nothing else but medicine on a large scale. Medicine, as a social science, as the science of human beings, has the obligation to point out problems and to attempt their theoretical solution: the politician, the practical anthropologist, must find the means for their actual solution. The physicians are the natural attorneys of the poor, and social problems fall to a large extent within their jurisdiction”.

–Rudolf Virchow

Dedicated to all the “Nobodies” who shared their stories, and inspired us.

Contents

about the book

Rural and tribal health in India fares far worse on all possible counts and parameters as compared to urban health due to a variety of reasons. People in rural areas suffer the consequences of adverse availability of the socio-economic determinants of health: food, poor environment and distance from health facilities, education and poor health systems. It is not surprising to see almost all diseases in much higher numbers and in more complex forms among rural and tribal people as compared to urban dwellers. Our work and our experience has taught us that *disease is the biological embodiment of deprivation.*

The Jan Swasthya Sahyog (JSS), literally the People's Health Support Group, is a collective of health professionals and workers, many of whom were trained at leading medical institutions in the country like AIIMS, has been running a health programme in rural Chhattisgarh in central India. A primarily service-based programme, JSS serves tribal and rural communities, covering over 1.5 million people in what could arguably be the epicentre of underdevelopment. We also train health workers at the village level and nurses and doctors at a higher level, conduct research on key health problems of the rural poor, and provide advocacy based on careful documentation to positively impact rural health care. The JSS also serves as a watering hole for those venturing into the uncertain world of public health for rural India.

Over the last 16 years, during which we have set up a modest community health programme in rural Bilaspur, catering to over 2,500 villages in north-western Chhattisgarh and south-eastern Madhya Pradesh, we have observed and tried to manage massive levels of hunger, malnutrition, resultant illnesses and much avoidable mortality. While we have tried to document disease patterns and distribution among the populace and occasionally published them in peer reviewed journals, we have also felt the need to explore and to understand their causes – not just their proximate biomedical causes but also the social, economic and cultural roots of these diseases.

As physicians and health workers interested primarily in the whys and hows of health, disease and with the primary objective of reducing inequity in health care among rural and tribal poor, we have also investigated regimes of political and economic values and policies that condition tacit aspects of sociocultural practices that in turn impact the cause and occurrence of disease – specifically, the role of structural violence. So in a sense, this book is also about the political economy of the ailments of the rural and tribal poor in India.

Of the wide spectrum of human ailments, we started with a list of 50 odd illnesses that we commonly see in our hospital and health centres at Ganiyari, Shivtarai, Semariya and Bamhani in Chhattisgarh. In trying to understand the causes of illness, we went back to the patient, to his/her family, hamlet and village, and thus we discovered the geographic, cultural, social and economic predicaments that lay behind the illness. We have tried to weave these together in the form of individual patient narratives, supplementing them with photo essays and commentaries on the causes of illness based on our understanding and experience.

Why do we call it an Atlas? Because it records the journey of specific ailments through time and includes graphics preferentially to highlight their causes. It tries to capture the complexity of ills in rural health in India in its right coordinates and perspective; for example, tuberculosis in Delhi is certainly not the same as tuberculosis in rural Bilaspur or any other rural area. The *Atlas* thus also emphasizes the need and importance of repositioning prevailing understanding of illnesses.

In this collection, there are **27 patient narratives** for a similar number of ailments. This is not an exhaustive list of ailments that we encounter, nor are these the most common ones. We plan a second volume that will include more narratives. We have also included over **40 picture stories** with short annotations, a few personalised **blog notes** that try to capture key aspects of the causes of disease, and several **disease maps** that represent the unequal distribution of diseases in the states of India. The 'state' may not be the only or the best axis to highlight the differential occurrence of disease, but we have retained it as a starting reference point. The disease maps included here capture just how unequal we are as a country. Finally, we have included a few poems and lists of books and films that capture inequity in health and disease prevalent among Indians.

Who would find this *Atlas* useful? Anyone concerned with human development and who views health as its essential component, and anyone working for greater equity and justice. Particularly, our co-travellers including those who are considering starting their journey in working for the health of the disadvantaged, whether they be medical and health professionals, social scientists, or those in a position to influence policy and practices in health care. We hope that these narratives will serve as a valuable compendium of rural health in India. We also hope that this synthesis of ideas based on a discussion of the socio-economic and biomedical causes of disease will allow for the development of a more inclusive perspective while providing fresh and innovative ideas for more equitable action. It could also be a resource base for developing training materials and programmes, advocacy strategies and a more nuanced perspective of rural health for all those interested in the health of the poor.

The making of this book, conceived about nine years ago, has been a labour of much love and sustained commitment to a vision. We would like to acknowledge all those people and their families whose stories and photographs are contained in this *Atlas* and who gave us permission to share them with you. Their names have been changed to maintain confidentiality. This print edition will be followed up with an online edition that will also include videos to supplement the text and pictures.

Yogesh Jain
for the Jan Swasthya Sahyog Collective

a worker's speech to a doctor

We know what makes us ill.
When we're ill word says
You're the one to make us well

For ten years, so we hear
You learned how to heal in elegant schools
Built at the people's expense
And to get your knowledge
Dispensed a fortune
That means you can make us well.

Can you make us well?

When we visit you
Our clothes are ripped and torn
And you listen all over our naked body.
As to the cause of our illness
A glance at our rags would be more
Revealing. One and the same cause wears out
Our bodies and our clothes.

The pain in our shoulder comes
You say, from the damp;
            and this is also the cause
Of the patch on the apartment wall.
So tell us then:
Where does the damp come from?

Too much work and too little food
Make us weak and scrawny.
Your prescription says:
Put on more weight.
You might as well tell a fish
Go climb a tree

How much time can you give us?
We see: one carpet in your flat costs
The fees you take from
Five thousand consultations
You'll no doubt protest
Your innocence. The damp patch
On the wall of our apartments
Tells the same story.

– Bertolt Brecht

small people
big problems

The Narratives

snake bite

Dal Singh and Aghani Bai

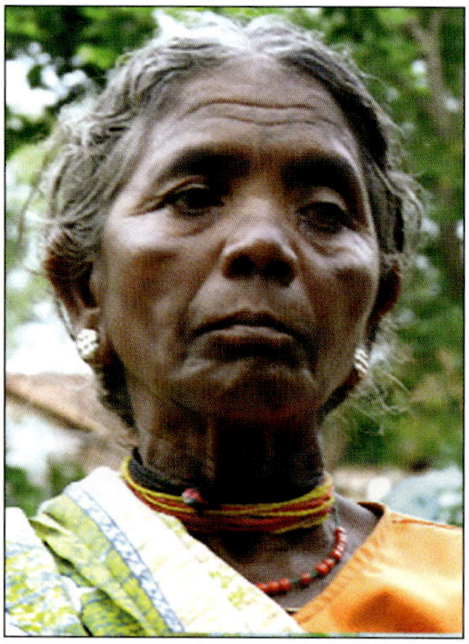

Aghani Bai lost her son on the day of Hareli, a festival celebrating the end of the planting season during the month of Saawan, at the height of the monsoons. She lived in a village in the remote Achanakmar Tiger Reserve area in a house neighbouring that of her son and his family. That day, after praying for a good yield and eating a hearty meal, her son, Dal Singh, went home with his wife and five children.

Sometime later that night, Dal Singh felt a cold sensation on his neck. Instinctively he put up his hand and his fingers closed in on something which bit him on the wrist. He immediately raised an alarm, calling for his mother who was sleeping next door with his three nieces. In the dim light of a lantern, his wound was revealed to be snakebite. A local belief held that if the snake that had bitten a person was killed, the person too would die. So Dal Singh carefully moved it away with a stick. The snake, which crawled into a hole in the brick wall, was revealed to be a common krait. The bite of the krait is often fatal.

Aghani Bai rallied the village elders and after the initial confusion, a party set out into the forest with lanterns to find a herbal plant that the Baiga tribals considered an antidote to snake venom. The roots were ground up and mixed with water and some of the mixture was given to Dal Singh to drink while the rest was plastered onto his wound. The local *jholachhaap*, an untrained village 'doctor', was summoned; he injected Dal Singh twice, once in the left arm and once in the right with what might have been saline solution, a standard treatment by such 'doctors'.

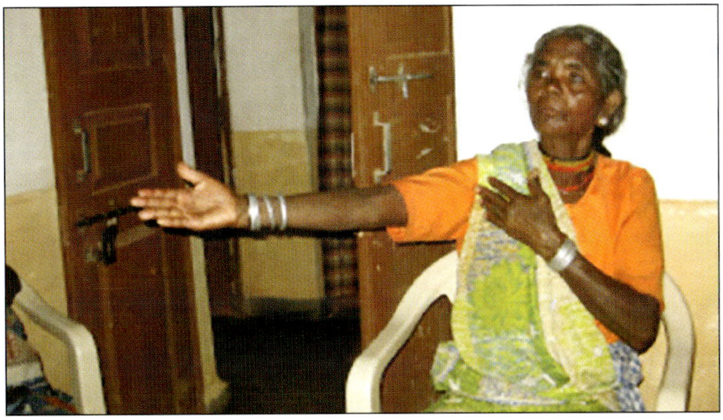

These 'remedies' did not work, and Dal Singh seemed to realize this. 'My mother and my brother: I know you will not be able to save me now,' he said. He put his palms together and with the words 'Ram Johar' bid farewell to all those present. His arm and fingers had swelled up, but he did not complain of the pain. His body turned the colour of turmeric. Aghani Bai and those present watched helplessly as the continued administration of herbal medicine failed to revive him. As the dawn broke, Dal Singh breathed his last.

Jan Swasthya Sahyog's snakebite awareness posters advise villagers not to waste time on traditional medicine. However, Aghani Bai was convinced that others who had taken the herbs had recovered. She believed that her son was the object of much jealousy, being educated up to class 8 and the vital point of contact for the forest officers and the village sarpanch. 'When my son was bitten, someone must have done *jaadutona* (black magic) on him and that must be why the herbs and injections didn't work,' she said.

Following her son's death, Aghani Bai was plunged into debt. She had to borrow Rs. 3000 from Dal Singh's in-laws for his funeral, repaying them with the harmonium with which he used to sing Chhattisgarhi folk songs. Her other son and Dal Singh's widow also shared part of the expenses, but Aghani Bai was left to shoulder a debt of Rs. 2000 after the ten-day funeral.

Soon afterwards, Dal Singh's widow, whom he had married after the death of his first wife, remarried and left the house with their two sons. Dal Singh's three daughters from his previous marriage were left with Aghani Bai. One of them also married soon and moved away. Aghani Bai was left to take care of a six-year old and a ten-year old. A widow herself, she was too old to work on her own land, so she hired some help to plough and sow it. She worked eight hours a day on the lands of others to earn Rs. 40 a day. Two of the five sacks of rice harvested from her land would go to pay the hired help and another two would feed her family. The last would be saved for seed. Aghani Bai also took up work as a *dai* or village midwife along with three other elderly women in her village. She would walk an hour and a half to the JSS sub-centre at Bamhani to be trained for this role, for which she received Rs. 150 per month. She scraped together a living with a will to educate her granddaughters until class 8, after which she hoped their education would help them get married into good families.

Aghani Bai also applied for a widow's pension to help supplement her income, an optimistic endeavour, as no one in her village had ever succeeded in getting it. Like them, she waited for five years, but the pension never came.

Dal Singh's death was not just an economic blow to the family, it took a psychological toll as well. 'I feel as if I have lost my soul,' says the bereaved mother, tears welling up in her eyes whenever someone mentions her son. She wonders when she will be reunited with him again and she waits.

Three years after her son's death, the first rains brought another krait into Aghani Bai's house. Her elder son killed it, but that night Aghani Bai could not sleep peacefully. She kept a stick under her cot and an ear alert to even the slightest sound. Even a mouse scurrying on the roof would disturb her and she would get up to shine a torch in every corner of the house. When the children asked why she had woken up, she would say she had been disturbed by the sound of an insect. Then she would crawl back under the mosquito net and wait for sleep.

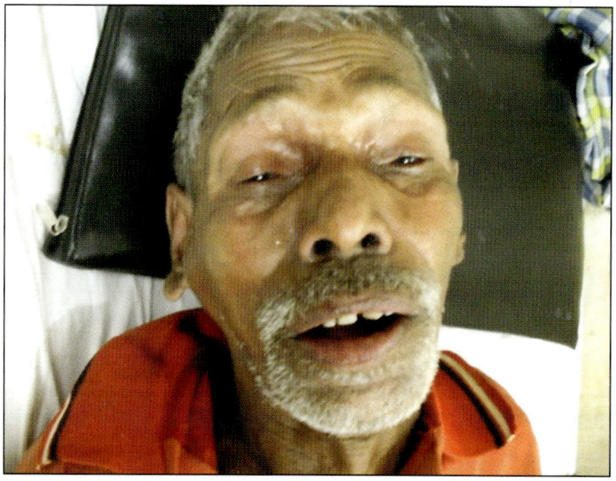

Deaths due to snakebites

Snakes will be present wherever there are rodents, and rodents will be there where food grain is stored and there are mud floors for them to make holes to live in.

And this controlling of the rodent population is in fact one great service that snakes do for us. However, the proximity of rats and snakes to human habitations, almost exclusively in rural situations where most houses still have mud floors even if the walls and roofs may be *pucca*, makes rural people vulnerable to snakebites due to accidental contact between snakes and humans.

This can happen at night while sleeping when humans may unknowingly obstruct the path of snakes that might be moving about in search of prey – rats and frogs – especially if people are sleeping on the floor. Or it may happen when people accidentally step on snakes while walking on the bunds, working in their fields, while harvesting, or when they put their hands into cool, dry, dark places where snakes prefer to rest.

There are four major poisonous snakes in India: the common krait, the saw-scaled viper, the cobra and the Russell's viper. Of this, the most important numerically is the common krait. This snake almost exclusively bites at night and produces neuroparalysis, which could appear as early as within an hour or two or may take up to twenty-four hours to show up.

Otherwise conscious, a person with a krait or cobra bite may show drooping of eyelids, an inability to pull out the tongue and may experience blurry or double vision as early symptoms much before their breathing gets affected. Someone might even mistake such a person to be drunk or having consumed some intoxicant. And often there is no bite mark or any significant local site pain.

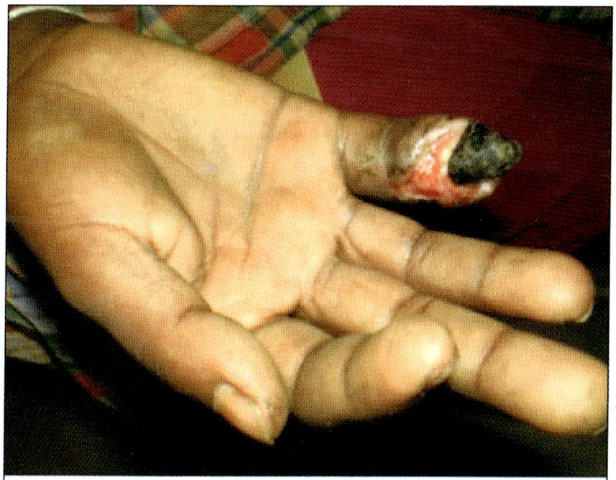

Blackening and gangrene of a finger due to a tight tourniquet tied at the base of the finger on which a bite of a snake had happened.

Since most if not all of these bites happen at night time, it is particularly important to ensure speedy transportation to a treating facility. We know that all transportation, especially from remote rural areas, is poor at night. No wonder that a large proportion of people with snakebites die due to respiratory paralysis even before they reach the hospital, as it happened with Aghani Bai's son Dal Singh.

The necessary first aid is to immobilise the bitten part or limb as one would do for a fractured limb by using a wooden splint held secure by bandages. This will reduce the spread of the venom to the bloodstream. There is no need to use a very tight tourniquet proximal to the bite in order to reduce the venom spread; inappropriately tight tourniquets can also be harmful as the stoppage of blood flow might cause gangrene of fingers or hands.

Thus, to prevent deaths due to snakebites, besides making people's homes safer by making pucca houses and using personal protection and precautionary measures to reduce the risk of accidental snakebites, what is needed is widespread awareness of how poisonous snakebites manifest and the need to quickly reach a health facility capable of treating them. Centres that can treat poisonous snakebite victims with anti-snake venom (ASV) and other treatment should be well distributed and no one should have to travel more than an hour to such a facility. Secondly, there should also be adequate and free availability of public transport to ferry victims from the remotest habitations to such facilities. An adequate stock of ASV and other drugs should be available, and physicians and nurses should be well trained to administer these life-saving drugs.

So while accidental snakebites will occur where there are snakes, if we have an equitable and efficient healthcare system, we can ensure that no one dies of snakebites or loses a limb or an organ. And this facility should be available to all people irrespective of their economic status, especially in remote rural areas. Snakebite envenomation is one of the neglected health problems of rural India owing to which so many avoidable deaths take place every year. Close to a hundred people die of snakebite every year in Bilaspur district alone, and almost all the deaths are preventable.

The Million Death Study showed that 0.47% of total deaths were assigned to snakebites mostly in rural areas, and more commonly among males than females, peaking between the ages 15 to 29. Snakebites also occurred more often during the monsoon season. This proportion represents about 45,900 annual snakebite deaths nationally (99% CI 40,900 to 50,900) or an annual age-standardised rate of 4.1/100,000 (99% CI 3.6 – 4.5), with higher rates in rural areas (5.4) and with the highest rate in the state of Andhra Pradesh (6.2). Annual snakebite deaths were highest in the states of Uttar Pradesh (8,700), Andhra Pradesh (5,200), and Bihar (4,500). Thus, snakebite remains an underestimated cause of accidental death in India today, causing about one death for every two HIV-related deaths. It is more than 30-fold higher than the number declared from official hospital returns largely because most deaths happen outside the hospitals. This study shows that only 23% of the snakebite deaths identified in our survey occurred in hospital.

How many cases of snakebites would there be in India every year? This study suggests at least 1.4 million non-fatal bites corresponding to the 45,000 fatal bites. The actual number of non-fatal bites in India may well be far higher as the community-based study in Bangladesh found about 100 non-fatal bites for each death.

This study emphasises three points: (i) hospital-based data reflects poorly the national burden of fatal snakebites; (ii) inadequacy of current treatment of snakebite in India; and (iii) vulnerability of snakebite victims outside hospital areas. Practical solutions include strengthening surveillance to allow a more accurate perception of the magnitude of the problem, improving community education to reduce the incidence of snakebites and speed up the transfer of victims to medical care, improving the training of medical staff at all levels of the health service including implementation of the new WHO guidelines, and deployment of appropriate anti-venoms and other interventional tools where they are needed in rural health facilities to decrease case fatality.

malnutrition & body mass index

Three stories: Rising GDP Falling BMI

Phagni Bai

Phagni Bai Baiga, a mother of four, had wrapped a shawl around herself as she waited for her two saris to dry. She was at her parent's home in Littikhola, a small village at the base of a mountain in Bilaspur district. When asked how she was doing, she smiled and said 'good'. She added that her son, too, was much better now and that the swelling of his stomach had gone down.

But in reality, things were far from good. Phagni Bai's husband had contracted tuberculosis two years ago, but with treatment and follow up by JSS, he was cured. A year later when Phagni Bai started to show symptoms of TB, she did not come to JSS because the family worried that they would have to arrange for Rs. 700 to meet expenses once again. So she wasted away in the remote village of Kurdar on top of the mountain. A few months later, her nine-year old son also began to waste away from TB.

The main source of livelihood for Baiga families in Kurdar is weaving baskets from bamboo collected from the forest. The baskets sold for rupees 15 to 20 each. One had to walk up to five hours one way to gather bamboo, evading the vigilant eyes of the Forest Department. When her husband fell sick, Phagni Bai was the only one fit to work, reducing their income to Rs. 300 a week. They could not afford to buy enough broken rice from the market to supplement the monthly subsidized 35 kg at Rs. 1 that they got from the ration shop. So when they had to buy rice, they ate less. As her husband recovered, Phagni became too weak to work, passing on the mantle of earning a livelihood to her husband.

At this time Phagni Bai aged 30, height 151 cm, weighed 25.7 kg and her body-mass index or

BMI was 11.3. Her son Raja, aged 9, height 91 cm weighed 10 kg with a BMI of 12. The disproportionately large appearance of Phagni's shoulder joints, her high collar bone lurking beneath her clothes, the swollen belly of her child tells of the vicious cycle of losing control over natural resources and livelihood, food security and health like nothing else could.

Ramkali Baiga

Ramkali's wrists seemed oversized compared to her wiry forearms as she tried to lift a handwoven cotton saree. She had been admitted at the JSS hospital in Ganiyari. At the age of 22, she weighed 24.6 kg, was 147 cm tall with a BMI of 11.38.

Married into a Baiga family across the border in Madhya Pradesh, Ramkali had to walk 10 hours to get to her in-laws. The landless family survived on broken rice bought from the open market, the cost of which severely restricted the intake of each individual. Her father-in-law had died of TB, followed by her husband. With an immune system severely compromised due to inadequate food, it was only natural for Ramkali to get infected by TB. 'He was emaciated like me' and had been treated with a 'suji-botel,' she explained matter-of-factly, referring to the quacks who pushed injections and administered saline water for most maladies.

Before coming to JSS, Ramkali had been living with her parents in the village of Bijrakachar. We caught up with Ramkali's parents Mahuku and Mangli Baiga, cooking dinner in the open field across the road from JSS. 'If we had more rice at home, we would cook more,' said Mahuku. Over the years they had lost access to the fruits, herbs and animals from the forest. 'Parts of the forests have been illegally taken over by some people who use it to rear cattle and sell milk in the cities'. Mahuku's agitation was palpable.

Although the family owned 5 acres of land, it yielded only 3 quintals of rice. A plot of that size in a moderately fertile area should have yielded between 40 to 50 quintals.

Mahuku remembered *bewar* (slash and burn agriculture) from his younger days in which they would scatter seeds of kutki, maria, salihar, bajra, makka, jhurga (kutki, ragi, bajra as millets, and maize and lobia as pulses) and many more varieties of grain. Such agriculture was not allowed anymore and the varied nutrition such grains provided has been replaced by a single type of rice. Traditionally, Chhattisgarh has had 22,000 varieties of paddy as well as a large variety of other grains.

In the ten days that Ramkali was in hospital, she did not gain any weight. The doctors were concerned. She was on a drip, one drop at a time entering her body, and yet another day that she wished she was home, taking care of her five year-old daughter.

Dhansaye Nagone

The headlights shone on a thin frame of a man in a blue fleece and a cloth wrapped around his head and ears. He was hanging on from the edge of a diesel auto-rickshaw, much the way he hung on for survival in an economic system that counted on his cheap labour but without letting him count on a decent survival.

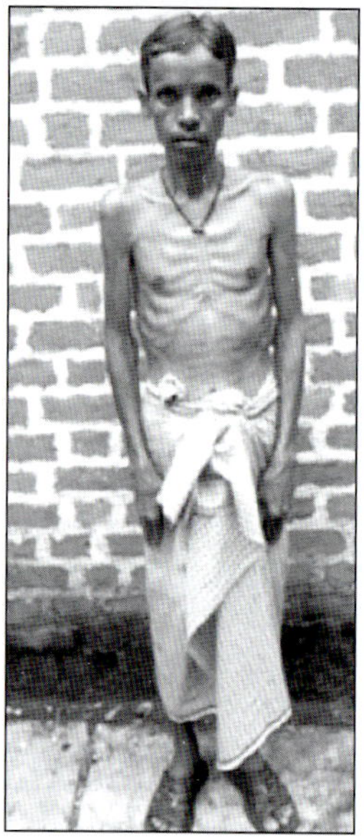

Thirty-six year old Dhansaye Nagone weighed just 43 kg in May 2010 when he was caring for his sister admitted with TB in JSS. 'At that weight he was already susceptible,' explained Dr. Jain of JSS, going through Dhansaye's history in the OPD. In the intervening ten months, Dhansaye lost another 8 kg. Despite such telltale signs, a major medical institution in Bilaspur had failed to diagnose his condition. Dhansaye spent Rs. 550 buying medicines which were completely useless for him.

'I asked the doctor to take a better look since my sister had already fought with TB a few months ago. But the doctor shooed me away,' Dhansaye had said with resignation. For the poor, we learnt, uncompassionate, expensive, exploitative, irrational and un-contextual healthcare were as much killers as the diseases themselves.

Dhansaye lived with his wife and three children in the city of Bilaspur and drove a cycle-rickshaw for a livelihood, earning up to Rs. 75 a day. The family, which paid a monthly rent of Rs. 400 and an electricity bill of Rs. 100, subsisted mainly on 35 kg of grain (15 kg wheat + 20 kg rice) bought at a BPL (below poverty line) price of Rs 2 per kg from the ration shop.

The poor of India, especially the adivasis, have been caught in the vice-like grip of a policy regime that transferred common property resources to private entities for profits to boost the gross domestic product (GDP), displacing the lives and livelihoods of all those who lived close to the land. The centralizing nature of the global economy fuelled by subsidized energy has displaced all forms of non-mechanized and decentralized production, eliminating millions of livelihoods and resulting in increased food insecurity. According to the economist Utsa Patnaik, the average Indian family's grain consumption had fallen by 110 kg between 1991 and 2005.

These stories are typical of cases seen at JSS at every OPD. In 2011, JSS treated 587 cases of TB with the average patient BMI of 16.17 – a substantial increase over 470 cases in 2010.

Nine per cent of patients had BMIs of less than 13 – a level below which is medically considered incompatible with life. In 2015, 58% of people with tuberculosis seen at JSS had a BMI of less than 16 – a cut-off for severe undernutrition and a level at which the body fat is zero. Despite the best treatment, the chances of dying at or below a BMI of 16 is at least three times higher than if it is more than 16. Mind you, the BMI is only a measure of wasting, i.e. losing weight after gaining weight. If you have low weight and height due to chronic or longstanding food deprivation from childhood onwards, you would be severely undernourished, and yet show a normal BMI.

A rising GDP at the cost of falling BMI certainly did not bode well for the health of the nation. In fact, it should be unacceptable to any civilized society.

rabies

Jethuram

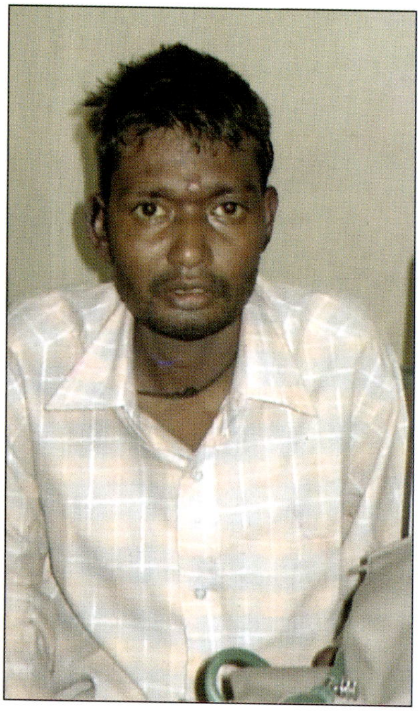

Jethuram was a Baiga tribal living in a forest village in Central Chhattisgarh, which was difficult to access at the height of the monsoon. While retrieving his cattle from the neighbouring village of Khudiya, Jethuram was attacked by a stray dog which bit his left thigh, just above his knee. His companions immediately sent him back to his village, where he swallowed an assortment of herbs and roots gathered from the forest. The pain lasted for a week, and then he forgot about it.

Three months later, his wife Sham Bai was witness to a frightening degeneration of her husband's physical and mental condition, and even more frightening, to the prospect of a life without him.

The pain in Jethuram's leg had returned and his behaviour began to change. He became prone to violent outbursts, trying to hit his wife and breaking pots and whatever else he could get hold of. Sham Bai and her four children began to fear him. When his behaviour escalated, someone they knew suggested they take him to Ganiyari for treatment. A call was made to the Jan Swasthya Sahyog sub-centre at Bamhani, and a vehicle was dispatched to the village.

At Ganiyari, the doctors confirmed that Jethuram had rabies. But there was nothing they could do for him now. Sham Bai was given permission to take him home to die.

Sham Bai likened her husband's behaviour in his last few hours to that of a dog, saying that even the family was afraid that he would bite them.

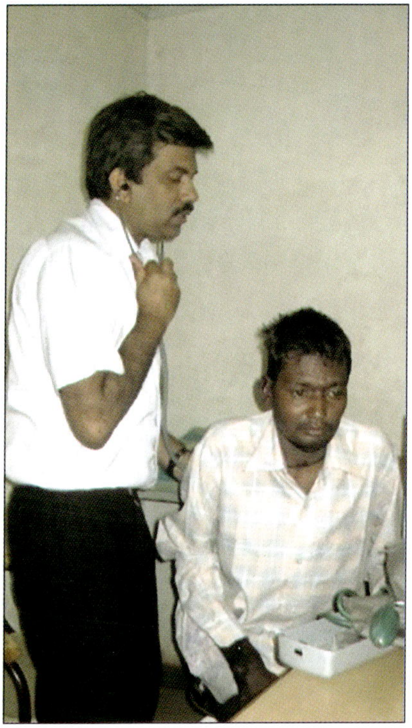

'He would shout and scream like a dog and come after us,' Sham Bai recounted. Jethuram ate his evening meal, but drank very little water. The next day he locked himself up in his room, but emerged when the family went out to work. On their return he made tea and served it to them, but Sham Bai was afraid to drink it, afraid of catching his illness.

When Sham Bai told her husband that the rabies was going to kill him, he said that after he was gone, his four daughters would be married off. 'You will find another husband and my son will be an orphan,' he said, 'So I am going to kill you'.

But Jethuram could not carry out his threat. Instead, in a sudden moment of clarity, he realized the predicament in which he was leaving his wife and children. He instructed his elder daughter to always go with her mother to the forest when she was collecting edible mahua flowers and told his wife to get someone to cultivate their land so that the family would be able to live off the crops. As he gagged, retched and vomited, he told her to make sure that their children would be fed. Jethuram attempted to walk out of the house, but collapsed. 'He vomited like a dog, lots of foamy vomit, and then he died,' Sham Bai said.

The incident scared and upset the family so badly that they did not want to live in that house any more. For three months, Sham Bai was too scared to even enter it. She eventually had the house brought down and moved her family into a single room nearby. And it was thereafter that all her troubles began.

First, she had to borrow Rs. 4,000 for Jethuram's funeral. Her land lay unused because there was no one to help her plough or till it. Jethuram's brothers were all dead, and her own brother in Boiraha did not want to shoulder her burden. Sham Bai went to work as a daily labourer, bringing home Rs. 40 every day. While eligible for subsidized rice from the ration shop, it wasn't nearly enough for the family. She had to make 12-16 km trips with her daughter just to collect the 35 kgs of rice that was due to them. When out of rice, she would buy broken rice from the market or borrow from the neighbours.

At her wit's end, Sham Bai went to find a proper term panchayat office with all her problems, and her realization: '*Mola koi posaiya nikko* [There is no one to take care of me]'. She submitted her identity card and other papers to the panchayat office for a widow's pension. Then she ran from pillar to post, getting documents from the block headquarters and submitting them at the Khudiya Forest Range office. The officer there said he would forward her papers to Bilaspur and inform her when her cheque arrived. That was the last she heard from him.

Circling back to the panchayat, Sham Bai found out that her village was apparently no longer under the jurisdiction of that particular sarpanch. So she went to another panchayat at Danganiya, where the new sarpanch wrote her name down amongst all the others who needed a nirashrit pension. That was the last that she heard from him, too.

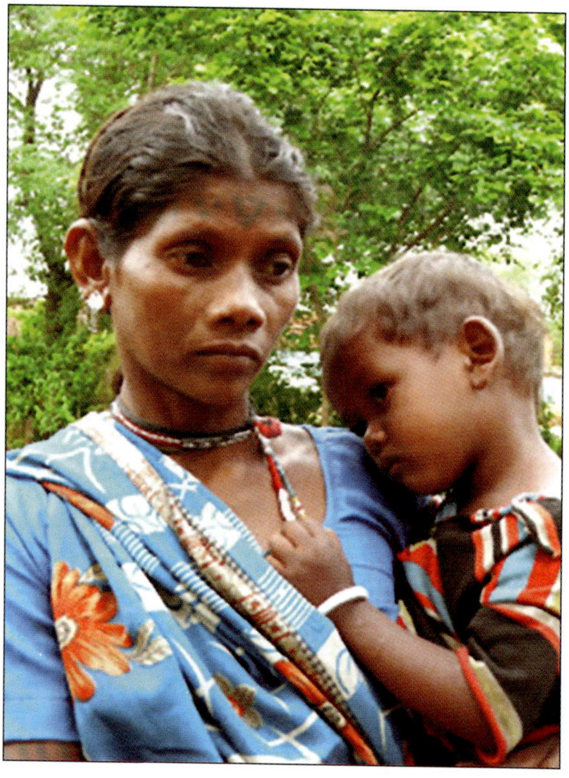

Rabies is one illness that is almost 100% preventable if correct and timely interventions are made, and 100% fatal if timely prevention is not done. There is no other human illness that we know that has a similar epidemiology. A disease of antiquity, rabies has been partially controlled in many countries and eliminated in a few. However, according to the World Health Organization (WHO), rabies continues to kill thousands of people in India each year, more than in any

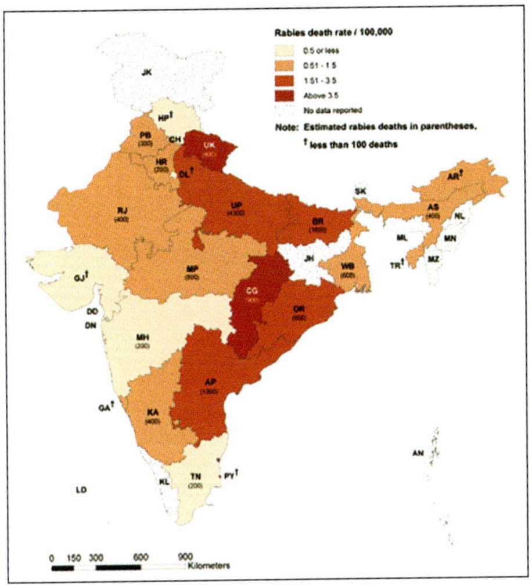

other country. Using a verbal autopsy to identify the causes of over 122,000 deaths on a large scale, (for a representative sample in India in 2001–03), the estimation in the Million Death Study (2005), approximately 12,700 people died from symptomatically identifiable furious rabies. Because verbal autopsy is not able to identify atypical presentations of rabies, our figure underestimates the actual number of rabies deaths in India. The Government of India's official figure of reported deaths, in the range of 244 to 556 per year between 2000 and 2009, is based on routine hospital surveillance. These reports of rabies deaths from hospitals are underestimates for several reasons. Most deaths in India occur at home, in rural areas outside medical care. There are large numbers of stray dogs in India. In many states, lack of community access to awareness and education about post-exposure rabies prophylaxis and adherence to traditional beliefs about the disease are likely to increase the risk of developing rabies after being bitten by a rabid dog.

The majority of rabies deaths occurred in males in rural areas and in children below the age of 15 years, (see figure). The concentrated geographic distribution of rabies in India suggests that targeting with preventive campaigns, including the vaccination of animals and post-exposure vaccination of humans, might achieve a significant reduction in the number of deaths or potentially, even elimination of mortality from this disease.

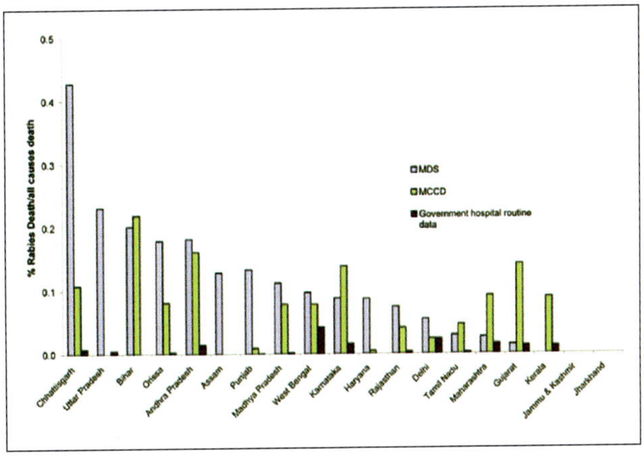

There is another issue. The clustering of rabid dog bites and subsequent rabies in humans makes a case for routine immunization of children prophylactically, which is still not done in India.

Typically, prevention after a rabid bite consists of three parts: (i) methodically cleaning the wound; (ii) administering the vaccine according to a schedule; and (iii) if the bite is of class 3, then administering the rabies antiserum in a standardised way. Tragically, there is a global shortage of rabies antiserum which threatens to disrupt preventive strategies in controlling rabies. And the poorest are likely to suffer the most from this artificial shortage.

In 2016, even a single episode of rabies is unacceptable, and is only a reminder of the poor public health provision and the inequity in health care in India.

More about rabies

Domestic animals infected with rabies may appear sick, crazed, or vicious. This is the origin of the phrase 'mad dog'. However, domestic animals infected with rabies may also appear to be overly friendly, docile, confused, or even completely normal. In the case of wild animals, any unusual behaviour, for example, seeing a normally nocturnal wild animal (like a bat or a fox) during the day or seeing a normally shy wild animal that does not avoid human presence, seems bold or even friendly should raise suspicion that it may have rabies.

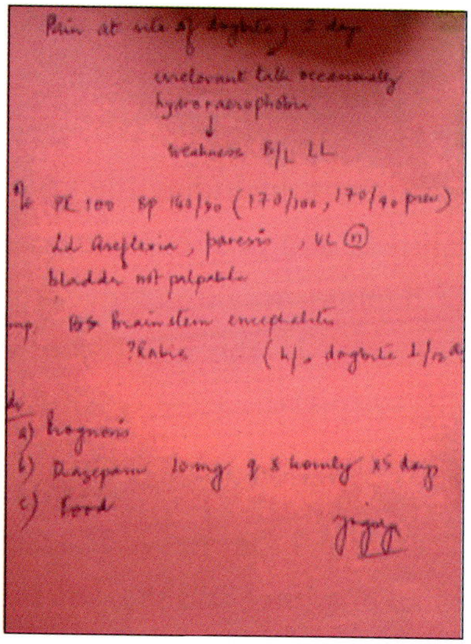

In humans, the average incubation period (the time from being infected till when the first symptoms appear) is 30–60 days, but it may range from less than 10 days to several years. Most people first develop symptoms of tingling, itching or pain shooting from the bite site (or site of virus entry). Nonspecific complaints of fevers, chills, fatigue, muscle aches, and irritability may accompany these complaints. In the early stages, these symptoms may appear similar to those of the flu, fever or similar virus infections, except for the shooting sensations from the bite site.

Gradually, however, the afflicted individual develops a

range of symptoms, including high fever, confusion, agitation, and eventually seizures and coma. Typically, people with rabies develop irregular contractions and spasms of the breathing muscles when exposed to water, a condition termed *hydrophobia*. They may demonstrate the same response to a puff of air directed at them, which is termed *aerophobia*. By this stage, the disease is greatly advanced. Eventually, various body organs are afflicted and the person dies despite support with medication and a respirator.

A rarer form of rabies, **paralytic rabies**, has been linked to vampire bat bites outside of the United States. In this form, one develops partial paralysis or inability to move the part of the body that was bitten. The paralysis gradually spreads throughout the body, ultimately leading to death. Hydrophobia is less common in paralytic rabies than in classic rabies.

Any serious animal bite should be cared for as soon as possible in a hospital's emergency department. In addition to the potential for transmission of rabies, other medical issues also need to be checked:

- Transmission of other infections such as bacterial infections from the mouth of the biting animal.
- Need for an injection to maintain protection or immunity against tetanus (another type of infection that can be transmitted by bites or to open wounds).

Always remember: even the most trivial bite can transmit rabies. Any bite or scratch by a rabid animal warrants the administration of rabies shots. Whether or not that animal is at risk for rabies depends on several factors including the region of the country and species of animal. Since it may not always be possible to determine whether the animal that bites you is rabid or not, it is always safer to take the rabies shots in the manner prescribed, the sooner the better, rather than wait for symptoms to develop.

malaria

Seven lives: The Mornings That Never Came

Between October and December 2010, an epidemic of falciparum malaria broke out in Chhattisgarh. The state government reported a statewide total of 32 deaths. In Bilaspur district alone there were 9 deaths, of which 7 cases were reported from the Jan Swasthya Sahyog hospital in Ganiyari.

While gathering evidence in an area where JSS did not have an outreach programme, the JSS Community Health team learnt of 250 deaths in the Kota block of Bilaspur district through a painful process of verbal autopsy. Of these, 200 deaths were confirmed to be from malaria. If these were the number of deaths in one block of one district alone, one could only speculate on the numbers statewide.

What follows are some first-hand accounts given by family members to the JSS team, in cases where at least one person had died.

Six-year old **Shyamlal Yadav** of village Rigwar had fever and headache for three days. He was going to the Anganwadi regularly where, it would have been his last year. When his body started turning yellow, his parents called a witch doctor to do *jhar-phook* (chase away the evil spirits possessing the boy), following which they took him to a quack who gave him an injection and the fever subsided for a day.

The day after, a Sunday, Shyamlal's father Anand Ram returned from the fields to find his son burning with fever and gasping for breath. Panicked, he wanted to take the child to the Primary Healthcare Centre (PHC) in Ratanpur, 25 km away. But the family had no means of transport and the last bus to Ratanpur had already left. The village Sarpanch was kind enough to arrange for a motorcycle. The doctor on duty at the PHC detected malaria and asked Anand Ram to take his son to Bilaspur, a distance of another 30 km. Anand Ram had only Rs. 200 with him and pleaded with the doctor to keep his son for the night while he went to arrange for the money, but he had no such luck. As the sun descended on a bone-chilling winter evening, Anand Ram made a last ditch effort to get medical help, but he got the same answer at another private hospital: he had to go to Bilaspur.

Catching the last bus to his village, Anand Ram returned home with a now gravely ill Shyamlal at 8 pm. The boy was coming in and out of consciousness. That night a frantic Anand Ram mortgaged one acre of his land along with the standing kharif crop. With Rs. 8000 in hand, the family waited with bated breath by the boy's side for the sun to rise. At 4 am, Shyamlal asked his mother for some water, and died soon after. The life of a 6-year old snubbed out due to reasons perhaps unimaginable to many frequent flyers, broadband users or anxious faces in the IPL galleries. While accurate estimates are available for projected GDP growth or an impending recession-recovery couplet, for Shyamlal's distraught family it would have been helpful to know an estimate of the time it takes for benefits to trickle down.

Three days later, Shyamlal's uncle's son, one-year old **Tilakram** showed the same symptoms. This family was better prepared with money and had rented a car to take him from the Community Health Centre (CHC) on Kargi Road to Bilaspur. But the parents could not convince the authorities to spare an oxygen tank for the breathless infant; Tilakram did not survive the journey to Bilaspur. Sickness and death has left the families of both Shyamlal and Tilakram in a debt of Rs. 10,000, and inconsolable.

Nandini (a year-and-half old) and Anjali (aged five) came from a landless family in village Porimohonda. Both sisters had fever and a PHC near the village detected both with malaria. The family was advised to take the girls to the Ratanpur PHC, 35 kms away, which had more doctors and besides a malaria camp was also running there. Since Anjali was less seriously ill, the parents took Nandini there. This went on for four days. Meanwhile, Anjali finished the course of medicines given by the village PHC, except that her belly was swollen. The parents thought she was better and left her behind to take Nandini to Ratanpur again. But this time, they were told to go to Bilaspur. The distance and the cost of transport, however, made the journey impossible for the family. While still at Ratanpur, they got the news of Anjali's death. In panic and grief, the parents rushed back home. One can only imagine the numbing effect of helplessness, hopelessness, angst and grief. A week later, before the mourning for her sister was over, Nandini, too, succumbed to the disease one night.

Bilaspur remained silent in the distance. The parents' lives are now caught between the grinding blocks of memories, and a debt of Rs. 15,000.

Manglu Ram Gond, aged 40, from village Berapat had fever for 8 days. His brother took him to the CHC on Kargi Road about 20 km away. He was detected with malaria, given saline, and asked to go to Bilaspur. His brother rented a car and took him to the medical college in Bilaspur where he was admitted and his treatment begun. The brother was asked to get some medicine from an outside pharmacy, but he did not have money. He tried to call people in their village to get money by morning. But Manglu Ram did not wait that long and passed away in the early hours.

His brother rented a car again, this time to take Manglu's body back to his four-year old son and his six months pregnant wife, who was also running a fever. She was taking paracetamol to control her fever, but by the time her brother-in-law returned, she and her unborn baby were dead. The brother took the two acres of land left behind by Manglu to offset the expenses incurred and raise the four-year old boy who found himself orphaned for reasons he might think were not preventable.

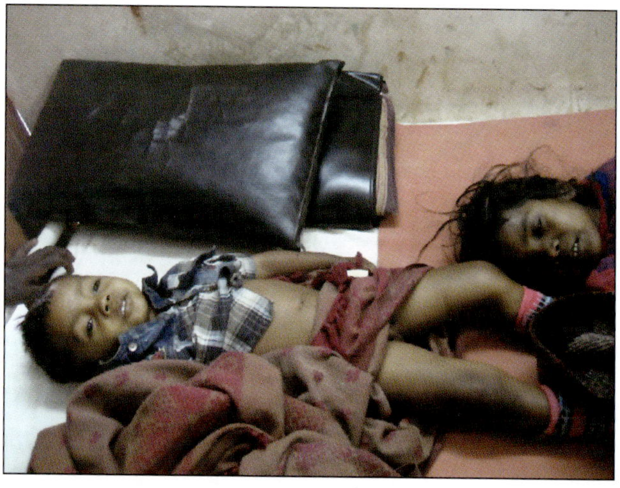

In official records, the causes for the above deaths would not be recorded as malaria, and certainly not poverty in an era of 10% growth, or the inability to travel 30 km in the age of 3G, or sub-standard PHCs when medical tourism is a formidable industry in India.

Malaria deaths start where political power ends, said a friend who works for malaria control among the poorest in our country. These deaths and many more are but grim reminders of the disempowerment that people far from resources feel and pay for with their lives.

Today, according to official figures in India, 2 million people get malaria every year in India and about 700 people die of it. The World Health Organization estimates 15 million cases in India annually, with 20,000 deaths every year. The Million Death Study estimate pegged the number of deaths at about 150,000 to 225,000 annually, though this was contested bitterly by the department of vector borne diseases control in India.

The majority of malarial deaths take place at home, and thus would not be counted as being caused by malaria. The government's figures are restricted to laboratory reports from its health facilities. Even if there is high likelihood of a death being malarial, unless there is a positive smear report for malaria, that death is not recorded as being due to malaria. But most people go to private doctors or other care providers for treatment and few suspected to have malaria actually get tested for it—treatment is usually presumptive. We are working without complete information. And little or no efforts are being made to improve the reporting of malaria cases and deaths.

In absence of correct information about malaria deaths, flawed and ineffective policy decisions are made. In 2010 when Chhattisgarh and other central Indian states witnessed a major epidemic of malaria with arguably over a few thousand deaths, of which at least 200 were reported by JSS from a single development block in Bilaspur district, the official statewide count of malarial deaths stood at 42! It is no wonder then that the Bilaspur Malaria Department's annual report for 2010 said that this was like any other previous year in terms of morbidity and deaths.

Map the worst-affected states in India, and you also map the poorest. Ironically, these states are rich in natural resources even as the people are desperately poor. Jharkhand, Chhattisgarh, Madhya Pradesh, Odisha and Assam are high-burden states for falciparum malaria.

This deliberate underreporting, and hence the subsequent flawed response to it, is not only unfair to those who have died but it also obfuscates facts about who are the ones who continue to die from malaria. The government's own data suggests that of all the falciparum malaria cases, 50% occur among the tribals—who comprise only 8% of the country's population—and they account for over 90% of all those who die of malaria.

In 1948, Rudolph Virchow had insisted that, 'Medical statistics will be our standard of measurement: we will weigh life for life and see where the dead lie thicker, among the workers or among the privileged'.

Among the diverse socio-economic groups in our country, tribals or adivasis bring up the rear on all social, nutrition and economic indicators. It is no wonder that this inequity and injustice expresses itself through a disease called falciparum malaria. Malaria is only a manifestation of the structural violence that adivasis, other forest dwellers and those who live on the fringes continue to suffer from.

eclampsia

Pushpa Bai

Pushpa Bai lived in Katami village, 2 km away from Bamhani, in Achanakmar Tiger Reserve area. Pregnant with her second child, Pushpa Bai had undergone all her routine check-ups and was taking her medicines regularly. She was on iron tablets and had taken chloroquine but could not take *choona namak* or calcium carbonate because it made her vomit. Her only problem was that her feet and her face would swell up, something her elder brother-in-law's wife attributed to cravings for food.

Three days before she went into labour on January 26, 2013, Pushpa Bai felt some back pain. She had her last check-up on January 10 when the village health worker had taken her blood pressure. Munni, the health worker, had said that Pushpa Bai's blood pressure was going up despite her medication and told her that she would speak to the senior health worker Manju at the JSS sub-centre. However, she failed to report this, and Manju did not hear of it until the seizures started.

On the night of January 29, Pushpa Bai was going about her daily routine. Her parents had come to visit and she was cooking a meal for the entire family, which included her parents-in-law, her husband's elder brother, his wife and their children. After food, she lay down to sleep. The first seizure gripped Pushpa Bai at 12 a.m. and was followed by a string of long seizures until 3 a.m. Munni had told Pushpa Bai that if her high blood pressure persisted, she was at risk for seizures. Pushpa Bai had not mentioned this to her family, who had never seen anything like this. Her father-in-law assumed that she had been possessed by a spirit and promptly called in other villagers and the *baiga*, a traditional village healer. Surprisingly, the baiga told them that Pushpa Bai had not been possessed, but was suffering from seizures.

The next logical step for the family was to take Pushpa Bai to the JSS Bamhani sub-centre for treatment. But her husband, Dev Singh, had no means of transport. All he could do in the meantime was try to straighten her legs, which were twisted from the seizures which came every half an hour. He uncurled her balled-up fists and massaged her arms and legs with mustard oil heated with garlic.

In the ensuing chaos, it did not occur to the worried family to summon Munni. Only when Pushpa Bai began frothing at the mouth did they call the health worker. A car was dispatched to get Pushpa Bai to the JSS hospital at Ganiyari. It arrived sometime after 3 a.m., an hour after the call was made. Santosh, the senior health worker and a nurse who came with the vehicle checked her blood pressure and gave her an injection of magnesium sulphate. The family was informed that high blood pressure had caused the seizures. But Dev Singh did not know what blood pressure was. Pushpa Bai was carried to the car on a cot.

Pushpa Bai's neighbours and Dev Singh accompanied her to Ganiyari. On the way she went into labour spontaneously. They rolled into the hospital gates at 5 a.m. Intravenous injections stopped her seizures, but she was disoriented. She thought she was still at home and was screaming and kicking at the nurses. Her records showed that she also had anaemia. Even after she delivered at 8.10 a.m., she was still confused as to where she was. She gave birth to a baby girl, later named Manvi, weighing 2.5 kgs.

After delivery, Pushpa Bai had joint pains and felt lethargic. Fifteen days after her discharge, her blood pressure was still high, but it became normal a month later. She then stopped her medicine but continued choona namak for a month.

After seven months, a team of three from JSS visited Pushpa Bai and her family at their home in Katami. The family did not know that her condition was called eclampsia or even understand what exactly blood pressure meant. Pushpa Bai remained remarkably unperturbed by her ordeal and told the team members that she didn't think about what had happened nor did she worry about future pregnancies.

Eclampsia is a condition in which there is an occurrence of new-onset, generalized tonic-clonic seizures or coma in a woman with preeclampsia. Eclampsia occurs in 1.6 to 10 cases per 10,000 deliveries in developed countries; in developing countries it varies from 6 to 157 cases per 10,000 deliveries.

Some factors which increase the risk for eclampsia are nulliparity, preeclampsia in a previous pregnancy, age more than 40 or less than 18 years, family history of preeclampsia, chronic hypertension, chronic renal disease, antiphospholipid antibody syndrome or inherited thrombophilia, vascular or connective tissue disease, diabetes mellitus, multifoetal gestation, high body mass index, male partner whose mother or previous partner had preeclampsia, hydrops fetalis, the woman being small for gestational age, abruptio placentae or foetal demise in a previous pregnancy, prolonged inter-pregnancy interval, partner related factors (new partner), limited sperm exposure e.g., previous use of barrier contraception, hydatidiform mole and susceptibility genes.

Two models have been proposed for pathogenesis of eclampsia. According to the first model, hypertension causes a breakdown of the auto-regulatory system of the cerebral circulation, leading to hyperperfusion, endothelial dysfunction and brain edema. In the second model, hypertension causes activation of the auto-regulatory system, leading to vasoconstriction of cerebral vessels resulting in hypoperfusion, localized ischemia and subsequent fluid leakage.

Most women have premonitory signs or symptoms like hypertension, headache, visual disturbances, abdomen pain etc. before the initial seizure. Ankle clonus is also a common finding. Most patients begin to recover responsiveness within 10 to 20 minutes after the generalized seizure. Foetal bradycardia for at least three to five minutes is a common finding during and immediately after the seizure. Ninety per cent of postpartum seizures happen within one week of delivery, but can occur till 6 weeks after delivery.

Some of the maternal and foetal outcomes in pregnancies complicated by eclampsia are abruption, disseminated intravascular coagulation (DIC), pulmonary edema, acute renal failure, aspiration pneumonia, cardiopulmonary arrest, liver hematoma, HELLP syndrome, perinatal death, preterm birth, intracerebral haemorrhage, transient blindness, cardiorespiratory arrest, hepatocellular damage, renal dysfunction, coagulopathy, hypertension, and neurologic abnormalities.

Eclampsia is a clinical diagnosis based upon the occurrence of new-onset generalized tonic-clonic seizures in a woman with preeclampsia. Neuroimaging findings consistent with reversible posterior leukoencephalopathy syndrome are the hallmark of eclampsia.

Management starts from keeping the patient in a lateral position to administering a good dose of safe antiepileptic drug. Oxygen therapy is almost always required to prevent hypoxia and subsequent hypoxemia. Blood pressure should be brought to a desirable level (both systolic and diastolic, though reducing systolic BP is found to be more effective).

The mainstay in the management of eclampsia is seizure control. The definitive treatment for eclampsia is prompt delivery.

Though not all cases of eclampsia can be prevented, majority of cases can be prevented by early detection and effective treatment of preeclampsia, for which good antenatal care services are needed.

Maternal mortality rates of 0 to 14% have been reported in pregnancies complicated by eclampsia. The incidence of eclampsia in India has been quoted as 1.56%. In a study conducted in India, eclampsia accounts for almost 43% of total maternal deaths, with case fatality of almost 5%. Majority of cases of eclampsia are young primigravidas and those with no prior antenatal care. Most of the cases belong to low socioeconomic groups from the rural population and are illiterate.

Maternal mortality rates are higher in Assam, Uttar Pradesh, Madhya Pradesh, Chhattisgarh, Bihar and Rajasthan, and least in Kerala and Tamil Nadu. Recurrent eclampsia occurs in 2% of subsequent pregnancies. Chronic hypertension develops in 24% of women with a history of preeclampsia/eclampsia. Women with a history of severe preeclampsia/eclampsia are at increased risk of obstetric complications in subsequent pregnancies compared with women with no such history.

pre-eclampsia

Tijabai Gond

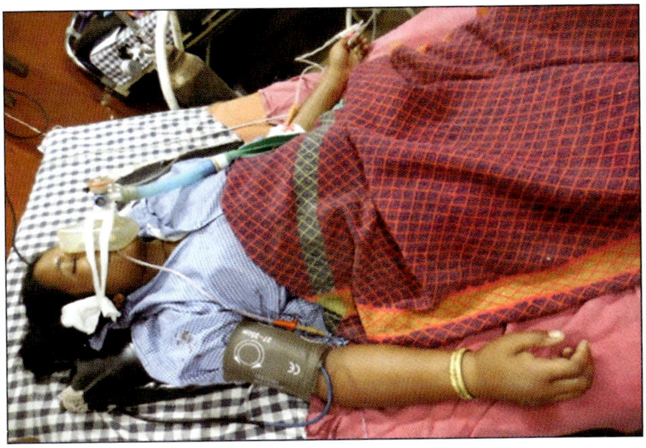

Tijabai Gond was rushed to the Jan Swasthya Sahyog hospital at Ganiyari in April with a full-term pregnancy, and severe shortness of breath. Her body had swollen with edema caused by the accumulation of fluid in her tissues, and her blood pressure was very high. She was immediately taken for a caesarean section and gave birth to a baby girl weighing 1.5 kgs.

Tijabai was from the village of Bade Berar in Kota block, 35 kms away from Ganiyari. Her husband, a daily wage labourer, was based in Bilaspur at the time. She lived with her mother-in-law, with whom she had less than cordial relations.

She first visited an antenatal care (ANC) clinic in her third month of pregnancy and had had a total of five antenatal check-ups. Her body began to swell in the eighth month of pregnancy, and when Tijabai visited the doctor, she was told to return for another visit and warned about the risks of hypertension and edema. When the swelling intensified in her ninth month, Tijabai did nothing about it, fearing she would be labelled fat. There was little family support to urge her to seek urgent medical attention and she barely understood the dangers of a high-risk pregnancy, either because it had not been well communicated to her or because she didn't think it could happen to her.

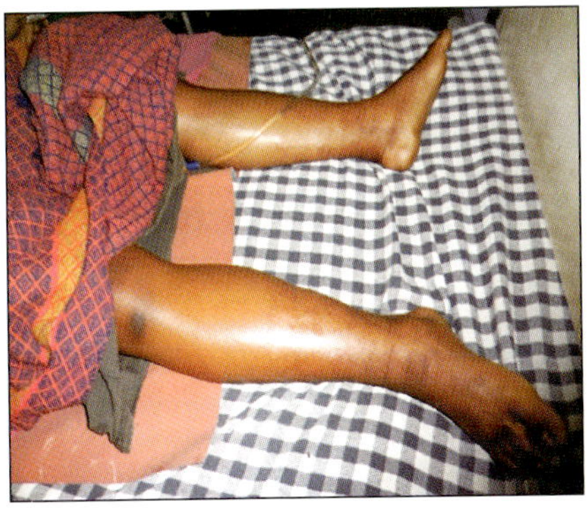

Even after the delivery, Tijabai continued to be sick. She was very swollen, was passing little urine and was also very breathless. Her blood pressure continued to be high, though she was conscious. She had to be given high-flow oxygen continuously to help her maintain her oxygen level in blood. She was given two medicines for hypertension and also continued on an infusion of magnesium sulphate which had been started soon after she arrived at the hospital. Blood tests were also performed, based on which a diagnosis of HELLP syndrome, a complicated form of pregnancy induced hypertension, was made. She had to be given three units of blood since she had developed severe anaemia.

Tijabai took more than three days to start showing improvement. First, her urine volume started to improve, followed by her kidney functions. Her oxygen requirements also started decreasing. She was kept at Ganiyari for six days until her condition normalised. At the time of discharge, while her liver and kidney functions and her breathing had normalised, she had to be sent home on anti-hypertensives. She told JSS staff that she hadn't given due importance to seeing a doctor and realized that her condition could have been avoided had she kept her appointment. She said that she would visit the clinic regularly in future.

Six weeks later, Tijabai still had hypertension, which necessitated that she continued anti-hypertensives for a longer period. This complication can follow any pregnancy induced hypertension.

HELLP syndrome is a life-threatening obstetric complication usually considered to be a variant or complication of pre-eclampsia. Both conditions usually occur during later stages of pregnancy, or sometimes after childbirth, like in Tijabai. Its incidence is reported as 0.5-0.9% of all pregnancies, but in 10-20% of women with severe preeclampsia.

'HELLP' is an abbreviation of the three main features of the syndrome, which are Hemolysis, Elevated Liver enzymes, and Low Platelet count. Tijabai's haemoglobin had dropped to 5 gram per cent from her previous haemoglobin of 10 grams per cent, and she required blood transfusion to maintain her haemoglobin status.

The serious complication of disseminated intravascular coagulation is also seen in about 20% of all women with HELLP syndrome, and in 84% when HELLP is complicated by acute renal failure. Pulmonary edema is found in 6% of all women with HELLP syndrome, and in 44% when HELLP is complicated by acute renal failure.

A woman with symptoms of HELLP can be misdiagnosed in the early stages, increasing the risk of liver failure and morbidity. Rarely, after a caesarean section surgery a woman may have signs and symptoms of a shock condition, mimicking either pulmonary embolism or reactionary haemorrhage. This is a scary obstetric emergency that we continue to see in many more women with pregnancy induced hypertension on preeclampsia. Managing it demands a well-equipped health facility, including intensive care, plus skilled physicians and nurses. If managed timely and well, the maternal mortality in this can be kept almost zero.

postpartum haemorrhage

Meena Bai

Meena Bai had delivered three children at home in her village of Saraipali, and at 36, she was expecting her fourth. She had experienced no problems with her previous pregnancies, had been for five to six check-ups and was administered three vaccines, one at JSS and two by the local auxiliary-nurse-midwife (ANM). Meena Bai would have delivered her fourth child at home as well, but the day she went into labour, there were no women around her to do the delivery. Her 'jethanis', the wives of her brothers-in-law, had gone to their own villages.

At about 10 or 11 a.m., as Meena Bai later recalled, she went into labour. Three people crammed themselves onto a motorcycle – Meena Bai, her husband Titra Singh and her sister-in-law – and sped over rutted roads to the Shivtarai Primary Health Centre, reaching at around 3 p.m. Meena Bai's waters had not yet broken, but the contractions had begun.

At the PHC, the attendant nurse did not check Meena Bai's blood pressure or anything else. She was given an intravenous injection to hasten the process of labour and put on a drip with some medicine injected into it. Meena remembered that she delivered just 10 to 15 minutes after she arrived at the PHC. The baby, a boy, did not cry, and she wasn't sure what 'they' did to make him cry. She was then wheeled into another room with an iron cot and a mattress. Her drip was removed and she was injected again, half an hour after delivery. She started feeling cold after a while. The nurses had left her to her own devices. She was forced to use a cloth for the bleeding because they had not given her a pad.

At 6 p.m., Meena Bai started bleeding copiously. She felt no pain but had to change cloth after cloth, and the bleeding still wouldn't stop. After alerting her family and telling them to call the dai and take her to the JSS hospital at Ganiyari, Meena Bai said that her vision was darkening and she couldn't see anything. Her family called Gayatri, the village health worker, to arrange for a car to take her to Ganiyari. By this time, the thick blanket beneath her was soaked.

The doctor at the Shivtarai PHC was, however, unwilling to discharge her. Meena Bai recalled that besides giving her an injection after delivery, the doctor had not touched her. He hadn't been present at the delivery either. No one had touched her abdomen to see whether it was rigid or soft, or to tell her if something was stuck in her uterus. She wasn't even given a drink of water.

Meena Bai finally reached the hospital at Ganiyari at 9 or 10 p.m, by which time her blood had darkened a blanket, a sheet, the shawl spread over the car seat cover, and seeped into the car seat. Her blood pressure could not be taken, it had fallen so low. The doctor and the nurse at JSS cleaned her up, gave her a couple of stitches and another injection. Her husband's blood was found to match hers, and he donated one unit of blood. The bleeding finally stopped by morning and she was given a meal. Meena Bai was discharged after three days with a month's worth of medication.

Meena Bai's cervix had been torn in two or three places, but she had not been given any stitches after the delivery at the PHC. This was repaired at JSS.

Titra Singh remained at home for two months after her delivery in the commonly held belief that it would take two months to replenish the blood he had donated to his wife. He was swayed by people saying one should not go out in the sun after giving blood, and was sceptical when Dr. Yogesh Jain told him that his blood would be replenished within 24 hours. But at least he was willing to give blood at a critical time, said Dr. Jain. Many villagers did not want to give blood or believed they were too weak to do so.

Titra Singh later recalled being struck by the callous attitude of the doctor at the government PHC. He called the PHC a living hell which did not even have a car and driver to transfer his bleeding wife. The doctors there would only administer medication that was purchased by the patient's family. Titra Singh said the PHC doctor did not even know what medication he was administering, he knew nothing. The three injections costing Rs. 1200 that he had bought for his wife had also been kept by the doctor.

Postpartum haemorrhage (PPH) or bleeding from the birth passages after birth of the baby is the most common cause of death in maternity, affecting up to 1 to 5% of deliveries. Between 250 ml to 500 ml of blood loss may occur in a normal vaginal delivery, and up to 1000 ml of blood loss may occur in a Caesarean section. More than that is dangerous and can be fatal. More than 500 ml blood loss in a normal birth may cause complications like worsening anaemia or haemorrhagic shock. When the blood loss is more than 1000 ml, it results in symptoms of hypovolemia such as cool peripheries, feeling weak and light-headed and low blood pressure. The first few hours are the most critical.

Nearly 90% of postpartum haemorrhage occurs due to partial retention of the placenta/membranes in the uterus or due to uterine atony. The possibility of PPH is increased by the presence of anaemia, multiple pregnancy or pregnancy induced hypertension. Such PPH can be largely prevented by active management of the third stage of labour by giving oxytocin 10 units immediately after delivery, or administering 4 tablets of misoprostol 800 mcg/sub-lingual or by rectal route. Reducing blood loss also has the added benefit of reducing postpartum anaemia in the young mother.

Up to 10% of PPH may be due to a tear in the cervix during the baby's descent. This has to be predicted and examined for, or else a mother may rapidly bleed to death. If detected, it requires expert suturing of the tear under good light with adequate local anesthesia.

If PPH ensues, then feeling for the uterus and if atonic, then administering oxytocin in higher doses including IV infusion of oxytocin plus removal of placental parts under general anesthesia may be necessary. These skills and necessary resources have to be available in institutions that call themselves capable of conducting deliveries. It is a fact that PPH can only be predicted in 50% of cases. The others may happen without any warning. Unpredictability of the occurrence of PPH necessitates preparedness for this most important complication in obstetrics.

Often PPH might progress to hypovolemic shock and needs intensive fluid resuscitation and blood products to maintain perfusion of organs. Such cases can occur at the peripheral centres and thus availability of blood is crucial for saving the patient's life.

When do we need blood in PPH? There is no straight answer to this question. We feel that any place that conducts deliveries must have a blood storage unit because PPH can happen to any woman in labour with or without high risk factors and it is like having a tap without a washer. However, the Government has declared 'Unbanked Directed Blood Transfusion' illegal, which means that in an emergency, a peripheral health facility can only transfuse blood given by the blood banks (which according to present guidelines, are very difficult to set up in rural areas. Even if the facility can test the blood, they cannot bleed a donor to give blood to the patient. Often the facilities might not have stored blood, and bringing blood from the blood bank is usually not feasible at that time.

If there is no arrangement of blood, the woman may lose her life. Those conducting deliveries, especially at remote peripheral/rural areas, at odd hours with no easily available transport may need blood at very short notice. It is also very difficult to transfer a woman with active postpartum bleeding. PPH is a critical condition in which all clinical evaluation and experience fails if one is not able to procure and transfuse blood at the right time. Thus, there must be a provision for Unbanked Directed Blood Transfusion if we want to prevent these clearly avoidable deaths.

cancer

Sonarin Bai

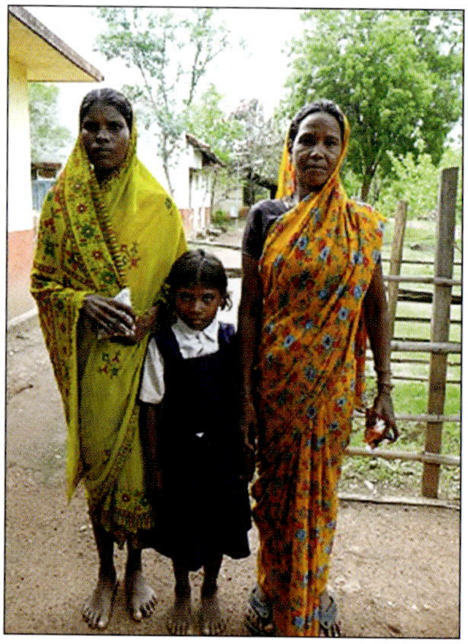

Sonarin Bai came to JSS in July 2010 with a swollen abdomen, a history of coughs and fevers, and two generations of worried relatives from her faraway village in Madhya Pradesh. She and her husband, both landless labourers, had borrowed Rs. 3,000 to make the two-day journey to the JSS hospital in Ganiyari on the advice of relatives and neighbours. Accompanied by her mother, an aunt and her 10-year-old daughter in a blue and white school uniform, Sonarin Bai told doctors of at least ten different episodes of cough and fever over three years. In January that year, she had begun to suffer from abdominal pain and swelling and began to lose weight. Her back had started hurting, and eventually, she had to give up working altogether as she could barely catch her breath even without exerting herself.

The JSS doctors diagnosed her with a rare form of bone marrow cancer called chronic myeloid leukemia (CML). The swelling in her abdomen was the result of millions of abnormal white blood cells teeming in her blood that had enlarged her spleen and, which now extended 15 cm below her rib cage.

CML occurs in about 20 per cent of all leukemias in children and appears as a painless abdominal swelling due to a swollen spleen and mild pallor. CML is diagnosed on the basis of very high white blood cell counts and a typical blood smear. Specialised tests may be needed, but are not essential for initiating treatment. The drug Imatinib can keep the disease at bay for years and has been a game changer in the approach to the disease.

Imatinib, also known by its brand name Gleevec, is manufactured by Novartis. It was the subject of an intense litigation as Novartis attempted to get a patent for the drug, which would prevent Indian companies from manufacturing and selling it at a fraction of the original cost. In April 2013, the Supreme Court of India ruled that the Novartis appeal was not valid as their new version of the drug did not provide significant improvement over the existing version.

Three years prior to that landmark judgement, however, the cost of Gleevec was prohibitive for a poor family like Sonarin Bai's. The company offered free treatment to patients at a few registered cancer centres located predominantly in metropolitan cities, including Delhi and Mumbai. Thus for her treatment, Sonarin Bai would have to go to the All India Institute of Medical Sciences (AIIMS), Delhi.

Sonarin Bai went home for about two weeks and returned to JSS on July 18 without her aunt and daughter. Her daughter had taken her mother's disease very hard. Along with seven other patients, their families and a coordinator from JSS, Sonarin Bai and her mother took a train to Delhi.

From there, everything went downhill.

AIIMS is thronged by thousands of poor patients every day and it can take days just to be seen by a doctor, and months for surgery. Sonarin Bai joined that throng, assisted by the JSS coordinator Jai Kumar. It took two days to get registered. The oncologist would not see her without a battery of tests being conducted. On the fourth day, only the blood tests could be done, by which time she was running a fever. The fifth day, Sonarin Bai made her way to the x-ray room, where a clerk advised them to go back and get the doctor's signature for a free x-ray. The sixth day was spent running from pillar to post in search of that doctor. Not finding him, they gave up and paid Rs. 30 for an x-ray the next day. On the eighth day, after waiting five hours in front of the doctor's office, Sonarin Bai finally met a medical professional. But he turned out to be a children's oncologist, who palpated her abdomen, prescribed some medicine and then referred her to an oncologist for adult patients. She was given an appointment the following week.

The next day, Sonarin Bai wasn't feeling well. She took the medicine prescribed by the doctor, but by evening she was racked with stomach cramps, diarrhoea and fever. She was wheeled to the hospital emergency room, where three physicians examined her – more in the space of a few hours than in the entire preceding week. Her mother waited anxiously in the hospital veranda as Sonarin Bai's condition deteriorated from 'seriously ill' to 'critical'.

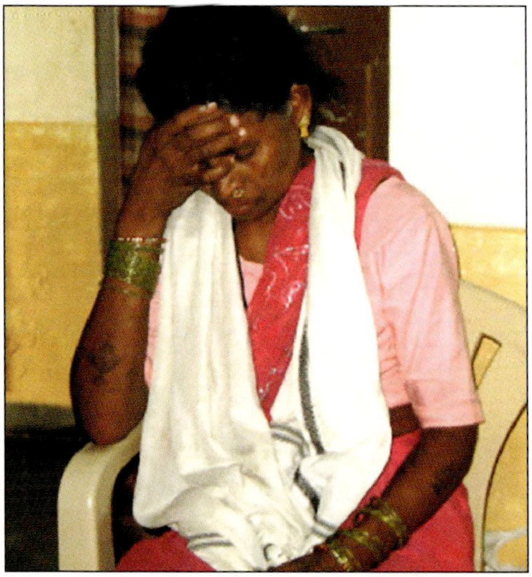

At four in the morning, a doctor told the JSS coordinator that Sonarin Bai had died. Jai Kumar went outside and told her mother, 'Mat ro mataram, Sonarin ab duniya mai nahi hai' [Don't cry mother. Sonarin is no more].

Chronic myelogenous, myeloid or myelocytic leukemia is a cancer of the white blood cells, characterized by the increased and unregulated growth of predominantly myeloid cells in the bone marrow and the accumulation of these cells in the blood. It is a clonal bone marrow stem cell disorder in which a proliferation of mature granulocytes (neutrophils, eosinophils and basophils) and their precursors is found.

It is a type of myeloproliferative disease associated with a characteristic chromosomal translocation called the Philadelphia chromosome. The most prominent risk factor involved in the onset of CML, irrespective of the Philadelphia chromosome, is exposure to high amounts of ionizing radiation. Increased rates of CML were observed in people exposed to the atomic bombings of Nagasaki and Hiroshima.

CML is now largely treated with targeted drugs called tyrosine kinase inhibitors (TKIs) which have led to dramatically improved long-term survival rates since the introduction of the first such agent in 2001. These drugs have revolutionized treatment of this disease and allow most patients to have a good quality of life as compared to the former chemotherapy drugs.

In Western countries, CML accounts for 15-20% of all adult leukemias and 14% of all leukemias, including those in children.

Before the advent of tyrosine kinase inhibitors, the median survival time for CML patients had been about 3–5 years from the time of diagnosis. With the use of TKIs, survival rates have improved dramatically. A 2006 follow-up of 553 patients using Imatinib (Gleevec) found an overall survival rate of 89% after five years. A 2011 follow-up of 832 patients using Imatinib who achieved a stable cytogenetic response found an overall survival rate of 95.2% after 8 years, which is similar to the rate in the general population. Less than 1% of patients died because of leukemia progression.

Most CML patients are asymptomatic initially. They are accidentally diagnosed during a routine laboratory check. Symptoms appear as the disease progresses.

The High Cost of Imatinib

The drug Imatinib, known by the brand name Gleevec, has proved so successful in chronic myeloid leukaemia that patients, who a decade ago survived only a few years, can now look forward to a near-normal life expectancy.

But the cost of Gleevec is high and has risen from £18,000 per patient per year to around £21,000 in the UK, and from $30,000 to $92,000 in the US. This is despite the fact that all research costs were covered by the original drug price, and the number of patients treated and the length of time they are on the drug have both vastly increased because of the drug's success.

Daniel Vasella, former chairman and chief executive of Novartis, the drug manufacturer, said the original price of Gleevec in 2001 was considered 'high but worthwhile' and was estimated to yield annual revenues of $900 million, enough to cover its development cost in two years. A decade later in 2012, its annual revenues were $4.7 billion (£3 billion).

In May 2013, more than a hundred CML experts published an article in the journal

Blood, stating that the price of drugs for CML was a reflection of the unsustainable prices of cancer drugs. The authors said that the revenue earned by Gleevec over the last ten years 'represent generous profits to the company'. But this has put heavy pressure on those who have to foot the bill. 'Grateful patients may have become the financial victims of the treatment's success, having to pay the high price annually to stay alive'.

In the US, even those with health insurance may pay an average of 20 per cent of drug prices out of pocket. Drug prices are the single most frequent cause of personal bankruptcies in the US.

Three new drugs have been approved for CML in the last year by the FDA but the prices are 'astronomical', the authors say, at up to $138,000 a year per patient.

Worldwide, only about a quarter of the patients with CML who could benefit have access to drugs because of the cost. 'A small fraction are rich enough to pay individually, and most are treated intermittently or not at all. The effects of these financial pressures on long term survival… are yet unknown.'

The article stated that in the UK, patients are shielded from the 'direct economic anxieties of illness'. But Professor Jane Apperley, chair of the Department of Haematology at Imperial College, London, and one of the authors, said high drug prices were still a cause of harm in Britain.

'The price of a drug heavily influences the decision of NICE whether we can prescribe it on the NHS. I am chief of service at Imperial College and we are constantly being asked to reduce our spending. We have to look very carefully at the cost of the drugs we use. Of course we need the pharmaceutical industry to go on developing new drugs. It is very exciting that a number of cancers are now becoming susceptible to these new drugs. But the rising cost is unsustainable. The drugs are very effective at keeping people alive. But if they are priced out of what you can afford, you know that you can keep people alive but you can't afford to do so. It is completely unsustainable for the

NHS because the costs are going up every year. We need a serious dialogue about whether we can sustain these costs,' said Dr. Apperley.

The authors have accused the drug industry of 'profiteering' i.e. making profits by unethical methods, and conclude: 'We believe the unsustainable drug prices may be causing harm to patients. Advocating for lower drug prices is a necessity to save the lives of patients who cannot afford them. We believe drug prices should reflect objective measures of benefit, but should not exceed values that harm our patients and societies.'

A spokesperson for the UK charity Beating Blood Cancers said: 'As a charity we want to see an ethical approach to drug pricing. There is no point in us investing in research if the pricing policy means drugs won't be available to patients.'

In a statement to *The Independent*, Novartis said: 'We recognize that sustainability of health care systems is a complex topic and we welcome the opportunity to be part of the dialogue. Our critical role, as one of many parties working towards improving cancer care, is to discover and develop innovative treatments.'

'Novartis innovation in chronic myeloid leukemia (CML) has changed the course of the disease. Before Gleevec (Imatinib) and Tasigna (Nilotinib), the five-year survival in CML was only 30 per cent. Today, nine out of ten patients with CML have a normal life span and are leading productive lives.'

The Supreme Court Judgement on Novartis's Gleevec

In a landmark judgment in April 2013, the Supreme Court of India rejected the patent application by Novartis for its cancer drug, Gleevec (Imatinib). This was a victory for public health, not just in India but across the developing world. The huge price difference between the Novartis drug and its generic version—and that it is a cancer drug—lent the case high visibility in the media and the public eye.

The judgment represented a firm-footed stance to protect people's right to health, in the face of stiff challenges from multinational drug companies. It built on a critical amendment to India's patent law in 2005 in the form of Section 3(d) that prohibits patents on new forms of known medicines unless they result in enhanced efficacy over the existing medicine.

This provision was introduced after India became a signatory to the World Trade Organization's (WTO's) agreement on Trade-Related Aspects of Intellectual Property Rights (TRIPS), which obliges countries to grant patents on technological products, including drugs. Indian drug companies must wait for a patent to expire before they can produce identical, quality copies of innovator medicines for use in India and for export to poor patients around the world.

Access to medicines increasingly depends on the use of 'TRIPS flexibilities', or legal measures enshrined in a country's laws to safeguard the right to public health. The Doha Declaration of 2001 emphasises 'that the TRIPS Agreement can and should be interpreted and implemented in a manner supportive of WTO Members' right to protect public health and, in particular, to promote access to medicines for all.'

India's patent law has been commended as a success story by the WHO and by health activists, doctors and patients across the world in widening access to HIV drugs and saving millions of lives. India is often called the 'pharmacy of the developing world' because of its generic drugs industry – and the April 2013 Supreme Court ruling is therefore vitally important.

According to Anita Jain, drug companies often use different 'evergreening' strategies, such as chemical tricks, reformulations, fixed dose drug combinations, changes in dosage regimen, and brand promotion among others, to prevent losses from sale of cheaper generic drugs and protect their market share.

So what determines how a particular brand of a drug is prescribed for a patient in

India? The person who presently determines the brand is the doctor who prescribes it. How does an average doctor in India, given the wide range of choices, choose to prescribe a particular brand? This is a difficult process to unravel and there is only anecdotal evidence. The brand that a doctor chooses for a particular drug could be based on perceived quality, efficacy, familiarity, marketing, availability, incentive, and perhaps the patient's affordability. Often it is a mixture of all of these, making the decision subjective and in a sense arbitrary.

Sanjay Nagral says that while the Supreme Court has partly cleared the way for the production of generic drugs, there is a need to understand the larger process of drug prescription and change it to a pro-patient one if the benefit of cheap generics has to reach patients. That change can also be pushed by making prescription by generic names mandatory, as well as by patients demanding cheaper alternatives. But perhaps a more difficult but effective shift would be for medical professionals to be sensitive to the cost burden their patients face.

References

1. Anita Jain, 'The Novartis Case: Weighing Innovation against Access'. *British Medical Journal*, UK, MJ 2013; 346: f2218.
2. Sanjay Nagral, 'The Cost of Drugs: Beyond the Supreme Court Order'. *Economic and Political Weekly*. April 27, 2013 Vol. 48 No 17.

cervical cancer

Bhaguri Bai

This is the story of Bhaguri Bai, a 35 year old woman from the Agadhiya tribe who lives in a forest village of Madhya Pradesh. To reach the JSS health facility at Ganiyari, she had travelled almost 150 km, first by bus, then train and then auto. When this frail woman entered the OPD, the room filled with a foul odour and people started making faces.

Examination revealed a large growth or tumour. Bhaguri Bai had cervical cancer, which had already reached an advanced stage (III b), and chemotherapy and surgical removal had a limited role now. She was advised radiotherapy which might help postponing death and improve quality of life. Such treatment was only available at centres in big cities like Raipur and Jabalpur.

The JSS hospital had very little to offer at this advanced stage of disease.

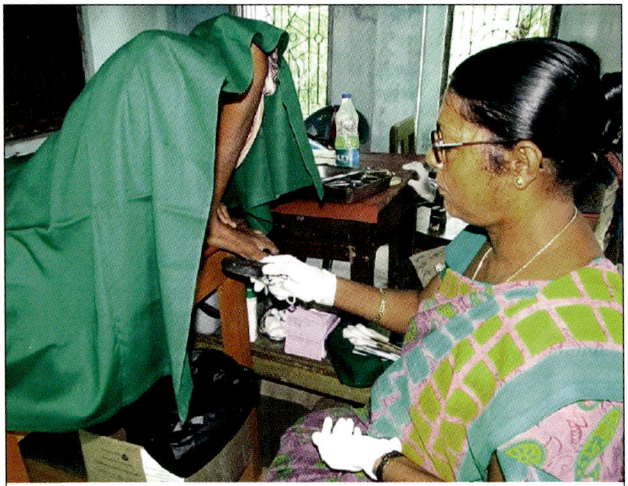

A woman undergoing cervical visual examination using Acetic Acid

Feeling helpless in a clinical job is quite common as one comes across many situations where medical science has no cure to offer. But this was not an anecdotal case. The JSS hospital gets an average of 20 old and newly diagnosed cervical cancer patients every month, with most of them at the late stage of cancer at the time of diagnosis.

The questions remained: why were so many of these poor rural women getting cervical cancer? And why were there

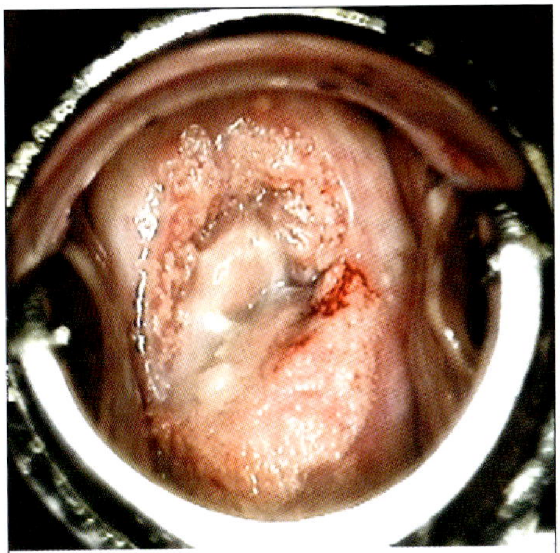

An abnormal growth seen after application of acetic acid

delays in diagnosis and treatment? Were these situations preventable?

Bhaguri Bai said, 'I am peeing so many times, and this smell...initially it was just a white discharge, now it is like pus...and this smell stays, even if I have had a bath, this smell stays...you can get it even from that corner. It's been two months that this foul smell is there. Then someone told us to go to Bilaspur to get my uterus removed. A woman from our neighbourhood got that done here a few weeks back. Hence we came.' Her face was filled with disgust and shame as she spoke because of the odour.

Bhaguri Bai had first tried some herbs available in their village, the usual local treatment for vaginal discharge. 'In our area, white discharge gets cured with wild herbs (*jangali jadijankadi*)...my husband knows...he used to get them for me. I was taking those...The baiga (faith healer) also gave me some.' She had taken the herbs for 7-8 months. When those did not help, she went to an uncertified private practitioner at the block level. 'There is one doctor from Bilaspur who has opened his hospital...Bangali doctor...*sooji aur botal lagave* [puts injections and saline bottle]'.

Did he examine you for your problem?

'No, it's not a big hospital...in the village that doesn't happen...He gave four-five bottles...Otherwise I was so weak I could not get up from the ground.'

In remote rural areas where qualified health care providers are either unheard of or inaccessible, quacks rule and their practice mostly survives on painkiller injections and IV fluids. This provides some degree of symptomatic relief. With no alternatives available, such malpractices are common and popular in rural areas.

Bhaguri Bai thus spent more than eleven months seeking herbal medicines and health care from unqualified practitioners.

'I thought usually older women have this watery discharge...I thought it might be the same what older women have sometimes...When it started smelling badly, I thought I have some disease. It's been four months now, I am not taking any medicine...Every day I have to change four-five clothes...whatever cloth we have, I cut those to make pads...then wash those with Nirma and use them again...what else?'

'I thought that women who have menopause, their menstrual blood stays in the womb and that starts flowing sometimes and stops by itself...or it sometimes comes suddenly...That is what I thought when I started having this (bleeding)'.

Symptoms like white discharge and abnormal vaginal bleeding were not recognised by rural women as something abnormal. This inability to interpret gynaecological symptoms correctly led to a delay in treatment.

When asked if she had ever heard of cancer, Bhaguri Bai said she had but did not understand it. In the villages it was known as 'dhat' (white discharge) or 'sujag', which she explained to us: '...where there is a vein of the womb (*bachchedani ki nassi*) that starts getting big...then because of that it starts melting the womb from inside and comes out drop by drop (*bachchedani ko gala gala ke girata hai*)... then there is swelling in the abdomen...yes that we call *singrahoni bimari*... in that the stomach starts bloating up (*pet phoolne lagta hai*)...then finish...death comes.'

This was a complete description of what her community thought was white discharge and where it could lead. Clearly, rural women thought of these problems, but ironically such reproductive health issues got very little attention from clinicians and public health policies.

An ethnographic study done a decade ago in rural and tribal regions of Gadchiroli had discussed similar findings about how women held considerable traditional knowledge about causes and treatment of white discharge. Because of this they often considered taking herbal medicines available to them or from a traditional healer.

Along with the inability to interpret these symptoms as illness, there was also a culture of silence around vaginal discharge and abnormal vaginal bleeding. The women felt unable to easily share their problems with their families and as one woman reported in the study: 'I felt shy telling them... They might make fun of me, saying, 'That old dame is having discharge from her vagina. That's why I haven't said anything to them....'

The poor status of literacy and specifically health literacy coupled with such unregulated health care practices were also reasons for the delay in reaching appropriate health care. Trained health care providers at the primary level were almost non-existent in rural and tribal areas.

Bhaguri Bai was also asked if she had shared her problems with a nurse, auxiliary nursing midwife (ANM), a health worker or Mitanin with the primary health services, or an ASHA worker visiting the village. But she did not know that she needed to be checked up in case of bleeding and also did not perceive the Mitanins or ANM as capable of solving her health issues. Women anticipated these situations based on their previous experiences and hence refrained from seeking public health services. But even coming to JSS was not easy for her.

Bhaguri Bai said: 'We are farmers...poor people...What work I could do with this (problem)?...I have a daughter...we arranged for her marriage...I thought I would always be able to work and earn...First I got her married. Then we arranged for a little (money) and came here.'

Then, in the midst of her narration, Bhaguri Bai suddenly asked: 'Won't I get better here?...Do something to make me better...We won't be able go to big hospital.'

Table 3: Incidence of cervical cancer in India (estimations for 2012)

Indicator	India	Southern Asia	World
Annual number of new cancer cases	122,844	145,946	527,624
Crude incidence rate[a]	20.2	17.1	15.1
Age-standardized incidence rate[a]	22.0	19.3	14.0
Cumulative risk (%) at 75 years old[b]	2.4	2.1	1.4

[a] Rates per 100,000 women per year.
[b] Cumulative risk (incidence) is the probability or risk of individuals getting from the disease during ages 0-74 years. For cancer, it is expressed as the % of new born children who would be expected to develop from a particular cancer before the age of 75 if they had the rates of cancer observed in the period in the absence of competing causes.

There was no answer. Bhaguri Bai sat there in her old slightly torn clothes, frail body, the foul smell of pus still lingering in the room, but her eyes full of hope…it was the cruel reality that lead to her present condition which was sickening to the core.

The global scenario

Cancer of the cervix is the second most common cancer causing morbidity and mortality in women worldwide: about 530,000 new cases and 270,000 deaths are recorded each year. Almost 85% of cases occur in low-income countries (WHO guidance note 2013).

Figure 3: Age specific mortality from cervical cancer in India, South Asia, and the World

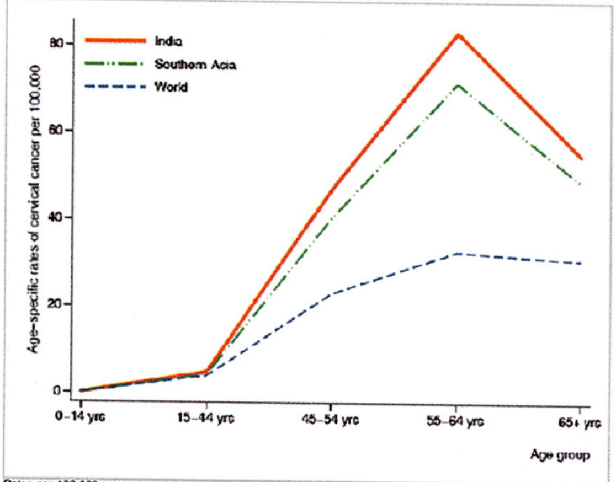

Rates per 100,000 women per year.
Data sources:
IARC, Globocan 2002 | WHO GBD 2004 (for WHO region estimates only)

Source: WHO/ICO Information Centre on Human Papilloma Virus (HPV) and Cervical Cancer (a). Human Papillomavirus and Related Cancers in India. Summary Report 2009. Available at http://www.who.int/hpvcentre/en/

Their socioeconomic status, access to care, and lack of financial security in form of health insurance have a significant relationship with delays in diagnosis, advanced stage, and impaired survival. An article by an international agency on research on cancer titled 'Social inequalities and cancer' brings the evidence from various studies that the socio-economic status of women and cervical cancer share an intimate relationship. In the Indian context, cancer of the cervix is the most common cancer among women.

WHO projects that the number of new cases will rise up to 226,084 by 2025. The prevalence and burden of cervical cancer is much higher among poor as well as rural women in India (Vallikad 2006; Kurkue and Yeole 2006). The reported deaths from cervical cancer every year are about 67,500. It also stands second among the major cause of death for women of the age group 15 to 44 years (Bruni L et al 2015).

The figure above shows the presence of excess mortality due to cancer of cervix in India, as compared to the Southeast Asia region and the world. Estimates suggest a 79% increase by 2025 (NCRP WHO 2004).

The bulk of population in India is rural, and ironically we don't have effective or adequate mechanisms to measure the magnitude of cervical cancer in these areas. It has been estimated that there are 100,000 new cases of cancer of the cervix in India every year, and 70% or more of these are Stage II or higher at diagnosis.

A descriptive study done in Bangalore states that: 'Clinical stage at presentation was the single most important variable in predicting survival'. Similar evidence is brought by a Malawian survey where 80% of women reached health care facility when surgical intervention was no longer possible.

Health care providers in India routinely see women with advanced, incurable cervical cancer. These huge discrepancies in cervical cancer survival rates in India and other developed countries are in fact preventable.

Determinants of Cervical morbidity and mortality

Social, cultural, economic conditions like poverty, education and health beliefs are underlying determinants that cause discrepancies in incidence and mortality. Lack of awareness of the risk factors and symptoms of illness, paucity of accessible and affordable screening and curative health services act as direct causes of excess mortality in India.

The disease gives a window of opportunity of approximately ten years in its natural progression, where early detection and treatment play a crucial role. But most often, the cancerous lesions go unnoticed until they reach an advanced stage.

At the household level, knowledge of disease and reproductive health, health beliefs around the aetiology of symptoms determine the recognition and interpretation of symptoms. Cultural notions of shame and sexuality often inhibit a woman from sharing these symptoms even within her close circle.

In-depth interviews done in rural Gujarat revealed that one cause of delay in seeking treatment for such symptoms begins by 'normalizing' or rationalizing the symptoms themselves. Rural Indian women tend to stretch their boundaries of endurance for pain and suffering as they consistently put their household, children and family responsibilities before their own health. Gender inequality, norms related to fertility and the lack of healthy spousal communication often results in this delay in seeking timely treatment in context of gynaecological morbidity.

Single women who were either widowed or divorced showed a higher risk of presentation at a late stage of cervical cancer (OR=2.08; 95% CI: 1.24-3.50).

As women refrain from sharing their symptoms openly, they use vague terms like weakness for complaints related to problems that are sexual and/or in the genital area. The health care provider often fails to understand these subtle hidden meanings.

A study done in Nepal on factors associated with late diagnosis of cervical cancer looked at a majority of rural women (77%), mostly illiterate (66%), where four in every five cases (80.9%) had delayed diagnosis. The study concluded that high rate of illiteracy contributes to delay in seeking treatment for gynaecological complaints. Women with education up to primary school or less showed a higher risk (OR=2.62; 95% CI 1.29-5.31) of reporting disease at an advanced stage.

The literature mentions that the lack of financial resources acts not only as an important barrier in seeking timely treatment, but is also an underlying determinant of other contributory factors. The lack of effective financial mechanisms like health insurance coupled with out of pocket expenditure involved in seeking treatment functioned as a major barrier which delayed timely diagnosis.

System delay

Lack of availability, accessibility and affordability along with poor quality of health care services, coupled with these societal determinants, function as barriers in the way of appropriate diagnosis and treatment.

A descriptive study from rural and tribal regions of Maharashtra found that of the 92% of women who participated in the study and who had some gynaecological morbidity, only 7.8% reached some kind of healthcare. For a rural woman, seeking treatment involved walking long distances in difficult conditions or paying money for travelling by compromising on their very limited means of living. Economic constraints mingled with travel costs involved in reaching health care stop people from seeking care.

Though public health services were meant to provide affordable and appropriate health care, they failed to. People were reluctant to seek health care from the public sector due to their poor quality. Often women coming with gynaecological symptoms were not examined appropriately. Addressing gynaecological complaints symptomatically without proper examination (per vaginal examination, cervical cytology) resulted in delay in correct diagnosis.

The public health response to cervical cancer and the provision for its screening is still at the conception stage. Amidst competing priorities like maternal mortality (MMR in Madhya Pradesh and Chhattisgarh is 310 and 275 respectively) and child health, other components of reproductive health are often neglected. Cervical cancer is one disease amidst various kinds of gynecological morbidities. Studies have shown that rural women often experience the huge burden of untreated reproductive health issues, and cervical cancer has a much worse outcome of untreated gynecological illness.

Despite the need and strong demand, by researchers and health activists for the provision of widespread reproductive health care services for gynecological morbidity (like cervical cancer), this has not received enough attention.

In rural India where primary health care services are often only focussed on achieving visible health indicators, gynaecological morbidities like reproductive tract infections, menstrual disorders, pelvic inflammatory diseases and gynaecological cancers are often not addressed at an early stage. That Bhaguri Bai, and so many like her suffering from cervical cancer, have to face the worst outcome of such diseases and premature death underlines the same urgent need.

vesico-vaginal fistula

Lachkunwar Bai

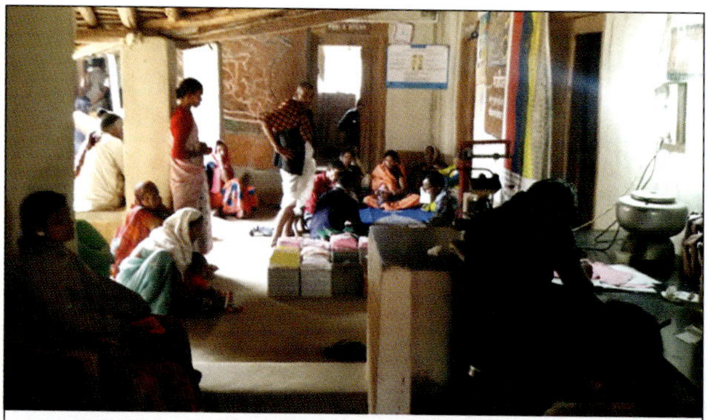

The Bamhani Clinic

As you drive down the road through the forest, the Achanakmar Tiger Reserve affords a picturesque view. The river Maniyari flows through the reserve, skirting the Bamhani clinic of the Jan Swasthya Sahyog. About 56 km from the JSS hospital in Ganiyari, the Bamhani clinic, which serves a cluster of 17 villages with a population of about 8,000, may well serve as a model for primary grassroots healthcare in India today. If you ever visit these remote and beautiful interiors, you will know why.

In one of those 17 villages, named Niwaaskhar, lives the family of Lachkunwar Gond, which includes her husband Dayaram and two daughters Bhagwati and Saraswati. They own three acres of land, which produces just enough rice for their own needs if the rain gods are kind.

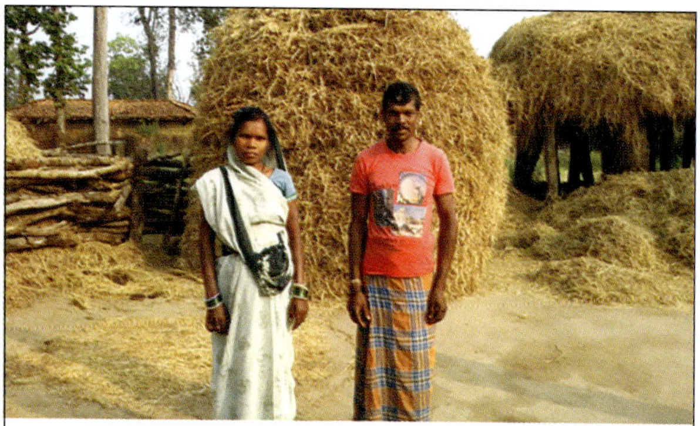

The Gond couple

'It was in 2009, 6 years ago, that the tragedy happened', said Dayaram, as Lachkunwar nodded in agreement. When we requested her to recite the story, Lachkunwar hesitated, her eyes reflecting the pain still fresh in her mind. Revisiting tragedies is never easy. She started from the beginning. 'I had 7 brothers and sisters, and I was married at the age of 18.

I was soon pregnant with my first baby, which was a girl. Later, I had another baby girl.

Both were uncomplicated home deliveries. The first one has dropped out of school because of financial constraints, while the second girl continues schooling.'

Manju, the health coordinator at Bamhani, asked her to continue and tell us about the third pregnancy. 'I started having pains towards the end of the term, and the baby died an intrauterine death by the time we reached the hospital', said Lachkunwar. Shaken by this death, they decided to take extra precautions and had regular antenatal check-ups at the Bamhani clinic during her fourth pregnancy. She was asked to get admitted at the JSS hospital 15 days prior to the expected date of delivery as it was a high risk pregnancy. But she did not take the advice seriously.

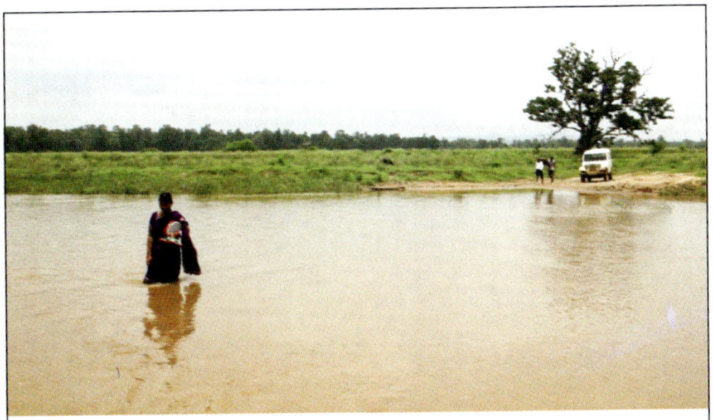

The Maniyari River

It was raining heavily when the labour pains started. Maniyari river, which separated the village from Bamhani, was flowing waist high. They decided to try a home delivery, a decision Lachkunwar still laments. 'The main delay was not because of the river, it was because of the delayed decision making on our part. We tried to get it done at home instead of reaching Ganiyari at the earliest, as I had been asked to do', she said.

As luck would have it, she went into obstructed labour as the baby got stuck at the outlet of the pelvis. Once the rains abated, with the help of local workers of Bamhani, they crossed the river with Lachkunwar on a cot. When she finally reached the JSS hospital at Ganiyari, it was too late. The baby had suffered an intrauterine death. And after about 8 days, she developed a vesico-vaginal fistula leading to a continuous dribbling of urine. Lachkunwar recalled, 'Those were difficult days. I could not move out of the house because of the continuous dribble. It smelt bad too.' Dayaram added, 'We still would sit near her. Even the neighbours would come for a few minutes and sit with her. No one wanted to hurt her.'

Lachkunwar talked about the day they travelled to Ganiyari. While in the bus, she was sitting with a small boy in her lap on the seat next to the conductor. The bus conductor's trousers got wet due to urine. 'He thought it is the boy who has urinated. It was embarrassing.'

There were times when she thought that her husband might abandon her for another woman. 'I had developed that constant fear and insecurity', she said with tears in her eyes.

She was advised surgical repair 6 months later. But she came to the hospital for surgery only after 18 months because the family could not arrange the small amount of money needed for the operation earlier than that. 'We were scolded by Yogesh sir for being so callous about my health,' said Lachkunwar. Manju explained, 'There is a mechanism whereby you can pay the operation fee in small amounts. Dr. Yogesh was angry because her family did not place her health as top priority.'

Lachkunwar Bai finally got operated in November 2010. She underwent the fistula repair and hysterectomy. There were episodes of mild stress incontinence thereafter, but she achieved a decent quality of life and, more importantly, became free from the social ostracism. She knew she would not bear children again, but it was a small price to pay considering the amount of mental trauma she was facing.

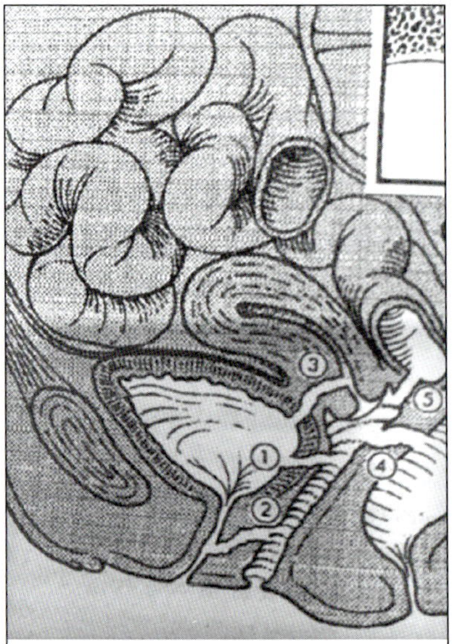

Fig: A VVF is an abnormal opening between the urinary bladder to the left and anterior and vagina which is behind the bladder.

For those of you not familiar with vesico-vaginal fistula (VVF), a fistula is an abnormal hole and VVF is a communication between the urinary bladder and vagina. It occurs due to prolonged obstructed labour when the lower part of the uterus presses on the posterior wall of the urinary bladder and the anterior part of thc vagina for too long and too hard. The lack of blood results in necrosis and the dead cells slough off to create a direct connection between the bladder and vagina, or in the worst case, the rectum and vagina. This abnormal opening called a fistula lets the urine from the bladder come out of the vagina. This over time may lead to vaginal stenosis which may lead to difficulty in having sex. The woman is never dry, day or night, so she smells of urine all the time. Her husband may not have sex with her, and her family may not have her in the house. Shemay be so unhappy that she may even be driven to kill herself.

A hundred years ago, VVF was seen everywhere because of poor antenatal care and lack of caesarean section facilities. But now it is seen only in some developing countries and that too in the underserved rural areas. Surgery is the only treatment for VVF, but the operation is always difficult, and sometimes impossible.

Even if a woman's fistula is repaired, she may be infertile. In most rural areas, women with VVF are not able to get the surgery done because surgeons who can perform this surgery are too few, too far away and too expensive. This is tragic. Some women leak urine for decades without knowing that their problem could be fixed surgically. Most women with this problem are very poor and deserve all support they can get. They may need more than one surgery.

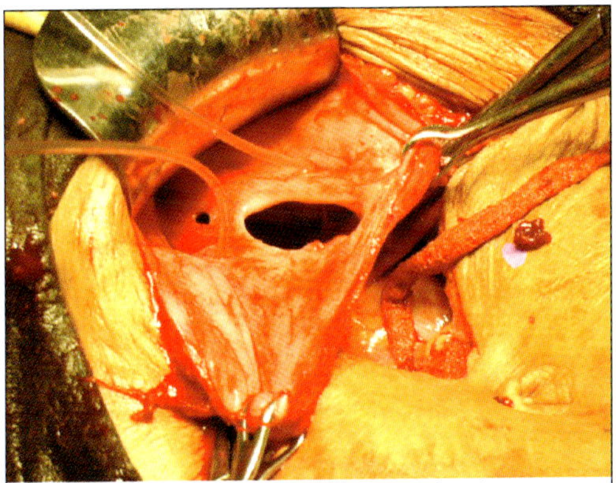

Fig: A large vesico-vaginal fistula getting operated.

We can do much to prevent VVF. Looking for high risk factors for cephalopelvic disproportion (CPD) such as short height and preventing obstructed labour are two things we must do. For preventing obstructed labour, using a partograph, a graphic depiction of the progress of labour, is an important intervention. As soon as there is a suspicion of VVF, a urinary catheter should be passed to relax the bladder which may hasten the delivery and relieve the obstruction.

Preventing fistulae requires preventing obstructed labour. This needs hospitals, health centres and antenatal clinics as close to women's homes as possible, all arranged in a hierarchy and following a timely referral system. Anything that obstructs the provision of these helps to cause VVF. It is imperative that all expecting mothers be warned of this complication and encouraged to have institutional deliveries, which lessens the rate of obstructed labour and VVF.

Six years on, Lachkunwar is content with her world and grateful to be alive. She wants her daughters and other women to be educated about pregnancy and labour so they do not have to face the problems she had to face. Though the couple is extremely poor and illiterate, they teach you that life moves on.

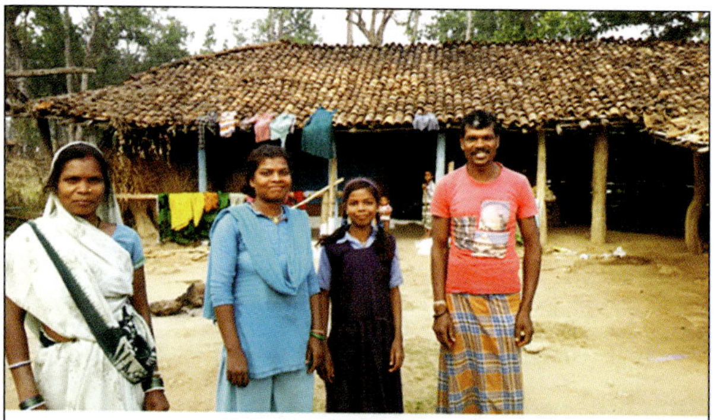

The Gond Family

diabetes

Dukhni Bai

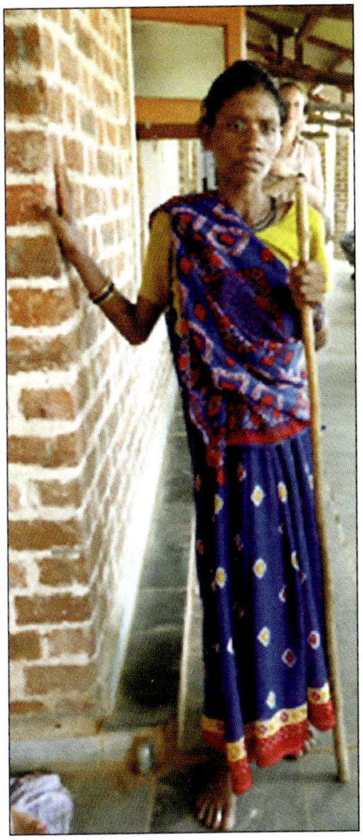

Dukhni Bai, a 36-year old mother of three, came to Jan Swasthya Sahyog, having lost both her health and livelihood. Two months prior to her visit, in November 2009, she had begun to feel a weakness in her legs and a weariness that would not allow her to work in the fields during the rice harvest. She was constantly thirsty and had to urinate frequently. Coupled with a constant backache and progressive weight loss, these symptoms put an end to Dukhni Bai's daily earnings of Rs. 40 as a landless labourer and cut her family's income in half.

Her husband, Jai Hari, managed to earn Rs. 50 a day by doing hard labour and agricultural work in and around their village of Nevra in Bilaspur. In July and August, he would be sowing seeds and ploughing the fields of landowners. Jai Hari had no livestock and would have to lug his massive plough on his shoulders to the fields of his employers. After the harvest in October and November, he would take up threshing. He also planted vegetables in others' fields, and when agricultural employment dried up between February and May, he would find digging work.

The loss of Dukhni Bai's income meant that feeding their three children and Jai Hari's 80 year old mother became more difficult. The family was barely holding its head up as it was; they lived in a one-room house with a single working bulb and no toilet. They did not have wiring for a second, now stolen, light bulb.

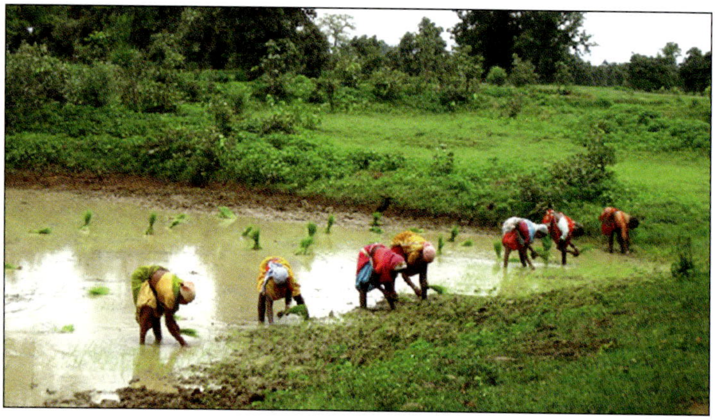

Dukhni Bai was diagnosed with diabetes and the cost of physician visits, lab tests and insulin kits was much more than the family could afford even if she had been working. Over five years, she had saved a few hundred rupees carrying headloads of grain, and that had gone to buy Jai Hari a second-hand bicycle. Now the family needed Rs. 1000 every month to pay for her treatment, but they did not even have enough money to get their bicycle repaired.

Since Dukhni Bai had stopped working, her husband was forced to take advances from the farmer he was working for. The family of six had barely been able to make do on the subsidized rice they were eligible for because of their 'below poverty line' (BPL) status. The rice usually ran out in two weeks and they would have to buy more on their own. The price of rice had shot up over three years, almost doubling to Rs. 35 per kilo from Rs. 19 in 2007. A kilo of dal would cost them Rs. 80, and as a result, they had cut it out of their diet entirely. Vegetables were eaten in minute quantities because they cost too much as well.

The World Health Organization has quoted studies that say that the treatment of diabetes in India could swallow a quarter of a family's monthly income. In the case of Dukhni Bai's family, it would have taken up nearly half of it. The management of a chronic condition would continue to push the family deeper into debt and when asked how he managed the family's finances, after pondering on it, all Jai Hari could say was: 'That's a good question.'

Diabetes: A disease beyond its medical perspectives

'What is diabetes?' Pose this question to any newly diagnosed patient or their relatives from rural Chhattisgarh and most often, you will get this type of reply: 'Don't know, but the local doctor told us that I am having 'sugar ki bimari'.'

This 'Sugar ki Bimari' is one of the least understood diseases in India, the new 'Diabetic Capital of the World', and it is slowly destroying the lives of more than 70 million people across the country. The challenges for people living with diabetes in rural India are even greater. First, many people have never before been diagnosed with diabetes in their lifetime. Of those diagnosed, many present for the first time one or the other grave complications related to the disease, for instance, 'diabetes foot' which can cripple the patient permanently and others such as nephropathy and cardiovascular which keep the patient under a constant risk of death.

Even after people get to know of the disease, many rural patients do not continue the treatment due to the high cost of medicines and related expenditure such as doctor's fee, expensive laboratory tests, travel etc. The high cost of healthcare is a major cause of forcing people into debt and poverty in a country like India. Due to their inability to seek timely and appropriate healthcare, many patients at risk end up with grave diabetic complications, leading to a much higher expenditure for treatment or a permanent disability. This further impoverishes them, and the vicious cycle results in multiplying their miseries.

Issues like poor availability of anti-diabetic drugs in government hospitals and the lack of understanding of diabetes among doctors and health professionals in rural India compounds the problem.

Undernutrition and low quality food are related to poor glycaemic control. Most poor people rely on the government subsidized carbohydrate rich food, such as wheat and rice that are cheap and the staple diet of a majority of Indians. Such foods have a high glycaemic index which leads to a derangement of sugar levels. Nor can many people afford footwear to protect their feet or do not use them as a regular part of their lifestyle. Going barefoot increases the chances of foot ulcers, cuts and poor wound healing which can result in the need for foot amputation. Unhygienic conditions also increase the risk of serious infections among the poor. One could say, 'misery breeds more misery'.

Counselling the poor and illiterate for diabetes is also a great challenge. Poor people are more concerned about their daily bread and butter and may not (or cannot afford to) appreciate the potential hazards of a seemingly less fatal disease like diabetes. Besides they may not have the constant availability of money and time to seek regular check-ups or afford regular medicines which a chronic disease like diabetes requires. Advanced or poorly controlled diabetes is even more difficult to treat. Most people dislike the idea of being pricked daily and poor compliance begins here. It can be difficult to explain the technique of administering insulin and incorrect dosages of insulin may be taken as a result. Insulin in this scenario acts as a double-edged sword with low therapeutic margin. The poor in rural India also do not have proper cold storage facilities to store insulin vials, and physicians are therefore also hesitant to start an eligible patient on insulin.

Diabetes-related disabilities are one of the major causes of DALY (disability-adjusted life year) losses in India. The burden of diabetic neuropathy, retinopathy, nephropathy and infectious complications is huge and currently we have very little to offer poor diabetics in rural India. This is certainly a 'double burden disease' as diabetes increases cardiovascular diseases as well as infections. For the rural poor to have diabetes is almost like death by slow poison which slowly devastates their families and destroys millions of dreams. While some people are striving hard to improve the understanding of this disease and its overall management, there is a lot to do to improve diabetes care in India for which we need both passion and compassion.

childhood tuberculosis

Anju

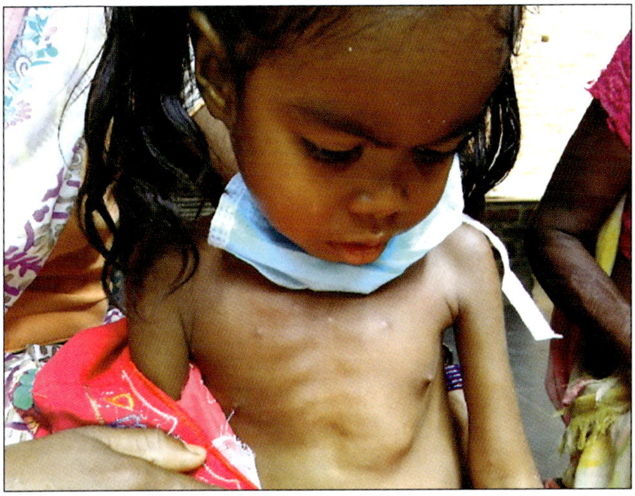

Four-year-old Anju Baiga was brought to the JSS hospital at Ganiyari with a mild cough and fever that had persisted for four months and a year-old protrusion on the left side of her chest. With a height of 85 cm and a weight of just 8.2 kg, she was severely underweight with signs of both wasting and stunting.

Anju came to Ganiyari from the forest village of Jhalapara, about 40 km away, where she lived with her mother, father, six-year-old sister, and three-year-old brother. The family's main source of income was the making and selling of brooms, for which they collected material from the surrounding area. The Baiga family used to farm on some nearby land, but two or three years earlier, the government Forest Department had claimed that land and begun planting trees on it. There was no significant medical history among the immediate family members. However, one relative who visited them regularly had been diagnosed with pulmonary tuberculosis and was undergoing treatment at JSS.

Anju's mother first suspected that something was wrong when one day about a year earlier she noticed a protrusion of Anju's chest, slightly more noticeable on the left side. She had also begun to notice that Anju didn't seem to be growing very well, in comparison to her older sister and other children in the village. She claimed that Anju was eating well until that time, although upon further investigation, the family's regular diet, both prior to and since Anju's illness, failed to meet the minimum standards for adequate nutrition.

A couple months after Anju's mother first noticed the chest protrusion, she decided to seek care at the local sub-centre, 4 kms from the family's home. The sub-centre was staffed by a local nurse, who told the family there was nothing she could do and that they should instead go to a Community Health Centre (CHC) or Primary Health Centre (PHC). With no CHC nearby, the mother decided to take Anju to the closest PHC, for which they had to walk one km before taking a bus that, when it ran, took 30 to 60 minutes. Upon reaching the PHC, they were again told that there was nothing anyone could do to help. The auxillary nurse midwife (ANM) told Anju's mother to take her to Bilaspur, where there was a hospital that could treat her.

At this point, the family had already invested much time, effort and money seeking care for Anju, yet they decided that travelling the 60-odd kms to Bilaspur was worth it if it could make her better. However, as they were planning their trip, a nurse in the village told them not to go to Bilaspur as there were no vacant beds at the hospital. Having no prior experience with the hospital system there, the family had little reason not to believe their neighbour and so decided to cancel their journey.

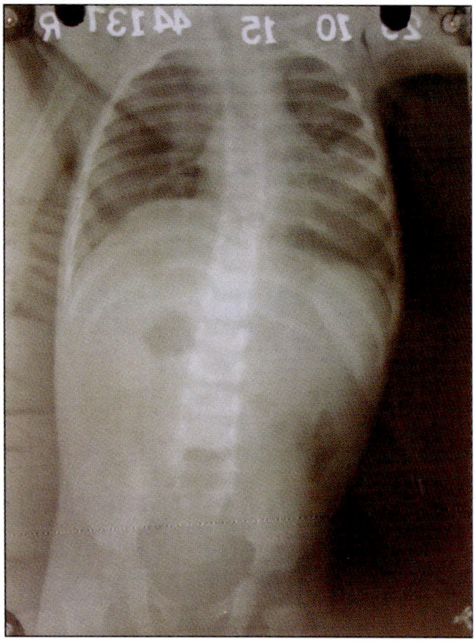

Instead, they took Anju to several traditional healers. Although the healers only asked for food as payment, the time taken to visit these healers only added to the family's burden, as Anju showed no improvement. Every four to five days, she would come down with mild to moderate fever and cough. Her appetite had begun to fall and she had lost weight. When weighed at the sub-centre, Anju was 9 kg. When finally brought to JSS at Ganiyari, she was 8.2 kg, having lost almost 10% of her body mass over the course of a few months.

As the family was running out of options, a relative

suggested that they go to the JSS hospital in Ganiyari. The relative's daughter-in-law was currently undergoing treatment for tuberculosis there and had made significant improvement. Anju's mother and grandmother thus made the 40-km trip to Ganiyari with her, which cost them Rs 80, and Anju was admitted with a suspected diagnosis of tuberculosis exacerbated by severe malnutrition.

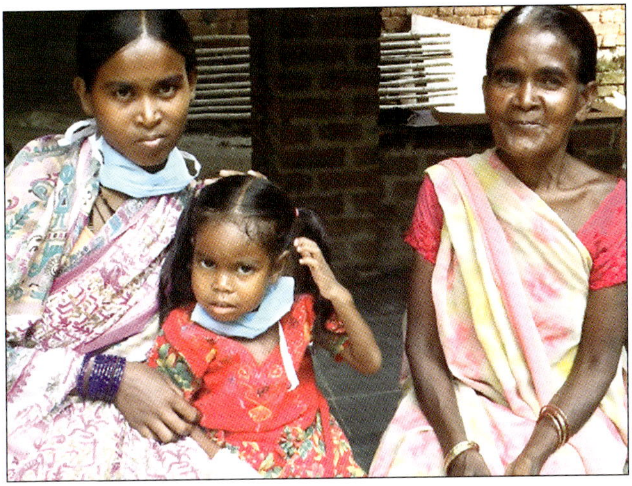

Anju was investigated for tuberculosis and found to have TB of the lungs as well as the urinary tract, especially the kidneys. This wide spread of the disease in more than one organ meant that the TB was disseminated. The accompanying severe undernutrition may have complicated the illness, which in turn would have worsened the undernutrition. Anju was put on anti- tubercular treatment with nutritional supplementation.

Anju's x-ray showed evidence of tuberculosis and some prior lung process, most likely untreated pneumonia. She was tested for tuberculosis using the tuberculin skin test, which came back positive. Because children are often unable to produce sputum, she underwent a gastric washing as an additional test. The gastric washing came back negative twice. However, tuberculosis was still suspected as literature had shown that severe malnutrition often causes false negatives in such tests. The results from the CBNAAT (Cartridge Based Nucleic Acid Amplification Test) showed the presence of mycobacterium TB (MTB). Anju had both pulmonary and renal TB.

Tuberculosis and malnutrition: a co-epidemic

Anju is one of 2.6 million people in India, and over 9 million people worldwide, suffering from active tuberculosis or TB. An infectious bacterial disease caused by mycobacterium tuberculosis, TB most commonly affects the lungs and is transmitted from person to person via droplets from the throats and lungs of people with the active respiratory disease (as per WHO).

In healthy people, infection with mycobacterium tuberculosis often causes no symptoms since the person's immune system acts to 'wall off' the bacteria. The symptoms of active TB of the lung are coughing, sometimes with sputum or blood, chest pains, weakness, weight loss, fever and night sweats. Tuberculosis is treatable with a six-month course of antibiotics.

However, in people who are moderately or severely malnourished, the progress of the disease and its treatment become more problematic as undernutrition has been shown to be both a cause and a complicating effect of tuberculosis. TB is often called a biosocial disease in that it is typically caused and exacerbated by social and economic factors, including poverty and malnutrition, and is more likely to spread among people living in crowded living conditions. Malnutrition both predisposes one to the occurrence of TB and is also worsened by TB, and is a factor associated with higher risk of death.

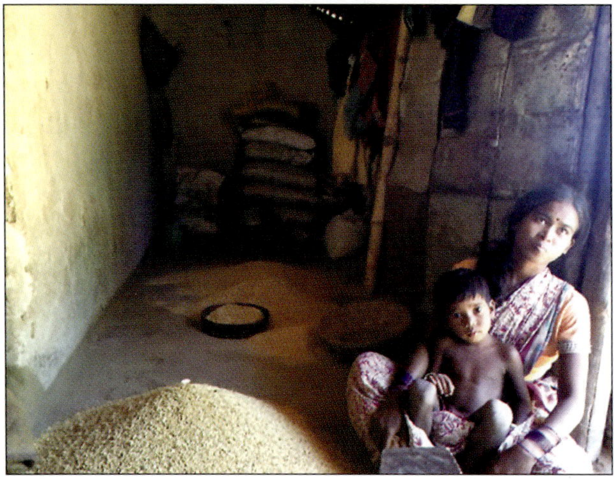

Undernutrition often complicates the diagnosis of TB in children like Anju by interfering with a delayed hypersensitivity immune response to the tuberculin antigen.

Thus the tuberculin skin test may turn out falsely negative. It also complicates treatment by predisposing one to drug-induced hepatotoxicity, which can lead to interruptions of therapy and even be fatal. In general, malnourished patients often do not respond to treatment for TB as they lack the necessary nutrients needed for adequate absorption. Finally, when not diagnosed and treated early, a TB patient can acquire a variety of complications due to malnutrition as undernutrition can lead to further infection caused by a suppressed immune system. To drive home this point, undernutrition-related diseases such as tuberculosis have rightly been called 'N-AIDS or nutrition AIDS'. It is no surprise that people with severe undernutrition present the same pattern and severity of TB and a similar immune deficiency effect as those with HIV coinfection. With over 55% of patients with TB in India moderately or severely malnourished, the co-epidemic of tuberculosis and undernutrition is a major public health hazard.

A social aetiology of undernutrition

The nutritional status of people in rural India is in a dire state. Over 50% of children below five are moderately or severely malnourished. Anju is just one of 44.61% of rural Chhattisgarh who live below the poverty line, which has been established by the Government as an earning of less than Rs. 738 a month. Anju's family earns about Rs. 24,000 a year, or $365, that is one US dollar a day for a family of five.

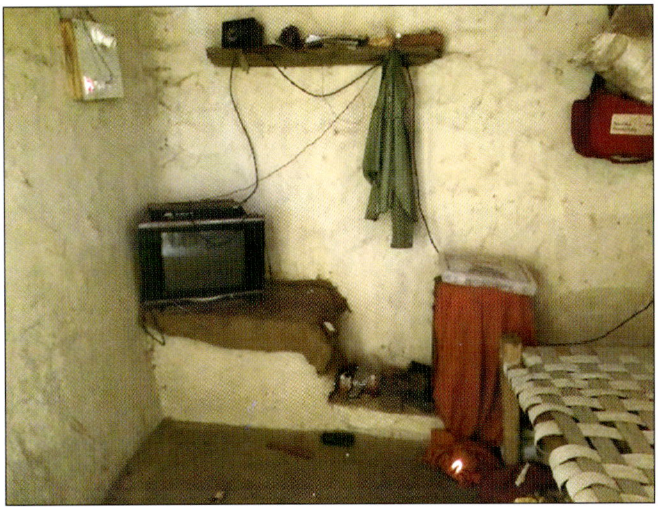

The uncertainty of income is aggravated by the fact that the Baiga family only has 2 acres on which to farm since the Forest Department had claimed a portion of their land two-three years ago. The fact that the Baigas are now forced to acquire most of their food from outside sources is a huge economic burden to the family. It not only greatly diminishes their ability to sell rice for cash income, but it means that in a year of poor rain like the one when this account was written, even with government rations, they were unable to produce enough crop to eat. They must use the money they make from their informal work of making brooms to purchase additional rice and other foods from the market.

Land rights among tribal populations is a major issue in rural India. Many like the Baigas do not have legal rights to the land they have lived on and farmed for generations. In 2006, the

Indian Government passed the Forest Rights Act (FRA), which aimed to correct this historical injustice and grant legal recognition to the rights of traditional forest dwelling communities. However, according to the Council for Social Development, which issued a report on the implementation of the Act in 2010, key features of the FRA 'have been undermined by a combination of apathy and sabotage during the process of implementation'.

Unfortunately, the Baiga family felt there was little they could do about the land situation except to continue to survive as best they could. When they found themselves short on cash, someone from the village loaned them food, with the understanding that they would eventually pay them back in kind. While there was no mention of debt, the family was unable to save any money at the end of each month. Rarely would they find themselves with a little extra, enough to buy some sweets or toys for the children.

Due to their BPL status, the Baiga family qualified for monthly rations of rice, salt and oil provided by the government. However, only the parents and Anju's older sister were counted in the government rations as children below 5 were not included. From this, the family received 21 kg of rice (7 kg per person and 1 kg of salt with which they must feed a family of five). According to the ILO, if someone was on a cereal predominant diet, the average food requirement per person per month was 18 kg. As such, the government rations often didn't last the family more than 15 days and they were forced to buy the bulk of their food from the local market. This mostly consisted of rice, for while they could scavenge for some greens and vegetables in the jungle near their home, pulses were too expensive to buy on a regular basis and typically, they only had dal once or twice a month.

The use of rice as the main staple of rural India comes from a history of developmental and agricultural policies supporting a low-cost, high-calorie diet for the rural poor. In 1970, a report declared, 'It is clear that the major deficiency in the diets of preschool children in India is calorie deficiency. Under these circumstances, the obvious approach would be to promote increased production and facilitate better distribution and utilization of existing conventional foods rather than a diversion of such foods for the preparation of sophisticated food formulations' (Gopalan 1970: 37). The emphasis on cheap calories was backed up by large government subsidies on rice and wheat. Since the 1970s, cereal production had more than doubled as families were pressured to grow rice due to the heavily biased economic support from the government. Yet, with such a monoculture, pulses and vegetables had almost disappeared from the diet of people like Anju Baiga's family. The Public Distribution Service (PDS) was created to fill the nutritional gap of BPL families. However, the rations mainly consisted of rice and a little salt and oil. According to Anju's family, pulses had recently been eliminated as a ration item. Such severe protein and vitamin deficiency was likely a major factor in putting Anju at risk for tuberculosis.

Despite repeated requests by the community, vaccines were not given to the children, and at the age of four, Anju had not received any immunizations. The sub-centre was not only poorly equipped to handle cases like Anju's, but also lacked a proper referral system to get her to a center that could give her the care she needed. Instead, Anju ended up at the PHC, which also lacked adequate staff and resources. As a result, the family wasted months seeking proper treatment. It was little wonder they were dissuaded from the allopathic medical system and turned to traditional healers.

TB of the spine (Pott's disease)

Kala Bai

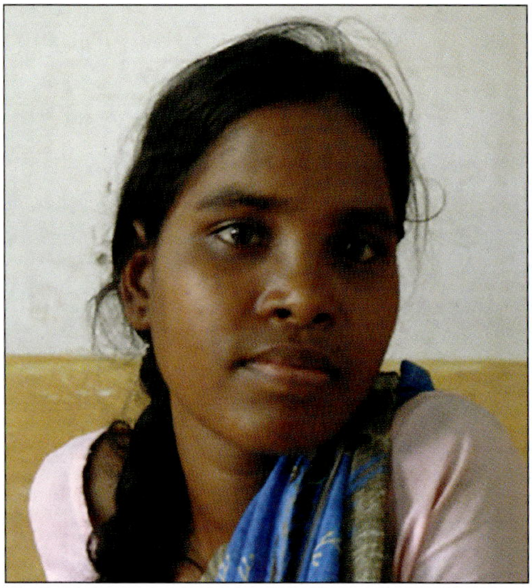

Kala Bai was in pain. It started in her mid-back, spread across her spine and pooled in her legs until they were so weak, she could barely do her daily chores. The root of her condition lay in poverty, in her inability to get enough to eat and the stress that early pregnancy and childbirth had loaded on her body. Kala Bai at 22 years weighed 32 kgs, a weight suitable for someone half her age. To add to her problems, she lived in the mountain village of Kurdar, where the roads were steep and uneven and her house lay at the end of a five km climb up the mountain. Kala Bai was in so much pain that she could barely walk a hundred metres.

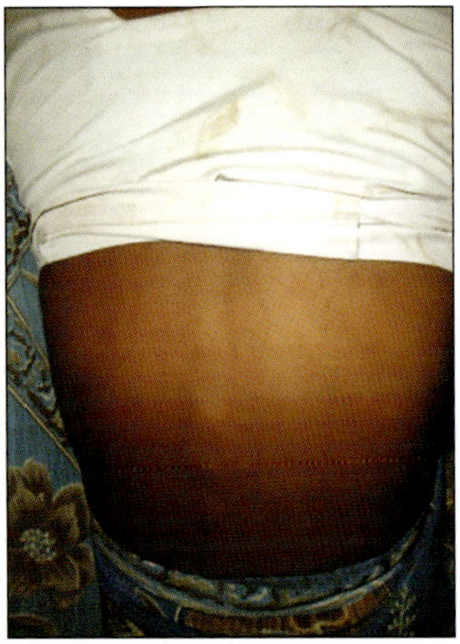

Getting to Ganiyari in the hope of treatment was an ordeal. It took Kala Bai four hours to descend the mountain and get to her parent's village of Aurapani. Three kms away lay the market village of Semariya, from where she caught the bus. It took her another three hours and Rs. 20 to get to Jan Swasthya Sahyog.

The attending physician found a walnut-sized lump on her spine and Kala Bai was diagnosed with Pott's Disease, a tuberculosis of the spine that is often found in rural India. Tuberculosis of organs including the stomach and brain is also found here. Kala Bai was started on a four-drug combination and would have to undergo nine to twelve months of therapy.

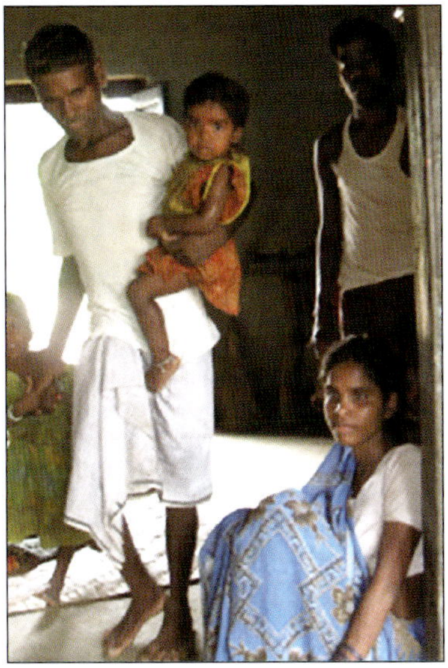

Her condition had caused major changes in her life and livelihood. She found it difficult to care for her two children and could no longer lift her youngest. Working as agricultural labour and even weaving baskets was now out of the question. Kala Bai and her husband earlier managed to scrape together Rs. 100-150 every day. But now with the fall in income and her lack of mobility, the family was forced to move to her parents' house in Aurapani.

Kala Bai's parents could barely handle the burden of their daughter's family. They wanted her to leave for want of space and resources. Her father said that her husband was an abusive alcoholic and would abandon his wife. Kala Bai could not help but be aware of what might happen to her with the months of treatment that lay ahead. JSS agreed to contribute to the cost of her therapy, but this too would not be enough. Her family depended on her income.

Pott's disease is one of the painful manifestations of tuberculosis and the patient usually complains of backache, which is mostly correlated with some trivial trauma or sometimes there is real trauma, causing fracture of an already weakened spine.

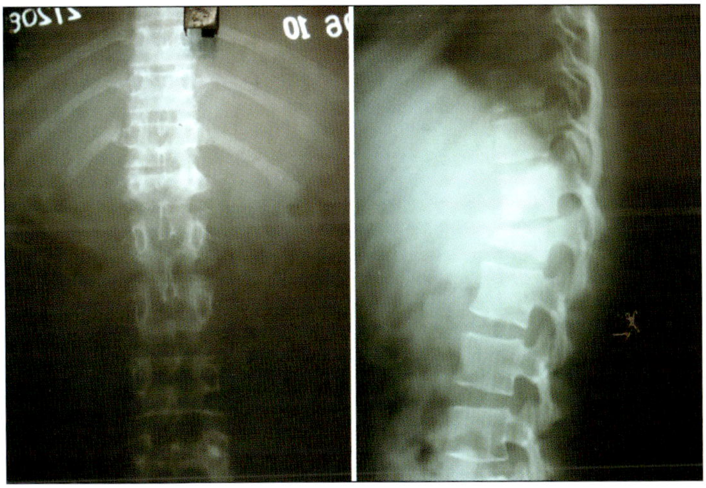

Although tuberculosis of the lungs is more common, tuberculosis of the spine is equally a cause for concern, having disastrous and often irreversible complications. Arguably, two lakh people in

India suffer from TB of the spine every year.

In more severe cases, the fractured spine compresses one of the nerves, leading to radiating leg pain, weakness of various grades, ranging from minor to complete paralysis. This may make the person bed-ridden for their whole life. The disease mostly starts with a mild cough with or without sputum. First this bacteria lodges in the lung, then it reaches the blood, and through the blood, to the spine.

Diagnosis is usually made based on a history suggestive of TB. Symptoms for spinal tuberculosis are localized back pain, painful movements, fever, a hump in the back, excessive weight loss, and in the worst cases, weakness of hands or legs. There are only a few physical examination findings, such as altered spine shape and prominent spine, termed 'Gibbus' medically. The diagnosis is confirmed with an x-ray of the spine, although an MRI scan picks up the disease much earlier. If the disease is confirmed on the x-ray, occasionally an MRI scan is still needed to see the exact level of nerve compression to forecast prognosis and determine the treatment plan of additional surgery, if any. The treatment includes anti-tubercular medicines to kill the bacteria, 4 to 5 medicines daily for a period of not less than 12 months and stabilisation of the spine to prevent or treat nerve injuries depending on the stage of disease. Spine stabilisation to prevent nerve injury can be achieved by posture education, physiotherapy, braces and traction. Spine stabilisation after nerve injury is a costly procedure (about 1 to 1.5 lac rupees) involving spine surgery.

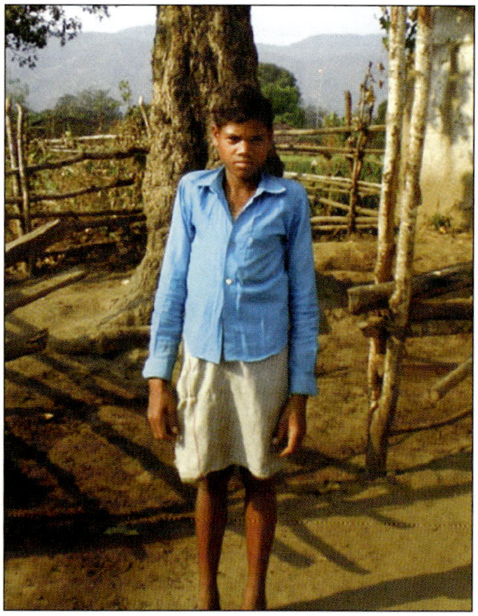

The thoracic region of the vertebral column is most frequently affected. Formation of a 'cold' abscess around the lesion is another characteristic feature.

Seeing a patient go through all these stages of disease and treatment is a long, painful journey. When a patient arrives, she has usually already travelled from being an erect, well-built, hardworking person trying to earn a sufficient living to a stooped, thin and depressed person moaning in pain. Pott's disease is seen more in poor people because of their poor nutrition status. Apart from the cost of treatment, the long duration of treatment really tests their patience as on one end, relief is either minimal despite taking many pills, while on the other, good relief gives the patient a temporary feeling of wellness. Both of these lead to stopping medicines in between and the worsening of symptoms. Those who complete the entire treatment may also have residual pain, weakness and disability for their remaining life. Daily activities such as walking erect and bending forward become difficult, and somebody's assistance is almost always needed. This means a loss of wages of one other person apart from the patient for a significant duration. With so much pain, doing physiotherapy and using braces is also challenging especially in rural households. Spine stabilisation is a good hope for those who can afford it but unfortunately that is not the case for many. Most live with pain killers, family support and physiotherapy for their entire life.

Persistent back pain present even during rest, fever and loss of appetite should alert one to a possibility of TB of the spine. No backache in childhood or a young adult should ever be ignored as there is a higher chance that this pain may be due to spinal tuberculosis. Controlling the spread of tuberculosis is the only way to prevent spinal tuberculosis.

epilepsy

Dashrath Baiga

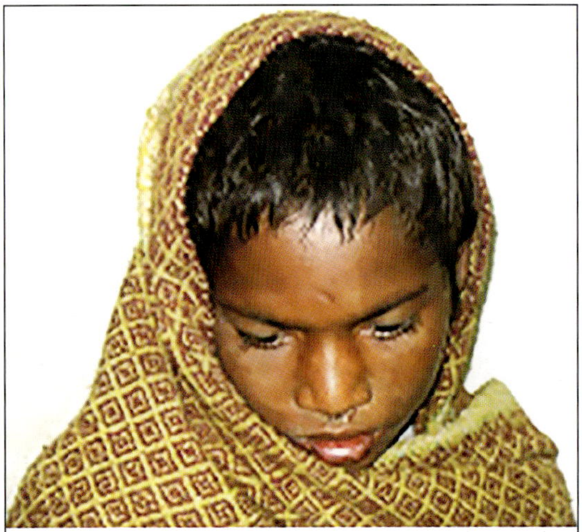

Dashrath, at age 10

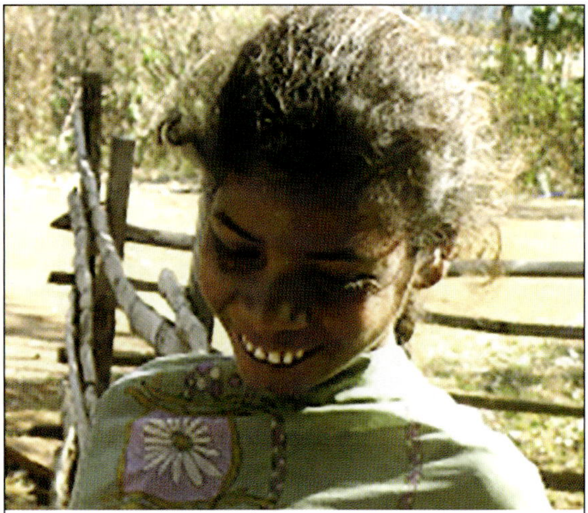

Jhum Bai, Dashrath's sister-in-law, age unknown

When ten-year old Dashrath first came to the Jan Swasthya Sahyog Outpatient Clinic, he had serious, infected burns in both legs. Dashrath had epilepsy. According to his sister-in-law Jhum Bai, Dashrath often wandered away from home, a matter of concern for her as his epileptic seizures were not controlled. His mother had died before Jhum Bai married into the family, and the boy had several seizures in a day. Four days before coming to the JSS hospital, while visiting another family in his village, Dashrath fell unconscious into a fire.

The next day, as the child's supply of anti-seizure medication had run out, a frequent occurrence, Jhum Bai asked the village health worker to help her get resupplied. It was then that the boy's burns first came to the attention of the JSS health worker, who organised for him to be taken to the JSS hospital in Ganiyari.

After his burns were treated, the doctors sat down in a quiet spot to hear Dashrath's story.

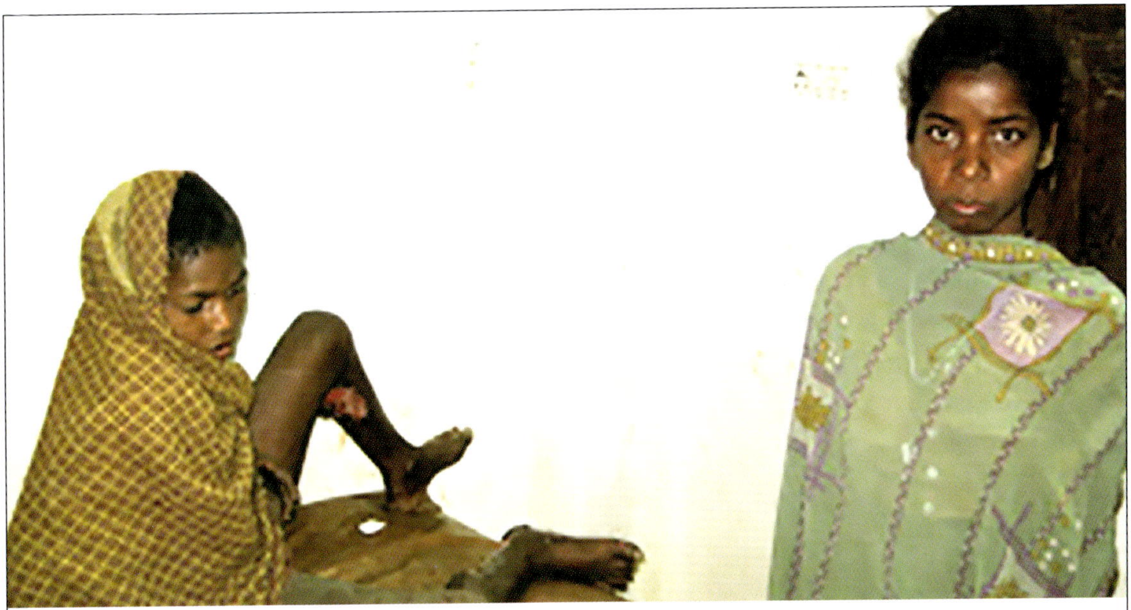

Dashrath and Jhum Bai in the JSS hospital at Ganiyari

Suddenly, without warning, Dashrath fell forward with a grimace, his eyes glazed over and he was motionless. He did not utter a cry. Dashrath recovered quickly but was listless.

This spell, Jhum Bai said, was how it always happened, several times a day.

A month earlier, Dashrath's father, aged about 50, was found dead on the road to the village. The police took the body away for autopsy, but demanded Rs. 2000 from the family, claiming it was a fee for the autopsy. Without paying, they would not release the body. There was no alternative but to sell the family's two oxen. The proceeds from the sale of Rs. 5,000 went to pay the police and the balance to pay for the traditional burial and a meal at a cost of Rs. 3,000, to which the whole village was invited.

On learning of his son's death, Dashrath's grandfather abruptly stopped eating and died two weeks later of a broken heart. This time Jhum Bai and her husband had to mortgage their small plot of land to pay out another Rs. 5,000 for the grandfather's funeral. The interest on this loan itself was 5% a month, or 60% per annum. By now they had depleted all their resources, and with no prospect of paying back the loan, they would still have to pay the interest, without which their property would be confiscated.

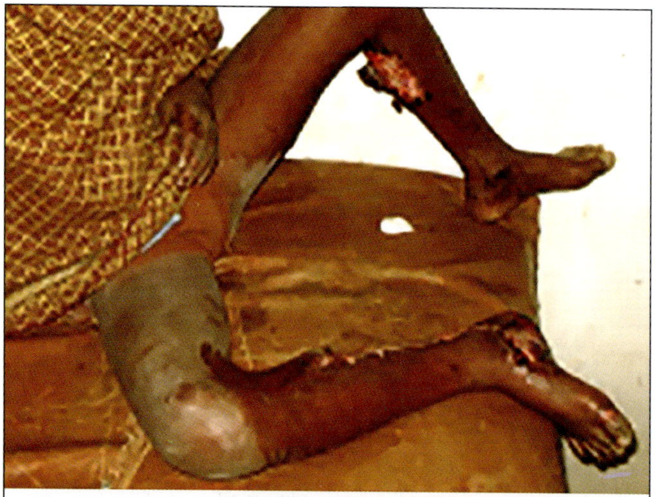
Dashrath's burned, infected legs. Burns are common complications of epilepsy in rural India.

The six surviving family members lived in a one-room house in Mangalpur, one of 54 remote forest villages where JSS had trained health workers. In Mangalpur, most families were below-poverty-line. Since her marriage, due t o Dashrath's frequent seizures, either Jhum Bai or her husband had to stay home with him on any given day. Jhum Bai usually stayed home to keep the boy from serious harm. She earned Rs. 100 a week by weaving baskets, she said, and working 'All day, every day'. Her husband and another brother each earned Rs. 50 a day, chopping wood in the forest as labourers. The boy's aunt and her son were the fifth and sixth members of the household. Sometimes the aunt gathered firewood in the forest as did Jhum Bai, making a three-hour trip by foot carrying the heavy load of firewood on their heads. Her aunt's son, though grown up, did not work. The six family members shared the one-room hut but the aunt, her son and Dashrath's other brother slept elsewhere. The government was supposed to provide electricity for one light bulb as it did for other BPL families, but the connection was out of order. So there was no light within the one-room home. The family had no radio or other electrical device. Drinking water was available from a bore well that served the entire village.

The family had three ration cards to purchase rice once a month at a subsidized price. But the rice ran out mid-month. To survive, they had to buy an additional 30 kilos a month on the open market, paying Rs. 20 a kilo that is Rs. 600, a sum they struggled to earn. A similar story was with dal or lentils, their chief source of protein. They were only able to afford a cup's worth of dal three or four times a month, enough for one meal for six people. The family ate something twice a day, but sometimes there was not enough food for a second meal.

This daily struggle to feed themselves is still the reality for many households in rural India. Jhum Bai said if they could double their combined income, they would buy more dal and rice. And if any money was left over, she would save it for emergencies.

In such a scenario, finding help even for a chronic disorder like epilepsy is a struggle.

About 1% of the world's population has epilepsy, that is, 65 million people. Roughly 20 million people are untreated or receive inadequate or inappropriate treatment. Fifty percent of people with epilepsy (PWE) can be treated with a single drug. The rest would require two or more drugs, and roughly 30% would not be able to gain seizure control.

India faces a chronic lack of specialists trained to treat epilepsy. For all of India, there are less than 1,500 neurophysicians for a population of 12 million PWE. Most people live in rural India, while most neurologists work in the cities. Access to specialists is a problem that cannot be solved without diversifying training to other physicians, health professionals and health workers.

Untreated or uncontrolled epilepsy is a serious problem. It results in accidents, as faced by Dashrath. Burns or broken limbs can become a cause of permanent disability and falling unconscious even in a few inches of water can be fatal, particularly for those with no easy access to emergency medical care. Even people with serious untreated epilepsy can become victims of sudden death. Sudden Unexplained Death in Epilepsy (SUDEP) is now recognised as a serious medical issue worldwide that requires urgent attention. Each year more than 1 in a 1000 people die of SUDEP. If seizures are uncontrolled, the risk increases to more than 1 in 150 PWE.

Dashrath's story was recorded in 2010. Recognising the need to treat epilepsy, in 2012 JSS started a unique programme to make epilepsy care and education available to people of rural Chhattisgarh living in the JSS village programme areas. The JSS Village Health Workers encourage those who stop treatment to continue taking medication and others to get their prescription renewed in time.

infertility

Jhum Bai

The Harshness of Village Life and Jhum Bai's Dream

The story of Dashrath, a victim of uncontrolled epileptic seizures, and his sister-in-law Jhum Bai of Mangalpur, unraveled, much like the road that led to their tiny village in the forest, with several twists and turns down narrow rutted paths. Their greatest suffering was the sense of helplessness which denied them the hope of a brighter future, free of the deprivations of poverty. Dashrath, then a ten-year old, lived from day to day, seizure to seizure. Jhum Bai, married close to the onset of puberty, remained childless six years later and faced the bleakest of all possible outcomes: abandonment. This was the fate of many

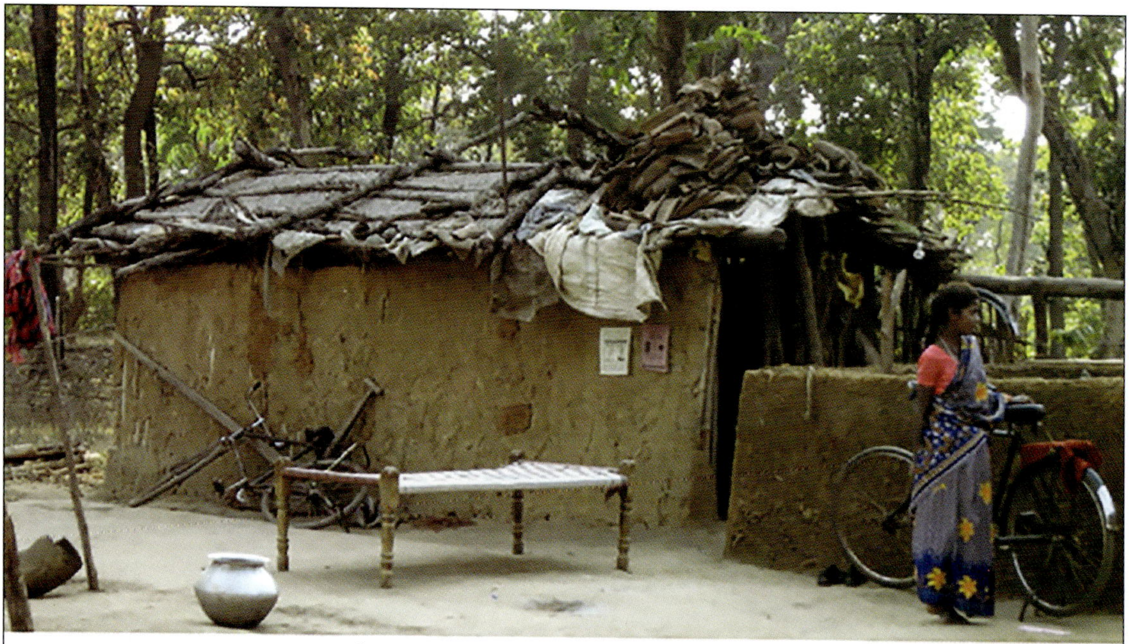

Jhum Bai standing in front of her home

childless rural women.

Mangalpur is a remote hamlet of 28 families and 150 individuals. Most single family dwellings had just one room; a few had tiled roofs; all huts were made of mud with dirt floors. None had latrines or running water. The primary school, too, was housed in a tiny one-room building adjacent to a newer structure that was never finished. At the time of writing this account, active electioneering for the first panchayat elections in sixty years was underway in the village.

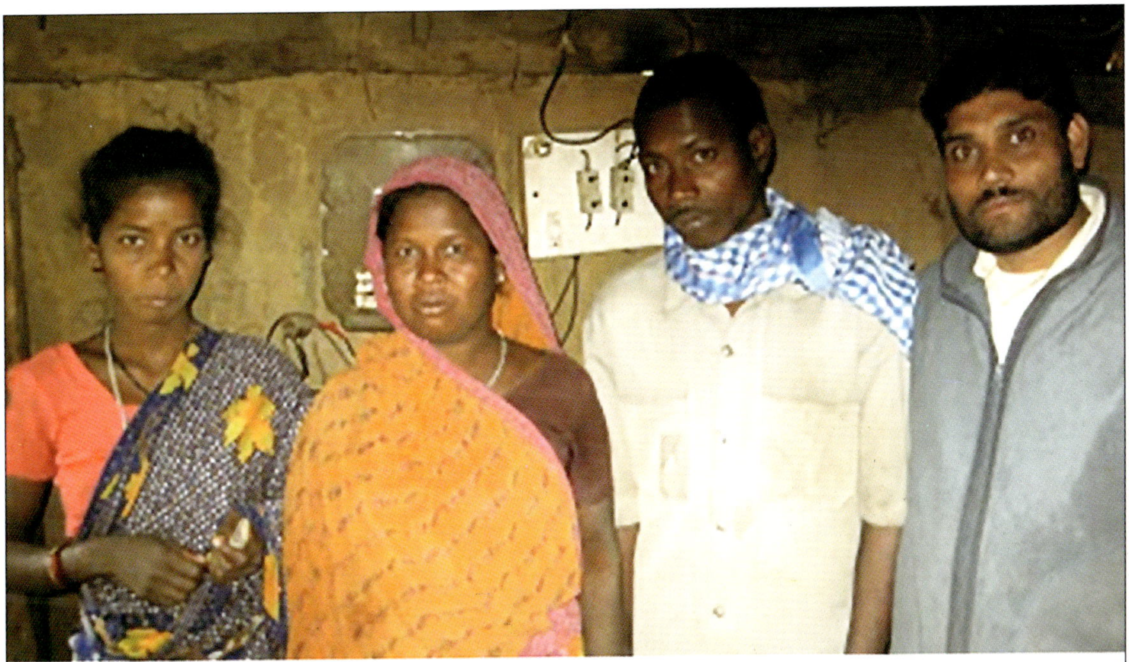

Left to right : Jhum Bai, Aghaniya Bai, JSS village health worker, Kunwar Singh, and Prafull, the JSS Field Coordinator

Jhum Bai's hut stood among a cluster of several others. Her husband Kunwar Singh and JSS' Senior Village Health Worker Aghaniya Bai were present.

The visit was to hand over a sum of Rs. 5,000, the balance required to pay off the moneylender and reclaim the family's small plot of land on which a single crop of paddy was harvested every September. News of this assistance from JSS had reduced Kunwar Singh to tears, Jhum Bai said.

The electrical connection, to the lone bulb inside the hut, had been out of order for months. The head of the panchayat, the local governing body, demanded Rs. 100 to get the responsible government official, based at the block headquarters in Kota, to fix it. Jhum Bai could not pay. Hence, it remained a useless relic. At night, the family depended on the dim light from a single bulb attached to the exterior of the hovel. Sometimes, a kerosene lantern was available. The battery of a torch, lying on top of sacks of paddy, had expired long ago.

Three large sacks of paddy from September's harvest were stored in the room. Since the failure of the monsoons in 2009, only about one-third the normal yield could be harvested. The family planned to extract seeds for planting on their plot of land at the onset of the monsoons in July. Hence, there would be no rice left from their own crop for the family to eat. They had to depend on the government-subsidized rice purchased with their BPL ration cards, but this lasted only part of the month.

As seen in the photograph, on the back wall of the hut hang some of the family's possessions: a few articles of clothing (Jhum Bai owned three saris), a mosquito net, and dried corn brought by Jhum Bai's parents who lived 40 kms away. Heaped on the floor were thin,

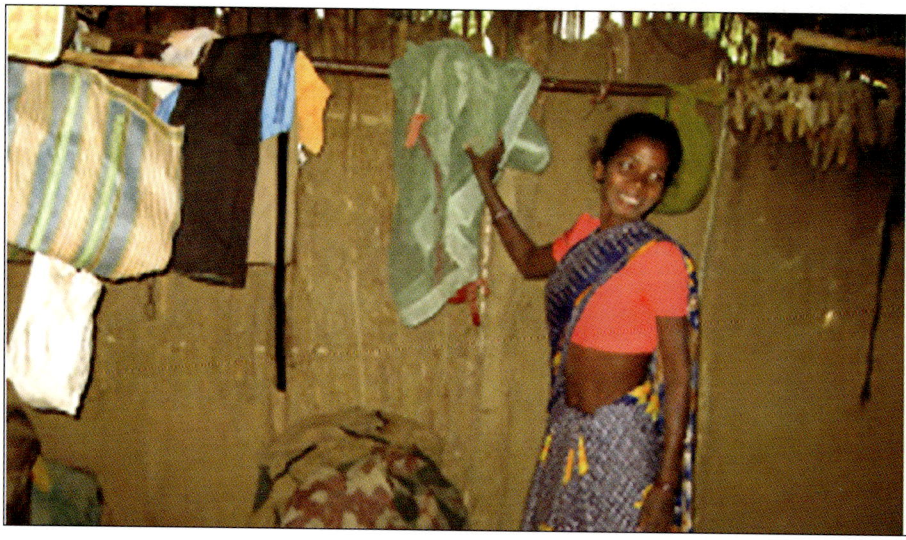

The back wall of the hut with clothing. Jhum Bai holding mosquito netting. Piled on the floor, flimsy blankets. Dried corn on upper right.

threadbare blankets and ground coverings. There were no beds or mattresses.

The family hoped to finish construction of a second room soon. When completed, Jhum Bai, her husband and Dashrath would live there. The current hut would be converted into an animal keep for the family's two remaining oxen and used for storage.

Life was unimaginably hard. During the winter months, November to February, despite the fire burning inside their hut at night, the family shivered from the cold. They had no woollen clothes and only the thinnest of blankets. Sleep was fitful. Often, Jhum Bai, her husband and Dashrath woke up by 2 a.m. and would sit around the fire to warm up before lying down once more to try and sleep. When in need, neighbours could not be counted on, nor the government. The bore well, the only source of drinking water near their home, had been out of order for a month. Two weeks earlier, each villager had paid Rs. 10 to the panchayat to get the bore well repaired, but nothing had been done.

The government had failed to install any latrines in this or other villages in the Achanakmar Forest Reserve. Four villages of the reserve had already been moved out and as yet, the government had failed to provide the displaced villagers with any amenities or compensation. A weak protest was slowly growing against overwhelming odds. These villagers, mostly of the officially protected Baiga tribe, were in fact scorned by officialdom as illiterate and were too few in numbers to be taken seriously.

The roof leaked badly; the best solution was tiling the roof, which was beyond their grasp. Even a new sheet of heavy plastic, to be covered with leaves, was unaffordable. Old and broken tiles hauled from another village could be used on the adjacent roof, but the quantity and quality was grossly insufficient.

For personal hygiene, bathing and washing up was done at the bore well pump, when it was functioning. But poverty dictated that soap could be used only every other day.

No one in the family owned a bicycle. Those seen in the photo belonged to Kunwar Singh's cousins who lived elsewhere.

When asked: 'If you were granted three wishes, what would they be?' without hesitation,

Jhum Bai replied: 'I would not have three wishes, only one: to have children'.

Her survival might depend on this wish coming true.

Back at JSS one day with Dashrath, Jhum Bai had talked about her life and childlessness.

There was resilience instead of despair. Jhum Bai explained: 'There are no children at home, except Dashrath. My husband's older brother is single and has made it clear he doesn't want to marry. So the burden is on me. I have one or two more years to have a child. If I don't, my husband Kunwar will take another woman…and I will leave, go back to my parents' home. There is further pressure from my parents. They remind me disapprovingly that my brother married about the same time as I did. He has two children while I have none.'

Adoption was discussed as a possibility. In rural India, it is customary to adopt within the family, for example, it could be a relative's girl child where there were too many mouths to feed. But this was not Jhum Bai's situation.

When asked if she would marry again if her husband took another wife, she said:

'No one will marry a woman who can't have children'. Nor, she added, would she consider living with another man. But this fate, feared by all childless women, was not sealed.

'Over the past two years, every time, I bring Dashrath for a visit to Ganiyari (the JSS hospital), my husband says: 'Why don't you have yourself checked up?' He has been urging me to get examined almost from the beginning.'

She had not she admitted, because the very thought of a gynaecological examination overwhelmed her with embarrassment, even if the doctor was a woman. But now that she was more familiar with JSS, she hoped to overcome her shyness.

There was a shroud of secrecy about vaginal bleeding, discharges or pelvic pain among village women. Further, itching, irritation or a white discharge from the vagina was so common, it was almost considered normal. Help was seldom sought and practically never discussed with others. Only when pain, as in the late stages of cervical cancer, became overwhelming did village women seek medical help. Mothers even avoided discussion of menstruation with their daughters. Jhum Bai has never talked with other young women in the village about her concerns. The doctor present, explained that in any case, the initial approach would be to determine if her husband was fertile and get a sperm count. Her husband would only have to go to Shivtarai, a JSS sub-centre close to their village. The idea of male infertility was a realm beyond. Jhum Bai promised to speak to her husband. To Jhum Bai and Kunwar, the idea of male infertility was novel. His response was not assured to be positive. In Indian villages, any hint of a man's lack of 'virility' would by itself bring shame and ridicule. So then why be tested?

Other than an explanation, at menarche, from her mother that menstrual flow would come monthly, and awareness that sexual relations may result in pregnancy, Jhum Bai had no knowledge of reproduction or the relevant female anatomy. That the uterus existed was news to her. Jhum Bai's education ended during the preschool years as her father had fallen ill and the family needed her to do the household chores and take care of the infants in the family. Even if she had continued through the primary grades, sex education had not come to the village schools of Chhattisgarh or, for that matter, to most schools in India.

She said her husband treated her well. 'He doesn't get drunk or beat me. I know he loves me as I do him. And I have friends my own age in the village. We go together to the forest to get wood. Sometimes I go with Kunwar to Kota, (the nearest village with a market)'.

'If I were better off, I wouldn't have to do all these chores. If I were rich, I would buy jewellery and some farm land.' Jhum Bai had a few, commonplace bangles and hardly any other jewellery, marking her as the poorest of the poor. Today, she had come wearing a sari which was in tatters.

Life would be different if she had a child she said. 'A child would give me inspiration to live – someone to live for and to build a future with'. It wouldn't matter whether it was a girl or boy, she said. 'I would devote my life to that child and do everything possible to see that my child receives a good education. Without an education, a child can't get anywhere.'

Jhum Bai added that the Mangalpur village school went up to the 5th grade. Then, two kms away in the nearby village of Karka, the school was up to the 8th grade. In Kota, 5 kms distance, there was a high school. Currently, three children from the village went there, two boys and a girl. They all had bicycles.

When asked if she would herself like to return to school, being still young, if JSS supported her financially, Jhum Bai replied: 'Yes, I would, if my husband agrees. I could go to school from eight in the morning until one, and then go home and work until eight in the evening. If not, and I don't have a child and am rejected, once I'm back with my parents, I will find work and then I will try to go back to school. I would not be interested in marrying again or living with another man.'

Jhum Bai added, 'Before I married, my family was better off. We had more to eat. When my parents decided that the time had come for me to marry, they considered three suitors. Two came from families with greater wealth. The third, Kunwar, came from a poorer family. My mother said: 'This will be a better marriage. The richer suitors will treat you with little respect. The poorer suitor is more likely to treat you well'.' So it had come to pass.

Jhum Bai was driven with a determination to improve her lot in life. After she married Kunwar Singh, she managed to save a little money over the years, so that they now had a few pots and pans. She told us that the other girls in the village used to make fun of her for marrying into such a poor family. Her tireless basket weaving brought in Rs. 100 a week, which not even her husband knew – she was keeping these savings in secret for hard times.

While the concern in reproductive health and fertility has been about high fertility and thus about contraception, infertility is a common clinical and social problem, especially in rural areas and thus deserves our attention. It affects 13-15% of couples, more so in developing countries where limited sources for investigation and treatment are available. One should start evaluation only after 12 months of the couple staying together.

The most common causes for infertility among couples are:

1. Male factor such as sperm abnormalities.
2. Female factors such as ovulation dysfunction and tubal pathology.
3. Combined male and female factors and unexplained infertility.

It is a major social problem and the feelings experienced by infertile couples include depression, guilt, shame and inadequacy with social isolation.

Some common causes of infertility which can be treated at a peripheral level if detected on time include:

1. Pelvic inflammatory disease.
2. Sexually transmitted infections.
3. Personal habits like smoking and alcoholism.

Male factors are equally responsible for infertility, a fact which is often overlooked. Semen analysis after 3 days of abstinence is advised. Recording the history of both partners separately and a good clinical examination are an important part of investigations in an infective couple. If none of the above mentioned factors seem responsible for infertility, early referral of infertile couples to a dedicated specialist infertility clinic may be indicated to increase their chances of conceiving.

Further investigations like hysterosalpingography, blood FSH and LH levels should be done only after a proper work-up omitting unnecessary investigations to reduce the total cost of treatment without compromising on their success rate.

Treatment options for infertile couples include three main types of fertility treatment.

1. Medical treatment (ovulation induction)
2. Surgical treatment (laparoscopy and hysteroscopy)
3. Different assisted reproductive techniques.

The choice of treatment is often related to issues of efficacy, cost, ease of use or its administration and side effects. Counselling of the infertile couple also forms an important part of the treatment. Management of infertility has always been a difficult task, not only because of the difficulty in diagnosis and treatment of reproductive disorders, but also because of poorly stated interaction between the partners' fertility potentials in achieving pregnancy.

epilepsy and special needs

Suman

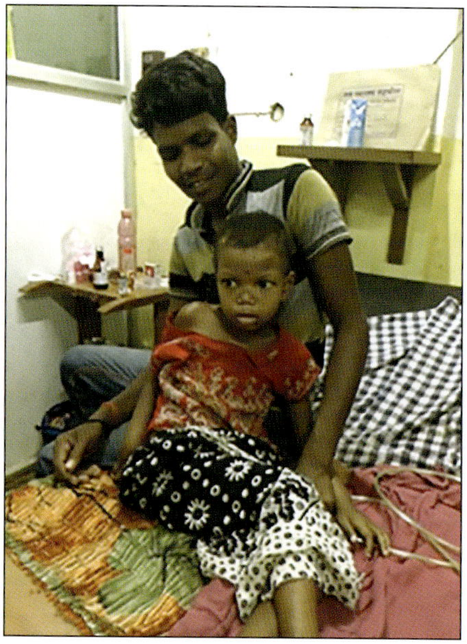

Suman was a six-year-old girl from Rathkandi village, in the forest area outside of Semariya. She lived with her father, mother, and nine-month-old sister. Suman came to JSS, Ganiyari, with a severe case of pneumonia, for which she was kept in hospital for 20 days. While pneumonia was not uncommonly seen at Ganiyari, Suman's case was unique in that she also had an extensive history of seizures which had left her weak, mentally challenged, and unable to care for herself.

By the family's accounts, Suman was a healthy child until she was a year and a half old. She weighed 3 kg at birth after a normal delivery and was exclusively breastfed until she was six months old. In 2011, at the age of 18 months, Suman developed a moderate fever that turned into a high-grade fever after three days. As her fever peaked, Suman had a seizure and became unconscious. With her father away in Bilaspur for work, her mother Draupadi was the only one at home. Their neighbours helped Draupadi take Suman to the government hospital in Belgehna, a few kms away.

The staff at the primary health centre at Belgehna said that they could not manage Suman's illness and that she needed to be taken to CIMS, the government hospital in Bilaspur town. Suman was admitted to CIMS, where she continued to have seizures. The seizure activity was more prominent on the right side of her body, particularly her face. After the seizures, she would have persistent weakness on the right side. The doctors ordered a CT scan of her brain

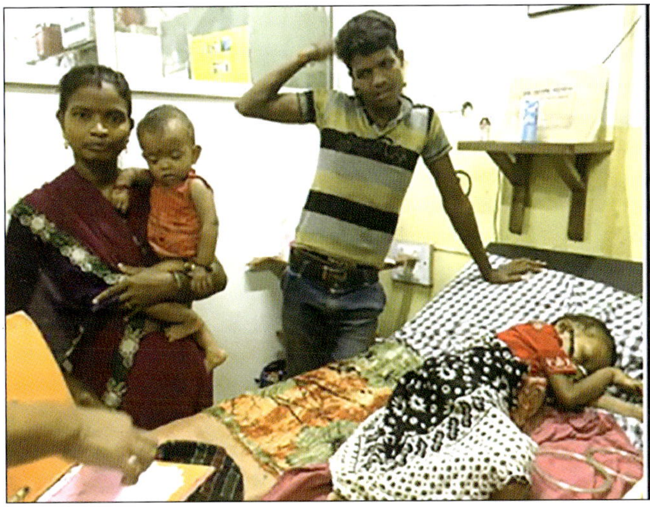 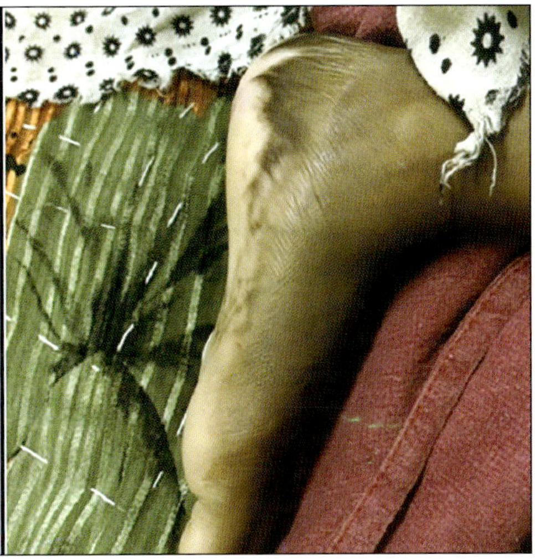

to see if there was any structural problem. The scans showed some abnormality in the brain, although the exact problem was unclear. There was no evidence of an abscess. Fifteen days after her admission, Suman was discharged and prescribed tablets for her seizures.

The family thought Suman's condition would improve, but she continued to have seizures, having about 10 such episodes a day. The family had to keep a close watch on her as Suman would often fall and hurt herself during a seizure. Her father was unable to go to work in Bilaspur, where he had a job as an electrician, because he had to look after her. This meant a loss of income. With allopathic medicines apparently not working, the family started to lose faith in modern medicine. Other villagers thought Suman's seizures might be due to ghosts or spirits and said it was important that she see a traditional healer. The family took Suman to three different traditional healers over the course of a year, spending between Rs 4000-5000.

In 2012, the family decided to take Suman to a peripheral clinic of JSS at Semariya, where Suman was started on sodium valproate, an anti-epilepsy drug. Her seizures dramatically decreased in frequency, but she was left with the debilitating effects of her frequent seizures. Her cognitive and physical abilities were slower than that of other children her age and she was quite frail. One day, when playing near the cooking fire, Suman got curious and reached out to touch the fire. She tried to pull away from the heat, but her reflexes being slow, she accidently fell into the flames and burnt her buttocks and foot. She was rushed to Ganiyari, where she was treated for the burns. Her epilepsy medication was monitored. Doctors also treated her for malnutrition as she was significantly underweight and suffering from loose stools. Suman was given nutritional supplements as part of her therapy.

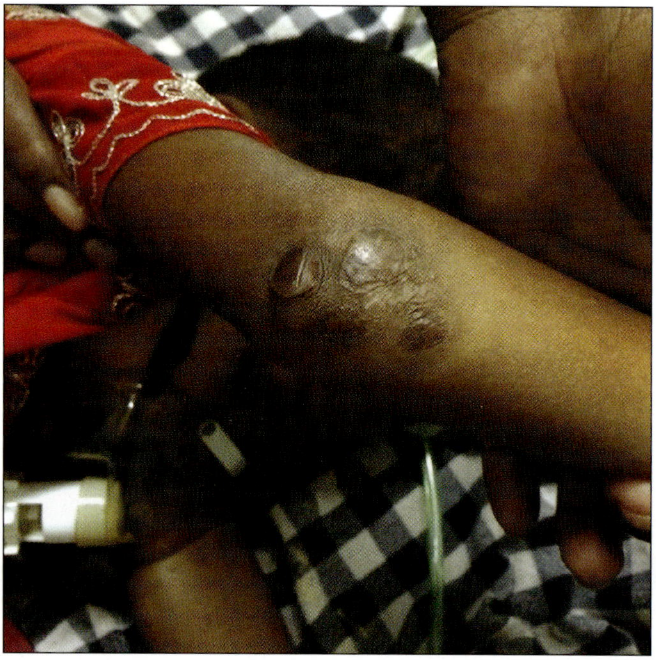

While Suman's seizures had dramatically decreased in frequency, she was still experiencing jerks on a daily basis. The sodium valproate dose she was receiving was causing extreme drowsiness. It was decided to put her on levetiracetam, an expensive medicine. With this, while the effects of prolonged seizure leading to brain injury could not be reversed, she could remain active and mostly seizure free.

The effects of Suman's disorder were a cause of constant stress on her family as her seizures were unpredictable. Suman also required extensive care on an hourly basis and her mental disability meant that she could not go to school.

Extensive rehabilitation was required for a semi-normal life, and for a family living in a remote forest village, the prospects of receiving such care were slim to none. With their own farming to take care of, money to earn, and a nine-month old who also needed care, the family was constantly pushed to their limits of endurance, emotionally and financially.

The planting of rice had already been done that year during Suman's initial 20-day hospitalization, allowing both her parents to stay with her at Ganiyari. The parents said they were barely able to manage financially with the harvest from both their farm and the farm in her mother's village, which they loaned out to farmers in return for 50% of the crop yield.

Rarely, when things were relatively stable at home, one of them would go and do daily wage labour on a nearby farm while the other stayed home with Suman and the baby. Yet despite being able to get by with what they had, there was no doubt that the time away from work and the cost of medication was a heavy economic burden on them. Since Suman's illness, the family had been unable to save any money and often had to resort to selling their stock of rice for money for her treatment.

Suman's medical condition was probably encephalitis, an infection of the brain caused by a virus. The exact virus is often not established, even in top hospitals. The encephalitis recovered partially but left Suman with two problems: first slowing of her mental processes due to brain damage; second, epilepsy which causes convulsions due to abnormal electrical activity arising from the damaged brain. There is no medical treatment for the brain damage that has taken already place, but the undamaged parts of Suman's brain will continue to develop; so there will be improvement as she grows older. But it is not possible to predict the extent and functional usefulness of this recovery with any great accuracy. There is medical treatment for the epilepsy and this has been quite effective. But for Suman's parents, this comes at a cost – the cost of not being able to afford other things because they have to pay for the medicines.

So what more can be done now for Suman and her family? Firstly, Suman needs to be in a safe place during the day so that her parents can resume work. Could she go to the phulwari village crèche if there was some extra support there? Are there any other girls like Suman in the village whose families could together share the costs for the crèche or a separate place of safety? Are there any villagers who would have the time to look after Suman at home? Secondly, are there any cheaper epilepsy medicines which would be as effective as levetiracetam for Suman? Effectiveness is the most important consideration in choosing a drug to abolish epileptic seizures, but it must be traded off with cost. Carbamazepine is about 2% less effective than levetiracetam but costs about 800 rupees less per month. For some, this cost difference outweighs a small loss of effectiveness.

Suman's story demonstrates that in all medical conditions there are two components: medical and social. For Suman both are important and interlinked, but not insoluble.

HIV

Santoshi

Santoshi's husband Naresh was admitted to JSS at Ganiyari with sputum positive tuberculosis in April 2015. He weighed a shocking 32.2 kg and was so weak he could not even stand, preventing the staff from taking his BMI. He was started on anti-tuberculosis treatment with first line drugs (HRZE), a four-drug regimen which was the standard therapy for TB. His sputum report later showed that his tuberculosis was resistant to rifampicin, a key antibiotic that was part of the regimen.

Three years before, Naresh had been diagnosed as HIV-positive and had started anti-retroviral therapy (ART) at the anti-retroviral drugs centre in the regional medical college, Chhattisgarh Institute of Medical Sciences (CIMS), Bilaspur. He had been off therapy for quite a while, but it was decided that once his condition improved, he would be sent back to CIMS to restart therapy. Naresh's cervical lymph nodes had enlarged and he had been started on a six-month directly observed treatment (DOTS) regime for TB of the lymph nodes at CIMS after being tested for it. He took this treatment for six months on a thrice weekly basis, and he was alright for one year, until he developed lymph nodal swellings again, which later led to a rupture of the lymph nodes. CIMS referred Naresh to the rural community health centre at Bilha near his home, and he underwent another six months of DOTS and streptomycin injections thrice a week (so called category 2 anti-TB drug

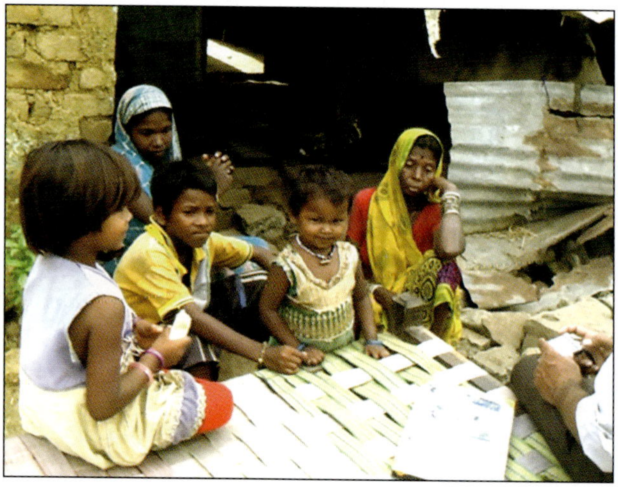

regimen which has one more drug in addition to the four drugs he took in the first treatment course).

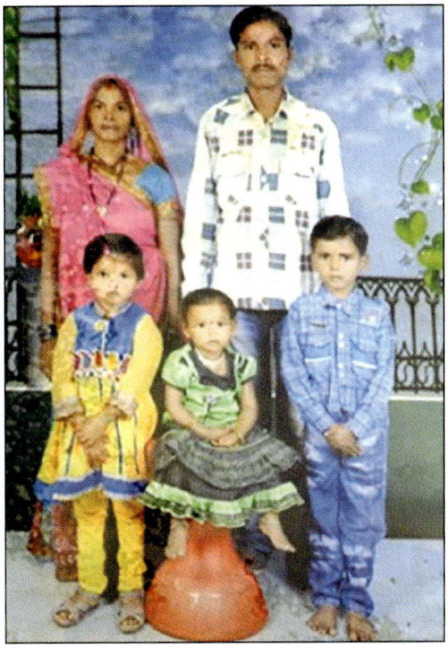

His wife later told JSS staff members that her husband was an alcoholic and a drug addict who often threw his medicines away in the past. He would drink alcohol like tea in the morning and was always smoking ganja (cannabis). He demanded chicken for dinner every night and it was often 12 a.m. before Santoshi would get to sleep. A year after his treatment began, he did not get better and it was a year before Santoshi could convince her father-in-law to take Naresh to the hospital. The old man was convinced that his son would improve slowly and it was only when Naresh had become extremely weak due to his cough that the family brought him to Ganiyari.

On his arrival at JSS, Naresh was found to have no appetite at all. He was given medication to induce hunger and convinced to eat, but he could not bring himself to do so. He was strongly opposed to the use of a nasogastric tube, but despite his objections, a tube was threaded through his nose and passed into his stomach. However, 15 days after his admission, Naresh died at the Ganiyari hospital due to persistent symptoms and progressive respiratory failure.

He left behind his wife Santoshi and three children. During a family screening, Santoshi was also found to be HIV positive. She had been running a light fever for two days. An AFB sputum test, which helps diagnose pulmonary tuberculosis, was found to be negative. Since AFB tests often show up negative in HIV patients, Santoshi's sputum sample was sent for a CBNAAT test, which was considered more sensitive and also detected resistance to rifampicin. A chest x-ray would show white streaks on her lungs (infiltrates), an indicator of tuberculosis infection. She was started on the antibiotic doxycycline and given preventive therapy of isoniazid, a second antibiotic. Santoshi had found out about her HIV status when she was three months pregnant with her third child. She had taken ART to protect her baby from HIV, but not for herself.

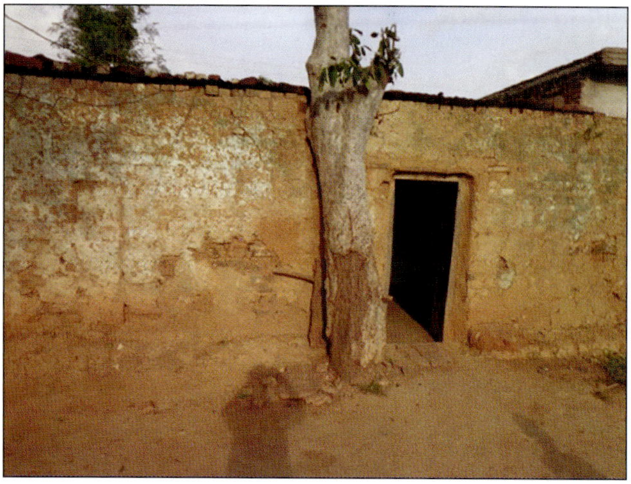

When the children were tested, they were all found to be negative for HIV. However, a Tuberculin test, conducted by injecting a TB antigen under the skin of the forearm, confirmed that her five-year-old daughter was infected with the tuberculosis bacteria.

Santoshi, now a widow, left Ganiyari with strict instructions to return for her preventive therapy and check-ups and treatment for her children. She would also have to go to CIMS to get her anti-retrovirals. Five days later, her CBNAAT test results showed a diagnosis of mycobacterium tuberculosis that was sensitive to rifampicin. A phone call was made to get Santoshi to return immediately to JSS. She never showed up.

A few days later, Santoshi told JSS staff over the phone that no one in her family was willing to accompany her to the hospital and she would not be able to come alone. Therefore, two social workers from JSS, Mannu and Saukhi, went to her house in the village of Hardi Kala to give her the drugs and to inform family members about Santoshi's condition.

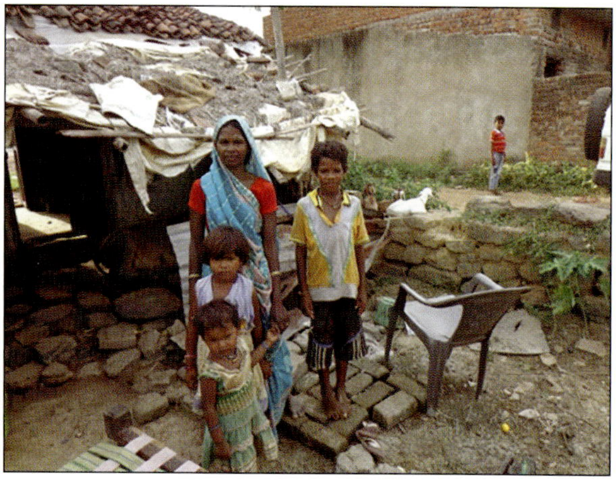

Hardi Kala village was 10 km away from Bilaspur city, and 30 km from Ganiyari, in the Bilha tehsil, a large cluster of permanent and semi-permanent dwellings equipped with a health centre, schooling until class 12 and an anganwadi.

After Naresh's death, Santoshi had been left in a two-room mud house adjoining her in-laws' four-room one. She had six goats, a cow that had come with her dowry and her husband's chicken shop. After her husband's death, she gave their calf away to her nephew and paid for the last rites out of her savings. One of her brothers-in-law looked after the chicken shop, the profits from which had been declining as the price of chickens rose. Naresh had been the oldest of seven children – two sisters were married and four brothers were not. His father was a mason and his mother worked in people's fields. Two years of heavy monsoons had made it difficult for her to find work. Naresh's mother said that no one in their family had ever had tuberculosis, and she was not keen to accompany Santoshi to JSS as she blamed the hospital for the loss of her son.

After speaking with the family, JSS staff suggested that Santoshi request the officials at the ART centre in Bilaspur to give her the TB medications she required, but her request was turned down. She was unable to meet the financial requirements of travelling to JSS Ganiyari for her treatment. So it was arranged that Santoshi would be given Rs. 800 every month for nine months to meet her travelling and medical expenses.

In September 2015, Santoshi came to take her second round of anti-tuberculosis treatment and brought her three children along. They were screened for TB and the two older children were started on isoniazid treatment. The following week, a doctor and a social worker from JSS went to meet the family and ask if Santoshi was having any side effects while taking her medicines or doing any work. They also wanted to educate the family on Santoshi's two medical conditions and on the importance of taking medication correctly.

Naresh developed HIV and because of his immunocompromised state, acquired TB in his lymph nodes. People living with HIV are 26-31 times more likely to develop TB than those without HIV. TB is the most common presenting illness among people living with HIV, including those taking anti-retroviral treatment, and it is the major cause of HIV-related death. The deadly combination of TB and HIV must have consumed Naresh to make him very undernourished.

The treatment that Naresh received, the thrice weekly frequency of anti-TB drugs, results in sub-optimal cure rates and thus had been abandoned as the treatment schedule for those with TB-HIV coinfection for several years. And yet he got this treatment, which expectedly led to a shallow cure that caused a relapse within a short period. As double damage, he was put on a therapeutically inappropriate regimen once again – that of five drugs now, with only one new drug added to the previous four. This is a completely wrong way of treating those who have been treated in the past and have come back with the disease. In the treatment of TB, we should never add a new drug to a failing regimen. Additionally, this wrong choice of drugs, called Cat 2 regimen in Revised National Tuberculosis Control Program (RNTCP) parlance, was also given thrice weekly. Due to this combination of misfortune and wrongs inflicted by the health system, Naresh got what is the worst possibility for a TB patient – a multi-drug resistant disease (MDR-TB), which in the presence of HIV has less than 30% cure rates despite the best treatment. Coupled with severe undernutrition, the outcome of death was almost predictable.

Who is responsible for Naresh's death? His poverty? His HIV? Or the poverty of public health systems? It is perhaps not wrong to say that he developed MDR-TB largely due to the amplification of drug resistance in the bacteria he carried, which occurred because he was offered suboptimal drug therapy twice from the public health system.

It was good and appropriate that he was started on anti-retroviral drugs when he developed tuberculosis. He is also likely to have been counselled to take his ART medicines regularly. But if a person defaults on his ART, there are no good community processes to ensure restarting of this most essential treatment. Discontinuation of his ART would have resulted in his immune status going down and that would also have resulted in his tuberculosis relapsing.

The HIV epidemic is exacerbating TB transmission, and that may be why his wife was not only infected with the virus through him, but also the tuberculosis that she developed.

As HIV generates a greater number of MDR-TB cases, the frequency of drug resistance among new cases may increase. At the institutional level, HIV has been associated with epidemic MDR-TB transmission in a number of countries. On a far larger scale, India has 1.7 million people co-infected with MDR-TB and HIV, and a multidrug resistance rate of 2% to 5% among previously untreated individuals with TB.

The reality is that the proportion of TB deaths attributable to HIV is 12%. Further, it is estimated that the overall Case Fatality Rate for HIV-related TB (including undiagnosed cases) is over 50% in many developing countries. Multi-drug resistant tuberculosis has been shown to be almost twice as common in TB patients living with HIV as compared to TB patients without HIV. Cure rates in those with HIV and MDR-TB have very poor outcomes in low resource settings.

What does it mean to be a poor widow with three young children, and have HIV-Tuberculosis? Even if the TB bacteria are sensitive to the drug rifampicin, it could still be an isonaized resistant disease. Santoshi needs daily anti-tubercular drugs for at least nine months, the appropriate regular ART and food supplements, plus family support for her to be able to come out of this. Life is going to be extraordinarily difficult for her.

childhood HIV disease

Mahi

Mahi was born to an HIV-positive couple on June 19, 2013. Her mother was being treated at JSS for tubercular lymphadenitis, a swelling of the lymph nodes caused by tuberculosis. While screening for HIV in tuberculosis, both parents tested HIV-positive. Mahi was called to the JSS OPD for screening in Sept 2013, and found to be suffering from a litany of complaints. She had had coughs and fevers for the past five months and showed marked wasting with a high respiratory rate. She had ringworm, a fungal skin infection, and oral thrush, a yeast infection in her mouth. Listening to her chest revealed bilateral crepitation, crackling and rattling noises whenever she inhaled, indicating that her lungs were inflamed. Additionally, she had an abnormally enlarged spleen and liver as well as generalised lymphadenopathy, which is swollen lymph nodes in more than two areas of the body. Her motor and development functions were also severely delayed. Mahi was unable to sit and roll down on her own, definitely abnormal for a child of one year, but especially for a child who was said to be normal till 6 months of age.

Based on her family history and their extensive examination, Mahi was diagnosed with paediatric AIDS and pulmonary tuberculosis, confirmed by an HIV TRIDOT screening test and chest x-ray showing lymph node enlargement in the right lung. The doctors at JSS prescribed anti-tubercular and anti-fungal drugs and sent her to the anti-retroviral therapy (ART) centre in Bilaspur in September 2014, to start treatment and to be considered for Dried Blood Spot testing.

In October, Mahi was back at JSS. The ART centre had decided not to test her for AIDS or begin any treatment because she was under 18 months of age. HIV antibodies are passed on from the mother to the infant in the womb and stay in the blood until the child is 18 months old. Until then, it is difficult to test the child for AIDS since commonly used tests detect antibodies in the blood, but which cannot distinguish if the antibodies are the mother's or the child's. Dried Blood Spot testing would have allowed the child's blood to be analysed for the AIDS virus (HIV) DNA rather than for the antibodies produced in reaction to it. However, the ART centre did not offer that testing service and could not provide the child treatment.

JSS then tried to make a case for offering Mahi empiric AIDS treatment based on clinical findings and arranged for a sophisticated antigen test called the RT-PCR test (reverse transcriptase polymerase chain reaction), which looks for the genetic sequence of the AIDS virus, to be conducted by a private laboratory. The result was positive. Armed with this information, JSS repeatedly followed up with the ART centre in Bilaspur, but to no avail. Mahi got no anti-retroviral treatment from the ART centre. Her condition marginally improved, and when she became 18 months old, another test was conducted at CIMS in Bilaspur. The ELISA test, commonly used to detect antibodies, showed no signs of an HIV infection in Mahi's blood. The result of the ELISA test done at JSS, however, showed that the test was reactive and that Mahi was indeed positive for HIV/AIDS. Yet she never received a single round of ART.

In February 2015, Mahi was brought to JSS for the last time, running a high fever, her breathing rapid and shallow. She was diagnosed with severe pneumonia and given antibiotics intravenously. Her medicine was later upped to a combination of the antibiotics piperacillin/tazobactam and co-trimoxazole, along with antifungal drugs. She had to be put on a ventilator and resuscitated. But six days later, at 8 a.m. on a Monday morning, Mahi died.

Had Mahi been tested for HIV by the Dried Blood Spot test at the very beginning, the outcome of her illness could have been very different. Caught in the tangle of erroneous tests, an unclear medical policy and a time lag, Mahi did not live to see her second birthday despite being clinically diagnosed with HIV by an experienced paediatrician. The diagnosis of tubercular lymphadenitis in the mother would have been fortunate for Mahi if only we had a sensitive and more effective health care system.

HIV in a child

Children are innocent bystanders in the vortex of HIV transmission and its epidemiology. They can get infected in the late fetal period, or at birth, or later through breast milk. Clinically once infected, most children show a more rapid and telescoped clinical course than adults. A lot of children would show opportunistic infections including tuberculosis, childhood pneumonia and gastroenteritis. But many children would show early involvement of the central nervous system (CNS) that would later manifest as developmental regression as well as evidence of other CNS involvement.

The diagnosis of AIDS is a little problematic, especially in the first 18 months of age. Since there is a passive transmission of antibodies of IgG and IgA across the placenta, the presence of disease-specific antibodies in this age-group cannot be assumed as evidence of HIV infection. Hence, several recommendations suggest that the ELISA or other antibody tests be deferred until the child is 18 months of age, by which time all antibodies from the mother should have become zero.

But what if an infection is suspected before 18 months? Disease symptoms of childhood HIV may be seen as early as 3 to 6 months of age, and if clinically diagnosed, deserves early initiation of antiretroviral drugs. At this early stage, one has to therefore test for HIV antigens such as P24 to confirm the disease. Unfortunately testing for the antigen is technically more complicated and also more expensive. Thus in the National AIDS control programme it is recommended that testing for HIV infection in this age-group would demand that a Dried Blood Spot (DBS) of the child's blood be sent to the regional laboratories competent in doing the antigen tests and analyses. Further, it is also mentioned that in absence of such confirmatory tests, the paediatrician is justified in starting ART on the basis of the clinical diagnosis.

It is very likely that Mahi had acquired the HIV infection from her mother, and also the tuberculosis. Additionally, she perhaps acquired a fungal meningitis as an opportunistic infection. And it is possible that she had a neurological involvement due to the HIV disease. The local AIDS control setup failed this child in not offering her the requisite antigen testing that she needed for her illness. A larger error was denying the ART to her at the age of 12 months when her antigen tests from a private laboratory confirmed her disease, quoting the specious excuse that this was a private lab report. Had she got the ART in time, perhaps Mahi would not have died.

Further, our efforts at convincing the national ART officer, based in New Delhi, and requesting him to reissue instructions to the states regarding principles of starting childhood ART medicines did not bear fruit. But we are still trying, and sooner or later, we hope to succeed. There is a urgent need to educate physicians and paediatricians in childhood HIV.

congenital heart disease

Meena

Sixteen-year old Meena Bai Gond had travelled with her parents all the way from her village in Dindori district of Madhya Pradesh to Ganiyari. On April 9, 2015, she came to the JSS hospital at Ganiyari with severe shortness of breath that her parents had been trying to get treated for three months, to no avail. Meena Bai had been complaining of shortness of breath ever since childhood. When her breathlessness started affecting her day-to-day activities, her parents decided to take her to a hospital. The first stop was a hospital in Dindori, where she was given medication which had no effect on her symptoms. Then they took her to the government hospital in the nearby city of Shahpura, from where she was referred to a hospital in Jabalpur.

Meena Bai was admitted at the Netaji Subhash Chandra Bose (NSCB) Government Medical College and Hospital in Jabalpur on April 4, 2015. A 2D echocardiogram was conducted, which uses sound waves to create an image of the heart to detect abnormal movements. The test showed that she had Tetralogy of Fallot, a complicated heart disease that comprised four heart defects. Meena Bai's heart had a hole between the lower chambers, which led to oxygenated blood from the lungs being mixed with deoxygenated blood from the body and then being circulated back into the lungs, putting pressure on the lungs to handle the extra volume of blood, and on the heart to pump harder. The main artery leading out of the heart was situated over the hole and conducted mixed blood out to the body. Coupled with that, a valve conducting deoxygenated blood to the lungs was constricted, so not enough blood was reaching it. The wall of the lower right chamber of the heart had thickened because the heart was working so hard to pump blood that it could have eventually led the heart muscle to stiffen.

Tetralogy of Fallot is treated with open-heart surgery. NSCB Hospital gave Meena Bai diuretics, steroids, bronchodilators to widen her airways and broad-spectrum antibiotics. She was observed for four days and then discharged. Even at discharge, she was breathless, but conscious. The next day after she reached home, her breathlessness worsened and she rapidly became drowsy and then unconscious. Sensing impending doom, the parents decided to rush to a hospital. But this time they decided to embark on a long arduous drive to Ganiyari, 150 km away, since Meena had not improved at the medical college hospital at Jabalpur where she had been less than 48 hours before. They hired a private taxi for a massive sum of rupees three thousand. That night, Meena was brought to Ganiyari with acute breathlessness. Examination showed her to be in a coma and she was breathing very rapidly but deeply and was intensely blue. Her blood oxygen content was 55% compared to a normal of over 93%. She had a clear chest. And thus a diagnosis of cyanotic spell was made. This complication is more common in children and not often seen in adults, and this may have been a reason why this complication was missed earlier. She was given oxygen, intravenous metoprolol and put in a knee-chest position. We wanted to give her intravenous morphine but could not because it was not available at our centre. This is because the license for morphine is extremely difficult to get for any size of hospital on the specious grounds and fears of making patient's dependent on opiates. And thus people with very painful problems such as advanced cancer, sickle cell anaemia crisis and post-operative patients are denied appropriate pain relief. After much struggle, our hospital at Ganiyari had managed to get the license for oral morphine, which is useful in palliative care of patients with cancer. But for life-threatening situations such as a cyanotic spell or acute myocardial infarction, an essential drug like intravenous morphine is not available in almost any health facility in central India.

We tried our best with other medicines but to no avail. And this girl died a few hours after reaching our hospital.

We talked to the physicians who were caring for her at the NSCB Medical College in Jabalpur about this. And they regretted having missed this classic complication of a cyanotic heart disease, which, if treated in time, could have been cured, and she would have been a candidate for corrective surgery of the heart, which would have given her a full life.

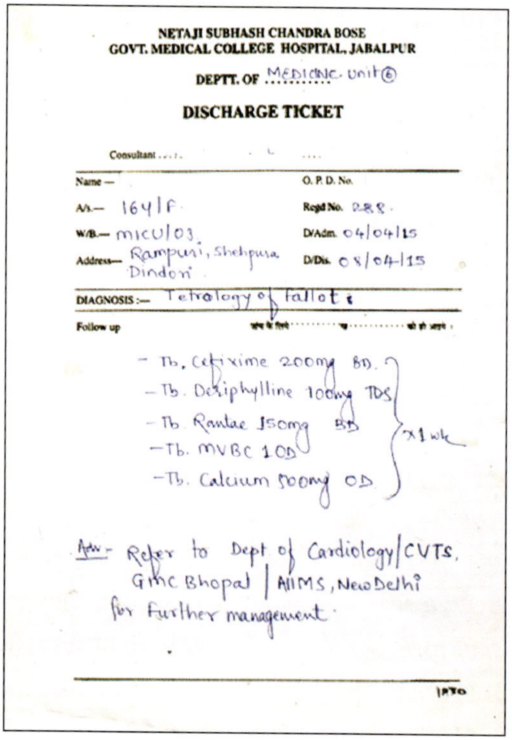
NETAJI SUBHASH CHANDRA BOSE
GOVT. MEDICAL COLLEGE HOSPITAL, JABALPUR

DEPTT. OF MEDICINE. Unit 6

DISCHARGE TICKET

Consultant

Name — O. P. D. No.

A/s.— 16Y/F Regd No. 288

W/B.— MICU/03 D/Adm. 04/04/15

Address— Rampuri, Shahpura Dindori D/Dis. 08/04/15

DIAGNOSIS :— Tetralogy of Fallot

Follow up

- Tb. Cefixime 200mg BD
- Tb. Deriphylline 100mg TDS
- Tb. Rantac 150mg BD
- Tb. MVBC 1 OD
- Tb. Calcium 500mg OD

× 1 wk

Adv- Refer to Dept of Cardiology/CVTS, GMC Bhopal / AIIMS, New Delhi for further management.

PTO

Who is responsible for this outcome? Inadequate skill sets among physicians in the largest referral hospital in central India, home to the poorest and most indigent in the country? Or the lack of public transport for people to access health systems? Or the completely irrational overregulation and licensing of opioid use, so much that it kills the basic utility of such vital and life-saving drugs?

Tetralogy of Fallot, a congenital cyanotic heart disease

This is one of the most common congenital heart diseases, and is often associated with cyanosis or blueness of the nails and tongue in childhood. This condition can be completely corrected surgically if detected in time, and the patient can live a full life.

The disease usually manifests when the baby is a few weeks old, and not at birth. The symptoms are blueness of fingers, tongue and lips. In severe cases, the child may have episodes of worsening blueness accompanied by rapid breathing and fast heart rate. If these episodes are not picked up early and treated or aborted, the problem may worsen and the child may lose consciousness and lose control of one side of the body, and subsequently die. It is critical therefore that these episodes called cyanotic spells are detected early and treated expertly, followed by preventive treatment for these spells, and then followed by planning of early corrective surgery. Such surgeries are done in regional cardiac surgery centres.

In Meena's case, her condition was not properly diagnosed until she had reached a relatively late age. And when she was taken in a critical state to the large regional specialty hospital, they mistook her cyanotic spell for pneumonia, and so treated her inappropriately. Then they made the next mistake of discharging her prematurely. When Meena returned home, the cyanotic spell or paroxysm worsened and she slipped into unconsciousness and into an irreversible condition. After she arrived at the JSS hospital and we had diagnosed the spell correctly, we still could not treat it adequately for lack of injectable morphine.

As mentioned, access to both injectable and oral morphine is highly regulated in India owing to fear of its misuse by those addicted to the opiate. The result is that most patients who desperately need morphine are denied this powerful and lifesaving drug. While at JSS Ganiyari, we have been able to get the license for storing and dispensing oral morphine, we still do not have intravenous morphine in our pharmacy. In fact we do not know if any other hospital in the entire Madhya Pradesh state of 32 million people has injectable morphine. Injectable morphine is irreplaceable by any other drug for episodes of acute myocardial infarction, bad cyanotic spells, and for severe pain as in a vaso-occlusive crisis in sickle cell anaemia.

Meena Bai need not have died, and could have lived a full life. For that, firstly, physicians must be better trained to correctly diagnose all common medical problems and emergencies. Secondly, the specialists in medical colleges should be answerable to the primary care providers in hospitals. Thirdly, public transport to health facilities in remote rural areas should be free or subsidised, even if it is for longer distances and across districts. Finally, the regulation of the sale of morphine, oral and intravenous, should be such that hospitals should be able to access and store it.

injection infection palsy

Kamala Bai

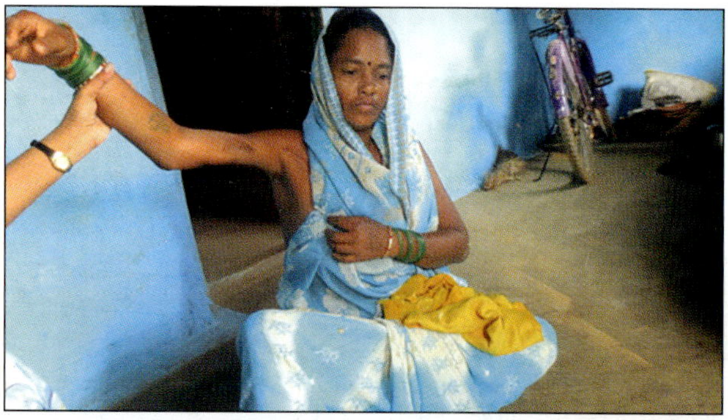

Kamala Bai, wife of Bahadur Gond of village Baigapara, gram panchayat Jhingatpur, block Kota, district Bilaspur, is today a disabled person, forced to live a miserable life, but she wasn't always.

Four years ago in 2012, Kamala Bai gave birth to her fifth child. Her family was poor and landless, and so Kamala Bai worried that she would have to go work soon after delivery. Because of this anxiety, she decided to see the local 'jholachhap' (an unqualified medical practitioner) in her village and asked him to give her an injection for strength. Kamala Bai thought she would quickly regain her strength with such an injection and be able to work as a manual labourer and earn something to meet the daily necessities of her growing family. But this was not to be.

The day after she got the injection, there was a lot of swelling at the injection site and Kamala Bai was in severe pain that soon became intolerable. Seeing her condition, the family contacted the Village Health Worker Ahilya Bai, who took them to the JSS hospital at Ganiyari.

At the Ganiyari hospital, it was found that there was weakness in her right arm as well as pus collection and other signs of infection at the site of injection. It was also clear that the injection had been given lower than where it should have been. Seeing the severity of her condition, the doctors at JSS operated on Kamala Bai's arm to remove the pus and other dead tissue where she had been given the injection. She was forced to stay at the hospital for one month for repeated dressing of the wound and grafting of new skin cover, and thus ran up an expenditure of Rs. 16,000.

After surgery, the wound healed, but there was not much improvement in the weakness in her arm primarily due to the nerve damage caused by the 'injection' being given at the wrong place. Even today, Kamala Bai is unable to work with her right arm. Her family has had to pay a high cost for this forced disability which has seriously affected their economic situation.

Kamala Bai tried to get help through government policies, but even there she only met with disappointment and neglect. She could not get a disability certificate issued in her name, and therefore has been unable to access any benefits. Yet, even today, Kamala Bai hopes someone will help her so that things might improve for her and her family.

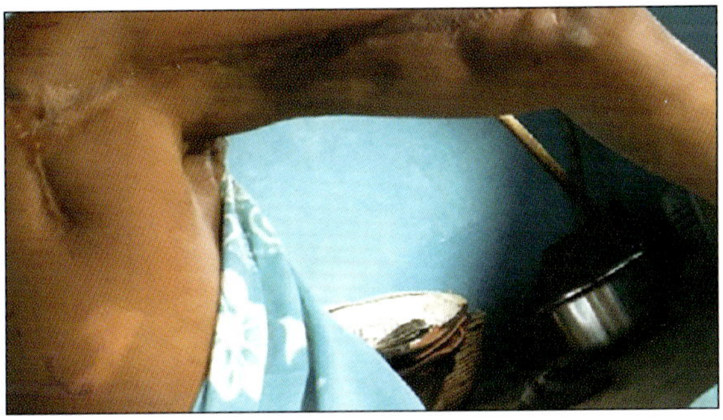

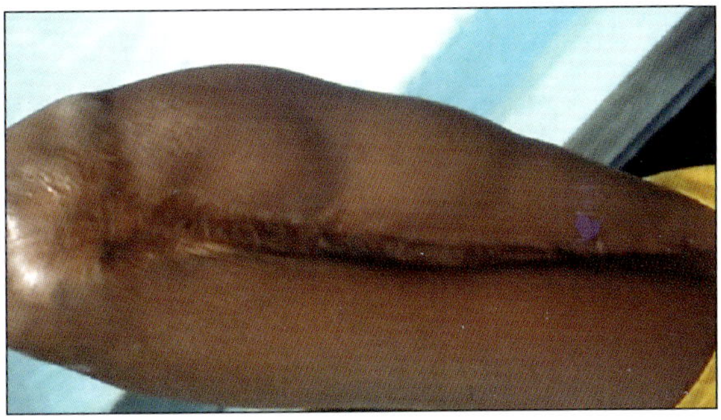

Injections, which are a common form of giving treatment, are sadly also associated with life-threatening blood-borne infections like HIV, local injuries and other debilitating infections. All these harmful effects can however be eliminated by safe practice and limiting injection use to only when necessary. Unfortunately, injection use is indiscriminate in developing countries, with an estimated 1.5 injections/person/year, and over half of these are unsafely administered (data from 1999 WHO Bulletin and 2001 NMJI).

Kamala Bai's case here tells many stories. There is the story of unnecessary and fake injections, compounded by unsafe use. There is the story of patients who are not empowered to demand correct treatment or recourse after medical error. And there is the story of how we as a society take care of the weak and disabled among us.

Why did Kamala Bai have to worry about returning to work soon after her delivery? And what support does she have now when she is disabled and in thousands of rupees of debt from a medical condition brought upon her by a quack?

The excessive and unnecessary use of injections cannot be addressed unless we have adequate access to public health facilities for poor people. Many private so-called medical practitioners in rural and sub-urban India indulge in excessive use of injections for higher profits since most injectable treatment is more expensive. They justify such unethical practice by attributing it to the 'demand' people make for injections even for minor illnesses where oral medicines would suffice. Community awareness and education about the risks that injections pose, more so if unsafely given, would work to reduce this demand. But at present, almost everyone who seeks treatment from unqualified practitioners in the villages gets injections, whether it is for minor coughs and colds, fever, weakness, or for some itchy skin conditions. Sadly, even in the public health facilities, especially in the sub-centres and primary health centres, there is indiscriminate use of injections. In contrast, at the JSS health centre where we see a significant proportion of more serious illnesses, the injection rate is about 3% of all patients at the OPD level.

Under what conditions and when should injections be given? These include illnesses where the patient cannot take medicines by mouth, such as when someone is unconscious, or is

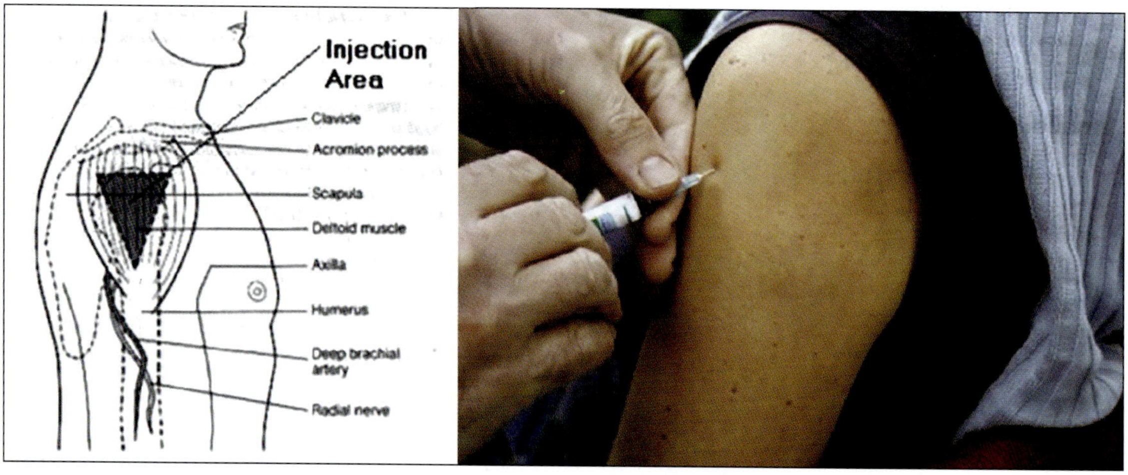

repeatedly vomiting, or is undergoing surgery under anaesthesia, or is in a post-operative drowsy state. Sometimes for quick and timely relief from an acute illness, injections may be required. Finally, certain medicines like vaccines and drugs which would get destroyed by the acid in the stomach need to be injected directly into the blood stream.

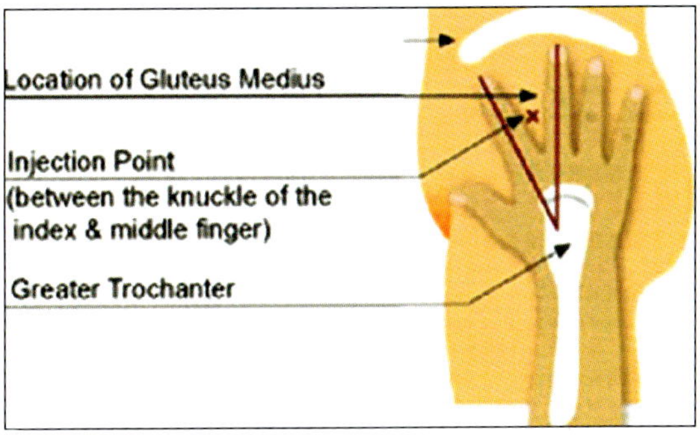

But taken together these should not amount to more than a few percent of all the illnesses that one sees at the outpatient level in a hospital.

Unsafe injections are an equally important issue. The lack of safety results from a lack of hygiene and from transmission of pathogens from one person to the next as well as from the flawed technique of giving injections in wrong sites. Not using sterile syringes and needles, reusing needles, not cleaning the local site before administering an injection are common mistakes. As in Kamala Bai's case, the injection was given too low on the arm, thus directly damaging the large nerve that powers the hand.

Similarly if given wrongly in the buttock, it could result in the paralysis of the entire lower limb, a condition that we see at least once every month at our small health facility at Ganiyari. And this weakness is irreversible. You can only offer some splints to make the foot drop, and decrease the handicap. Some complex surgeries can give some relief, but they are difficult to arrange for the majority of the affected people.

It is not unsuspecting and desperate patients but the public health and medical system that need a shot in the arm, to wake up its conscience.

mental health

Siya

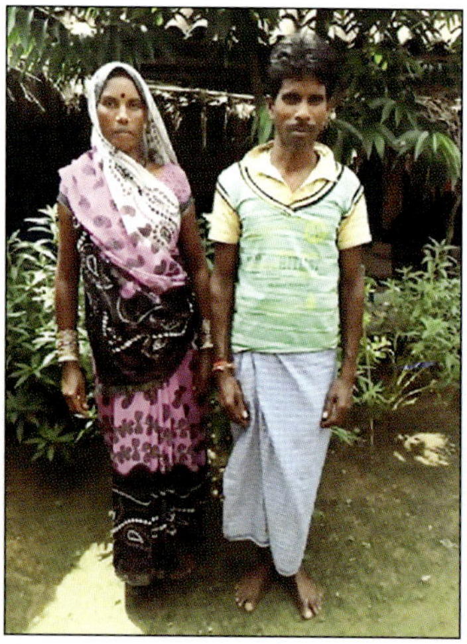

Siya Bai lived in Bamhani village with her husband, three sons, and a daughter. Both Siya and her husband grew up in Bamhani, where they fell in love and decided to get married against the wishes of her husband's family. They had a relatively large land holding of six acres, which produced enough to save some money each year.

In 2013, Siya Bai's son came down with chicken pox. Many communities in rural India, like Siya's, consider getting chicken pox a pious event and believe that it is a sign of god visiting one's home. Religious prayers are often performed and the house kept immaculately clean. Yet when her son fell ill, Siya Bai was menstruating, and therefore was unable to go near her sick child or conduct pujas for his well-being. In many parts of India, across caste, class and community, it is still commonly believed that menstruation is an impure condition during which the woman is not supposed to perform any religious rituals, cook food for the family, touch various household objects and so on. The stress of not being able to care for her sick child set something off inside Siya Bai. For seven days, she was unable to sleep or work and she began to have panic attacks with tremors all over her body.

When Siya's husband took their son to a traditional healer, he also expressed his concern over his wife's condition, and told them to go to the local sub-centre as he was unable to treat her. Thus, Siya Bai was brought to the Jan Swasthya Sahyog Bamhani sub-centre, where she was seen by a senior physician during one of his weekly visits from JSS' main referral hospital at Ganiyari. He diagnosed Siya Bai with a form of anxiety and depression and treated her with diazepam and citalopram. She was also detained at the centre overnight for monitoring until her condition stabilized. When her condition did not improve overnight, Santosh, one of the local health workers, gave Siya Bai an injection of diazepam, which seemed to help. She returned home the next day with a month's supply of citalopram.

Although she started to take her medication, she found issues with citalopram as she was not too comfortable with the way it made her feel. She therefore only took it periodically, and when she needed more, she would go either to the sub-centre or directly to Santosh for treatment. This pattern continued for about a year during which she continued to have panic attacks on and off. After a year, Siya Bai was reevaluated, and it was determined that she should be given diazepam to take when needed. She then reported that she typically took it once every two to three months as she had been feeling much more stable.

When Siya Bai first showed signs of a panic attack, her family thought she had gone mad and that was why she was not able to sleep. 'But I went to the doctor and whatever they are treating me with has made me well, so they don't say that anymore.' When asked about some of the possible triggers that set off such episodes of panic, she claimed that she didn't have any issues until her son got chicken pox in 2013. However, when her husband left the room, she admitted that he had been a heavy drinker, and the stress his alcoholism inflicted on the family had weighed mightily on her. During the worst of his alcoholic days, he would suddenly become angry and often beat Siya. On several occasions, she ran away to her relative's house, where she would stay for several weeks at a time in order to escape his wrath.

In addition to worrying about her safety, she also began to worry about her family's economic situation. They had always been relatively well off as their land produced 12,500 kg of rice per year, which brought in close to 40,000 rupees. Of that amount, they were able to save between 5 to 6,000 rupees by the year's end. Yet, the more her husband drank, the scarcer both money and food became, as there was no one to harvest the crop and any money earned was spent on liquor.

Fortunately for Siya Bai, her life then changed for the better. Her husband an alcoholic, who abused her physically and neglected his family, took help, joined the de-addiction programme started by JSS and quit drinking. Siya Bai's anxiety and depression were also treated, and she could now talk about her worries, stressors and worked to find solutions.

But how many women are there who are still struggling to survive, take care of their families more or less alone, and who live with the fear: 'How is he going to be this evening when he comes back? Will he be violent?'. This fear coupled with other worries over a long period of time seems to play a key role in the development of anxiety, depression and psychosomatic complaints like generalized body aches, sleep disturbance and so on.

According to the Indian government's figures, around 37% of Indian women have experienced some form of abuse by their husbands – pushing, slapping and hair-pulling, punching, kicking, choking or even burning. The actual figures could be much higher as many of them are not willing to come out and talk openly about the violence they face day-to-day from those with whom they share their lives.

Women victims of domestic violence lose interest in household activities. If employed, they fail to work with full capabilities in the workplace. Other features of depression like sleep disturbance, bodily weakness and aches and pains are common. In order to deal with this repeated physical and emotional trauma and still be able to function, women often cut off their emotions and feelings – bad ones but also good ones, leaving them functioning like machines. The trauma returns again and again, verbal, physical and sexual. Around one-fourth of Indian men admitted in a survey to having committed sexual violence at some point during their lives.

Domestic violence is a common hidden problem for women attending the clinics and is likely to be a major cause of mental ill health globally, not just in rural settings. Domestic violence affects children as well, even if it is directed only against the mothers. Children are traumatized watching their mothers being abused and grow up with a fear of losing their family if the parents separate. Helpless spectators, they love the abusive parent and sometimes hate him, which often leaves children confused, lodging silently in them the unvoiced feelings of sadness, anger, loathing and fear. They find it difficult to concentrate on studies, often drop out of school and do not get the education they otherwise might have got if they were not disturbed. Thus the country loses its most productive and valuable asset to domestic violence. Growing up as witnesses of domestic violence, many children with such hidden anger end up repeating the same unfortunate patterns in their own relationships or are unable to form any lasting relationships.

The Indian Government has taken measures to try and address domestic violence through legislations such as the Protection of Women from Domestic Violence Act 2005, which was brought into force from 26 October 2006. The Act provides for the first time in Indian law a definition of 'domestic violence', with this definition being broad and including not only physical violence, but also other forms of violence such as emotional/verbal, sexual, and economic abuse. It is a civil law meant primarily for protection orders and not meant to penalize criminally. To take the extreme example of violence, rape is not considered a crime when it occurs within a marriage.

Domestic violence is now being viewed as a public health problem of epidemic proportions all over the world. Sometimes, men are also victims of such violence and abuse, but in the vast majority of situations, men are the perpetrators. At JSS, we often see women who come with psychosomatic complaints and depressive features, and when specifically questioned, report physical abuse at home. It is also a common subject of discussion in women's groups and in support groups for mental illness. Quite often, alcohol abuse and domestic violence are directly linked as men act violently under the influence of alcohol.

For the women, children, caregivers, and sometimes even for the abusive men themselves, it is a situation of desperation and helplessness. Increasingly, support groups against domestic violence are being formed in villages which hold discussions, conduct rallies and even punishment rituals for men. In some instances, these groups have also taken up alcohol abuse and have tried to ban cheap country liquor from being sold in their villages. But these efforts are difficult to sustain when the husbands feel ashamed and forbid their wives from taking part in such activities. There is still a long way to go and the men, too, need to join in such efforts, assuming that the wellbeing of their family is also important to them.

psychosis

Luman Baiga

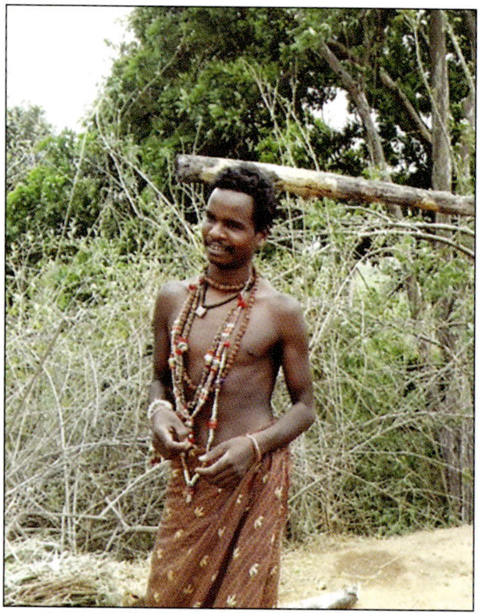

There was a festive atmosphere at Luman Baiga's house in Mangalpur village. It was Thursday, and the villagers were expecting many people to arrive from another village. In preparation, some were already busy cooking since morning while others arranged for vegetables from the neighbouring villages. Aghaniya Bai could not understand anything, but she took pride in the fact that people from another village were coming to see her son Luman, and despite her worsening finances, she had borrowed money to arrange for food for everyone.

Luman Baiga's brother-in-law Ramnath had asked the villagers to celebrate this day as a festival. He had even hired a tent and loudspeaker from the nearby Kargi village. All the villagers were happily dancing to the music from the loudspeaker, when there was a power cut and the music abruptly stopped. But they kept on dancing despite that to please Luman Baiga. People who had come from nearby villages to offer him coconut and rice also joined them.

Luman Baiga, whom the people worshipped like a god and danced in front of, looked on uncomprehendingly at the festive bustle around him, his eyes vacant. He looked emaciated; he had not eaten for weeks. No one could get him to eat. There were garlands in a polythene bag and some other things placed on top of his head. If this fell off his head, he would get anxious and quickly put them back again to feel at ease. He was not bothered about his clothes.

When Prafull, the JSS health cluster coordinator for the area, asked Luman Baiga if he recognized him, Luman did not reply. So Prafull asked him again, 'Luman, I am asking you something'. And Luman replied, 'I don't know brother, where are you going'?

Luman Baiga liked to go to Bilaspur. Many years ago, he had asked Prafull to go to Bilaspur with him, so Prafull had taken Luman there and brought him back the next day. After that Prafull started visiting him regularly in Mangalpur village.

Luman was worried about the miserable condition of the villagers. He tried in many ways to take control of the Panchayat so that he could improve conditions in Mangalpur, even making his wife contest the Panchayat elections, which she lost narrowly. But now he no longer recognized his own wife and told the villagers to idolize her as Goddess Saraswati.

When Prafull went to Mangalpur again after a gap of three months, on seeing him Luman started laughing, just as he used to, and so Prafull was sure that Luman would talk to him that day. He told Prafull that he no longer lived in the village but lived near the Naktabandha pond, in a small hut which he had built with the help of a few villagers.

Prafull tried to revive Luman's memory of some old incidents, like the time he was put in jail for four months for encroaching upon forest land, and asked him who would go for the next court hearing. But Luman said he no longer took an interest in these things, and that he was now arranging for a hut for the village. He said he could show Prafull a snake and high ocean-like waves in the middle of the lake, which could wash them far away. Prafull said, 'Okay, show me,' and in reply, Luman asked him to come the following Thursday.

It had been five months since that meeting and Luman had started talking to some people more freely now. He had been asked to take some medicines, and he had agreed. The JSS senior health worker had started giving him medicines for his mental disorder as prescribed. But even now, Luman does not take his medicines regularly but only when he feels like it. He does not do anything consistently. And he has only the villagers and his family members to look after him.

We chose the story of Luman Baiga because his was a case of a psychotic illness of moderate severity, with manifestations not unusual for manic psychosis, with a community response quite peculiar to the rural setting. In his manic grandiose state, Luman believed that he had achieved supernatural god-like powers. He saw a snake in the pond and thought he could create a flood and walk on water. These were not unusual delusions of grandeur, considering our mythological stories. Although his family was quite sure that he was suffering from some kind of mental illness, they still gave him the benefit of doubt and arranged for people to come and pay obeisance to him and to feed them as well, spending a huge sum of money, which pushed them into debt.

Psychosis is a major mental illness that is characterized by a lack of insight. Luman was suffering from a mood disorder with an exaggerated or euphoric state, with ideas flying in his mind, a lack of concentration, a lack of need to sleep and a feeling abnormally strong or endowed with supernatural powers. Coupled with fixed ideas (delusions) that he had god like powers, he behaved like one and the information spread like bush fire and people started collecting from distant villages. Psychodynamically it was as if Luman had for the time being taken respite in a state of power away from his stress and worries. It might sound pleasant but most of the time irritability accompanied this state of mood. Sooner or later it became difficult for the client to live with it as the client loses touch with the reality.

Another type of psychosis is that caused by schizophrenia. Here the affected person is usually more suspicious, guarded, and may fear that others are trying to harm him in some way. A schizophrenic person may hear voices talking about them or to them, stealing their thoughts or inserting thoughts in their mind. These experiences can be scary and disturbing for the person and it can be difficult for him to integrate the two worlds and clearly differentiate between them – the one outside and the other within his own mind – which is why this condition is called schizophrenia, or split personality. The mechanism of this disorder is an abnormal increase in the nerve transmission of certain pathways in the brain using dopamine as neurotransmitter. Individuals suffering from schizophrenia give a specific and often bizarre and extraordinary interpretation of things and events in their immediate environment, which to others may seem perfectly ordinary. For instance, watching a woman in a red sari, a person with schizophrenic psychosis might suddenly give a special meaning to the red colour and, in addition, might develop ideas of reference to himself like: 'The red colour of the sari is meant especially for me to give me the following message...'.

This inability to distinguish between the real and unreal and over-involvement with the inner world is likely to induce strange behaviour in the person, which can easily be observed by others, who may then label the person as mad or deranged. Often, the schizophrenic individual finds it difficult to perform everyday routine tasks, and is thus more or less dependent on the family or caregivers.

Psychoses of mood disorders come and go, sometimes with long symptomless periods in between. Psychoses of schizophrenia on the other hand can often be of longer duration and despite treatment, often only partial remission is possible. The treatment is primarily by medication, typically with drugs that block the transmission of dopamine to the brain.

In a rural context, however, where extreme poverty and disempowerment go hand in hand with illiteracy, lack of awareness and superstition, the strange and inexplicable behaviour of the suffering individual is often attributed by traditional healers to supernatural phenomena, and rituals, prayers, sacrifices and exorcisms are offered as treatment. Patients of schizophrenia in particular need regular medicines. For lack of availability of or access to regular treatment, families look for a one-time treatment. This is often done in an unregulated manner, using injections of long-lasting antipsychotic preparations, which may initially appear to do wonders. Unfortunately, high doses of antipsychotics administered like this can lead to serious side effects. Moreover, the beneficial effect is shortlived, lasting only a few weeks to months, and as the effect of the drug wears off, the full blown psychotic state can return in case of schizophrenia.

In acute psychotic states, the person can behave in completely unpredictable and peculiar ways and may even turn violent; this has given rise to the stigma of 'madness' associated with such mental illnesses. The financial strain apart, it can be a tremendous emotional burden for the immediate family and community to manage a patient of psychosis, and they may need counselling to help them cope. But the awareness that such mental illnesses can also be managed well with regular treatment and follow-up needs to get across. One of the methods we use at JSS is support groups for patients and their families. The other method we plan to start is using outreach services to go to patients who do not come to the health centre due to lack of awareness or resources. Telepsychiatry services are also available at JSS, Ganiyari, for patients for whom a psychiatrist's expert evaluation is needed for diagnosis and treatment.

rheumatoid arthritis

Shakun

Shakun Gond, 51, is a resident of Bamhani village, which is located deep inside the Achanakmar Tiger Reserve in rural Chhattisgarh. He was a small farmer and daily wage labourer with a land holding of about 1.25 acres. He lived with his wife, three daughters, two sons, and three grandchildren. The Jan Swasthya Sahyog team had visited Shakun at his home after hearing that he had a case of rheumatoid arthritis but was no longer taking treatment.

We first met Shakun and his wife in the evening as Shakun's wife was eating her twice-a-day meal of rice. Shakun was sitting on the bed; his wife said he was unable to get up due to the pain in his knees. In addition to being hard of hearing, Shakun appeared disoriented and had trouble responding to questions. It was obvious that both he and his wife had been drinking, which they openly admitted upon asking.

What had led to Shakun's current condition? It seemed that there was more than the inflammation of joints that was affecting this man and his family.

Nine years earlier, Shakun Gond began complaining of pain and swelling in both his knees. At times, the pain and stiffness was so bad that he was unable to walk. His wife took him to a traditional healer in Ratanpur, about 40 km from their home. Shakun saw the healer three times. The second time was when the healer had come to a nearby village to conduct religious healing ceremonies. Shakun's family decided to pay the one thousand and one rupees for Shakun to participate in the healing ceremony, with the hope that the healer's magic would be able to cure him of his ailment. Things appeared promising at first, as according to Shakun's wife the healer's powers could be visibly seen during the ceremony. However, in the weeks and months that followed, Shakun's condition failed to improve and the family eventually gave up on the healer's ability to cure him.

The entire family was affected by Shakun's inability to work and his condition was only getting worse. Even basic activities like using the toilet were becoming extremely difficult and painful, as he often found himself unable to bend his knees. In 2013, the family decided to again try and seek another form of treatment. In December 2013 Shakun visited the JSS sub-centre at Bamhani. He was diagnosed with rheumatoid arthritis and prescribed a month's treatment of Methotrexate, low dose prednisolone, ibuprofen, and folic acid. He was provided a hundred percent discount for his medication from JSS's poor patient fund. However, Shakun did not return to the sub-centre again until March, where he was given another month's dosage. He returned once more in April for another refill of his medications, each time receiving them free. However, after April, Shakun discontinued his treatment completely. When asked why, the family replied that Shakun's condition was not improving, so they assumed that the treatment was not working.

To understand the family's apparent apathy or carelessness toward Shakun's treatment, one must look beyond the clinical record. Upon visiting Shakun and his family at home, it became apparent that there were other major problems that the family was dealing with in addition to Shakun's chronic and crippling arthritis.

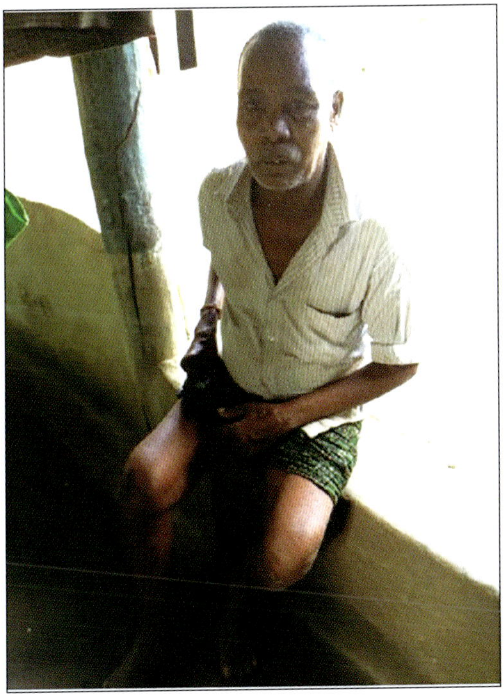

The family was in a state of extreme poverty. With Shakun unable to farm, his son was the one who

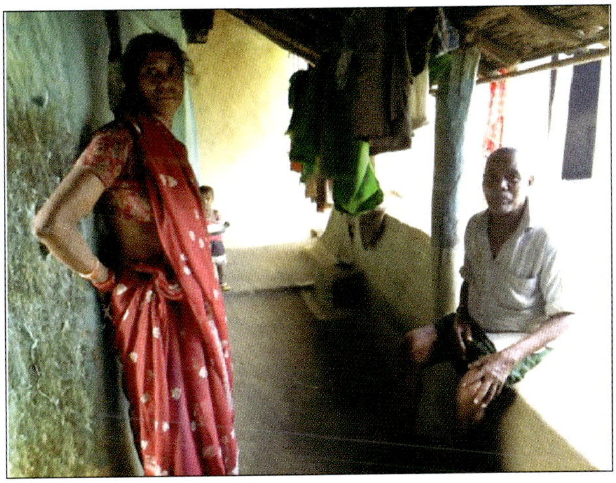

Shakun's house and their living conditions:

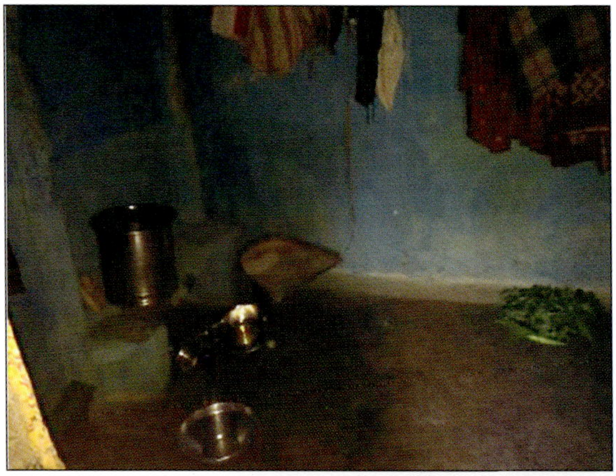

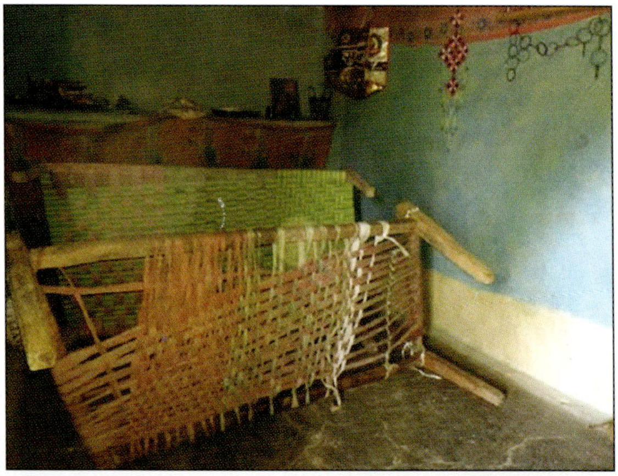

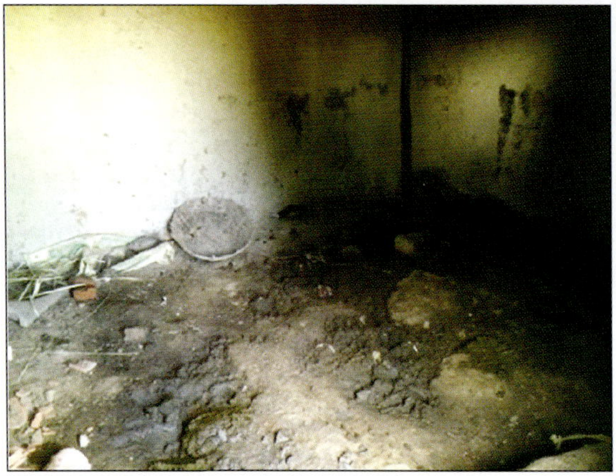

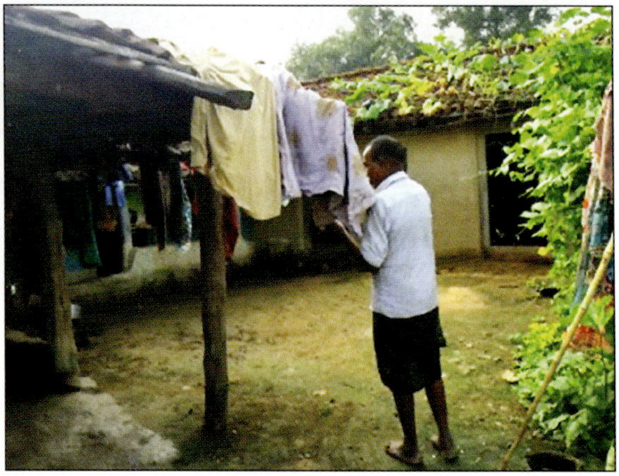

took care of the 1.25 acre crop. However, the food he was able to harvest first went to feed his own immediate family – his wife and three children, including a 15-day old infant. In a good year, the crop yielded about 1000 kg, which was usually enough for the remaining four adult Shakun's house and living conditions: members of the family – Shakun, his wife, and their two daughters. However, that year, the family was expecting only 10% of the ideal yield. Hundred kilos was nowhere near enough to feed the entire family, and even with the 28 kg of rice per month that was rationed to them by the government, they were often forced to buy rice from the market.

Without a stable source of income, Shakun's family had to come up with creative ways to survive. Five years earlier, when Shakun's daughter was in the 7th standard, she stopped attending school in order to help bring in money. She and her mother began doing daily wage labour on neighboring farms. In addition to such work, Shakun's wife sometimes also traveled to Bilaspur to work for two to three months at a time, where she was able to save Rs. 2,000-3,000. The family also made and sold brooms, which earned them up to Rs. 300 a week depending on demand. They hoped that through their daily wage work and by selling brooms, they could make up for the deficit in rice production. However, much was uncertain.

What was certain was that despite all their hard work and efforts, there was not enough to go around for the family to maintain a healthy diet. When asked about their eating habits, they reported a diet of rice with small amounts of vegetables. Lentils and other sources of protein were almost nonexistent in their diet as they could only consume pulses four to five times a month. With such small amounts of protein and other vital nutrients, it was a wonder that anyone was able to work at all.

Apart from rice, alcohol might be considered another staple of their diet as they regularly bought a bottle of locally made brew for Rs. 20. Shakun's wife was also often gifted alcohol as a form of appreciation for her services as a local dai or midwife. It should be noted that JSS ran a training programme for traditional midwives, which she was initially a part of.

The use of alcohol was both a cause and a symptom of the Gond family's current condition. While it perhaps could be argued that the 20 rupees used to buy alcohol could be better spent on lentils, the family's choices become a lot harder to criticize when seen in the context of their socio-economic situation. For Shakun, frequently bedridden and living in constant discomfort, alcohol may have been the drug that best dulled his pain. For his wife, who constantly worried about bringing in enough food and money for her family, the choice to consume alcohol might be one of the few choices she could make when so much in her life remained outside of her control. Unfortunately, these symptoms of poverty often became part of the cause, further throwing individuals and families into cycles of poverty and ill health.

Rheumatoid arthritis (RA) is a chronic inflammatory disease of unknown aetiology marked by a symmetric, peripheral polyarthritis. It is the most common form of chronic inflammatory arthritis and often results in joint damage and physical disability. Because it is a systemic disease, RA might result in a variety of extraarticular manifestations, including fatigue, subcutaneous nodules, lung involvement, pericarditis, peripheral neuropathy, vasculitis, and hematologic abnormalities.

The incidence of RA increases between 25 and 55 years of age, after which it plateaus until the age of 75 and then decreases. The presenting symptoms of RA typically result from inflammation of the joints, tendons, and bursae. Patients often complain of early morning joint stiffness lasting more than an hour that eased with physical activity. The earliest involved joints are typically the small joints of the hands and feet. The initial pattern of joint involvement might be monoarticular, oligoarticular (4 joints), or polyarticular (more than 5 joints), usually in a symmetric distribution.

The clinical diagnosis of RA is largely based on signs and symptoms of a chronic inflammatory arthritis, with laboratory and radiographic results providing important supplemental information.

In Shakun's case, the diagnosis of RA was based on clinical findings and a raised ESR.

Rheumatoid arthritis is a biological disease entity and has been studied extensively in that light. But we have many questions. What might be the non-biological determinants of this chronic disease? What does it mean to have RA in a state of poverty and social deprivation? How much could the disease advance in such conditions? How do this biologic phenomenon and the associated failure of our social structures in bringing equity lead to a poor quality of life?

A cycle of deprivation and disillusionment

While discussing the reasons why poor people fail to access health care, questions of culture and accessibility often arise. Shakun's culture seemed to play a major role in his decision to seek a traditional healer, as well as his lack of belief in allopathic medicine. It also helped to explain why the family seemed to take Shakun's illness in their stride when so much more could be done. It seemed to be part of the culture of rural life that whatever happened, whether poor rains or illness, one must simply accept it. Yet what is culture but a set of beliefs and practices built up over time, practices that were directly influenced by the social and economic conditions? We must ask ourselves whether it was people's culture that needed to change, or the social and economic conditions that fed into and influenced that culture?

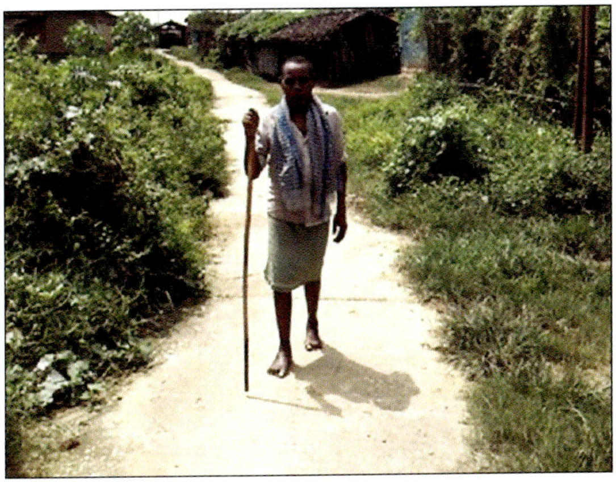

Similar questions could be asked about access to health care. We came to see in Shakun's case that access must be thought of as more than just physical access. Shakun lived only a few houses away from the JSS sub-centre at Bamhani; even with his limited mobility, it would not have been difficult for him to seek care there. Besides, there was daily transportation provided to Ganiyari should he have needed a higher level of care. We also saw that access must be more than an issue of money, as JSS provided treatment to poor patients like Shakun free of cost.

So then what did access to health care really mean, and how was it still a problem for people like Shakun? Perhaps one cannot ask about access to health care without first asking about access to education, or access to a steady income, or access to food. Perhaps if someone in his family had been educated on the benefits of allopathic medicine, they would have been more likely to seek treatment from JSS earlier, and perhaps would have been less likely to discontinue treatment. Or perhaps if the daughter was not forced to drop out of school in the 7th standard, she would have felt empowered enough to begin to take more control over her own life and work to lift her family out of poverty. Perhaps if the family had a stable source of income and could afford to eat a balanced diet on a regular basis, they would not feel the need to turn to alcohol as a coping mechanism. Perhaps then they would be in a better position to make choices concerning their own well-being.

Shakun Gond's story may thus have been more about deprivation and disillusionment than it was about rheumatoid arthritis, although his debilitating disease no doubt played a significant part.

silicosis

Rinki

Rinki, a 25-year old woman came to Jan Swasthya Sahyog on 8 October in 2014. She was very thin weighing only 30 kg, with a BMI of 14. She had been suffering from acute shortness of breath for a year. Day by day her problems were increasing: she was losing weight, not eating well, and her tolerance for physical activity was decreasing. She had severe wheezing which worsened at night and a bad cough with phlegm, but there was no history of fever.

Rinki's was a family of brick-makers and this was their main source of earning. Rinki worked till she became ill, but others in her family continued doing the same work without any precautions and perhaps were not aware of the harmful effects.

Tests, including a chest x-ray, were highly suggestive of silicosis. There was some improvement with bronchodilator drug inhalers, but Rinki soon stopped coming to JSS for a follow up. A JSS community team member reported back that her weight was now around 25 kg and she had a cough and was on anti-tubercular treatment provided by a government hospital for the last one and half months. She could do some household work but most activity made her very tired.

Silicon comprises 28% of the earth's crust. It combines either with oxygen to form silica or with other elements to form silicates and these contribute to the bulk of rocks, clay and sand. Quartz is the most common type of crystalline silica. These together form a major component of the environment, and silicosis is not only a problem for large industries but especially prevalent in rural areas in developing countries. The major industries prone to silicosis are: stone quarries and crushers, quartz mining, foundries, sand blasting, ceramics, gem cutting and polishing, slate and pencil, construction, mining, and glass manufacturing where unwary workers may inhale the fine crystals of silica and the damage starts in their lungs, causing fibrosis of tissues. Labour in these sectors is unorganized, so any government policy related to silicosis never reaches them. It is estimated that there are more than 12,000 stone crushing mills in India.

A person suffering from silicosis is additionally vulnerable to develop tuberculosis, as in Rinki's case.

As per the report of the Indian Council for Medical Research (1999), about 30 lakh workers in India are at a high risk of exposure to silica. Of these, 17 lakh are in mining and quarrying activities, 6.3 lakh in the glass and mica industry, and 6.7 lakh in the metals industry. In addition, 53 lakh construction workers are also at risk of silica exposure. Experts say this number could be much higher as detection is low and workers are often diagnosed and treated for tuberculosis, which aggravates the situation for them.

Rajasthan, Gujarat, Madhya Pradesh, Haryana, Delhi and Karnataka are some of the worst affected states. The victims are mostly poor migrant workers employed as casual wage labourers who suffer or die for lack of specialised treatment.

The National Human Rights Commission in 2011 said that the occupational hazard of silicosis is preventable if the working conditions are properly regulated and proper warning and protective equipment are used. Once a worker or any other person is afflicted by silicosis, it becomes a constitutional obligation on part of the State to take appropriate short-term and long-term measures in order to provide medical facilities and rehabilitation to the victims. However, there has been little or no implementation of the NHRC recommendations and the existing laws, both at the Centre and the State level, putting lakhs of workers employed in these hazardous jobs at risk.

Silica enters the human body in an invisible, silent and painless manner. It does not cause any irritation, is odourless and its entry goes unrecognized, and hence unchecked. It does not manifest for a long time, and by the time it shows its hostile nature in the form of symptoms, it is too late to do anything.

Classic silicosis usually manifests after 10-20 years of exposure, as in the case of Rinki who had been working at the brick kilns since childhood, and was now a victim. Accelerated silicosis on the other hand manifests after a much shorter duration of exposure, as rapidly as within 1 to 10 hours, and follows a very aggressive course.

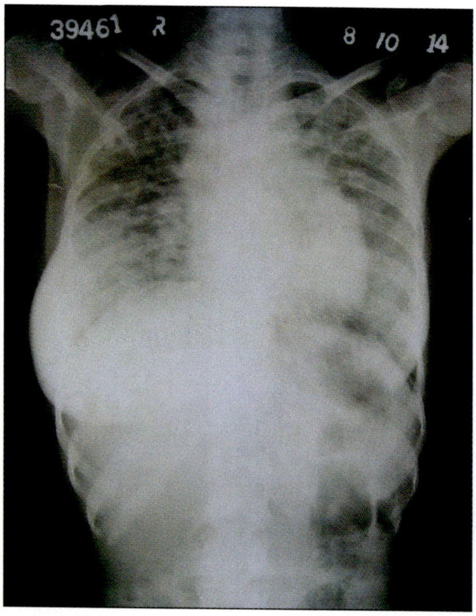

Intense exposure of very fine dust can cause acute silicoproteinosis within weeks to months.

Silica is highly fibrogenic, and so silicosis is a progressive illness and protection at this stage is not going to help much. It starts with tiny nodules and can progress to massive fibrosis. It looks very much like miliary tuberculosis, with early mottling followed by cavitation on the chest x-ray. Silicosis predisposes one to chronic bronchitis, so patients have obstruction of their lungs from the phlegm as well as restriction from the silicosis and suffer acute breathlessness. Silicosis also predisposes one to cancer and autoimmune diseases such as scleroderma. Chronic kidney disease can also be caused by prolonged silica exposure.

The attached x-ray looks almost the same as we see in malignancy or tuberculosis in our routine clinical checks, and we are often in a dilemma what to do next. We send patients for bronchoscopy when they test negative for tuberculosis bacteria, and if we don't get clues for any other lung illness, we empirically start anti-tuberculous treatment. But if there is no response to the TB treatment and the chest x-ray is the same even after completion of treatment, we suspect silicosis. Silicosis is therefore a big problem, both in terms of morbidity and mortality.

However, there are things we can do: we can make the public and health workers more aware of its causes and presentation. We can advocate for the provision of safety measures at the industrial site which can be easily followed, like using tight-fitting masks or tying a wet cloth to cover the nose and mouth while working; daily washing of clothes after work; cleaning the hands, face and mouth properly before eating or drinking anything and doing so in a less dusty place. We can emphasise that smoking, active or passive, worsens silicosis.

Prevention of silicosis is far easier and far more effective than its treatment. Once the disease develops, except for monetary compensation, there is scarce little that can be done for improving the quality of life except taking steroids, bronchodilator drug inhalers, and supportive therapy. Therefore, the government surely has a role to play. Even so, it is an uphill task getting compensation. The establishment is often bent on denying the diagnosis of silicosis, failing which it is difficult to contest for any compensation.

Is silicosis nature's revenge on us for disturbing the earth? Do we have to have so much of construction? Even so, why should the poor have to pay that price with their lungs and their lives?

fluorosis

Ved Prakash Gond

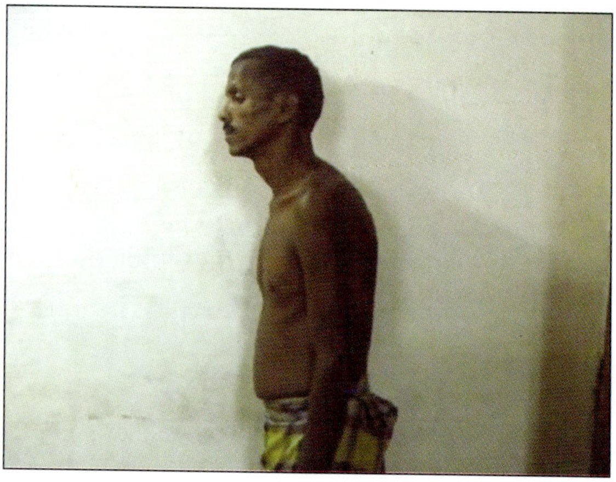

Ved Prakash Gond, 45, came to the OPD at JSS Ganiyari from his village Amatikra, in Podi Uproda block, district Korba, on 23 April, 2013, with severe pain and stiffness in his back, which he had been suffering from for the last four years. To begin with, the pain was in both feet, but later it spread to other parts of the body and also increased in severity. He also developed stiffness and it became difficult for him to stand straight. There was some abdominal tenderness on both sides of the umbilicus as well.

On examination, his weight was 59.3 kgs, and his height with his stoop was 165 cm. An X-ray of his spine showed very dense looking bones that were highly suggestive of fluorosis.

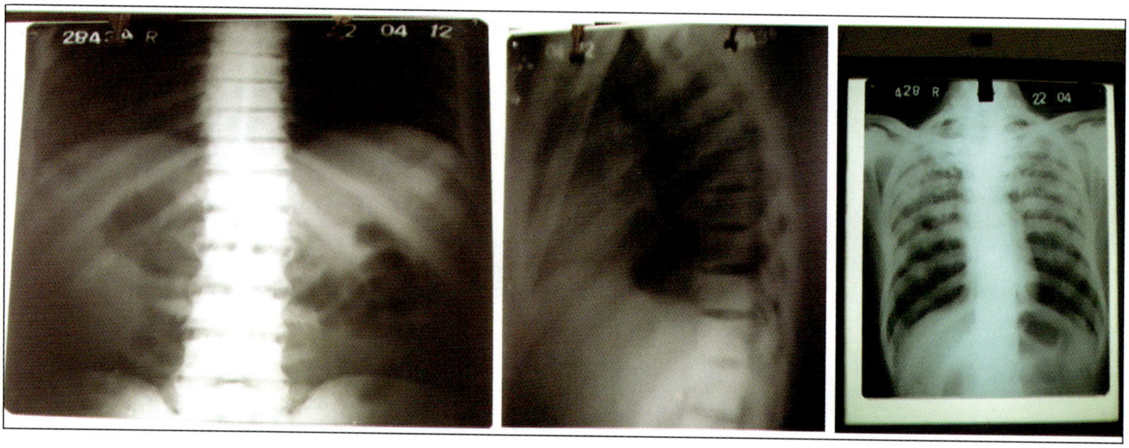

On questioning, Ved Prakash told us that the teeth of most children in his village seemed discoloured, and until then he had thought that either they had not been cleaning their teeth properly, or that they were consuming gutka. He also said there were many not so old people whose back had grown bent.

We asked him if the villagers would be interested in a visit by a team from JSS, and he answered in the affirmative. On the same day, his brother Bhola Ram, who was suffering

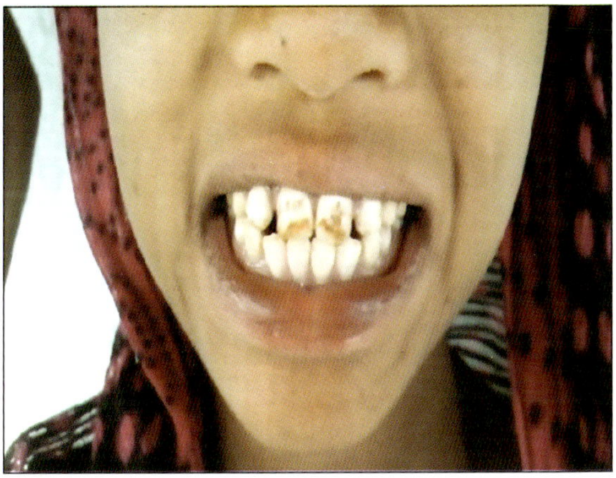

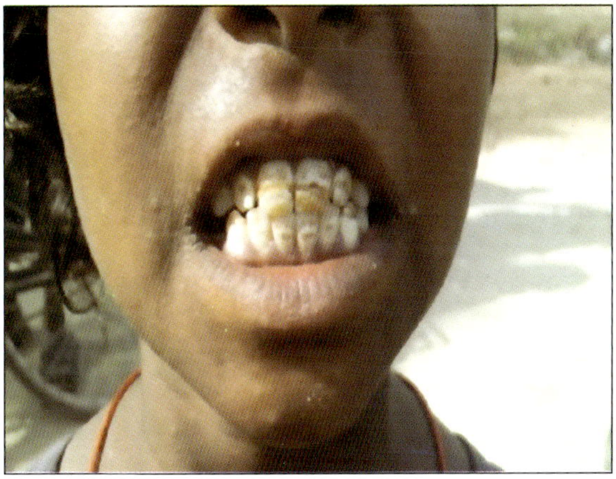

from cough and fever for two months, was diagnosed with tuberculosis and also found to have skeletal fluorosis.

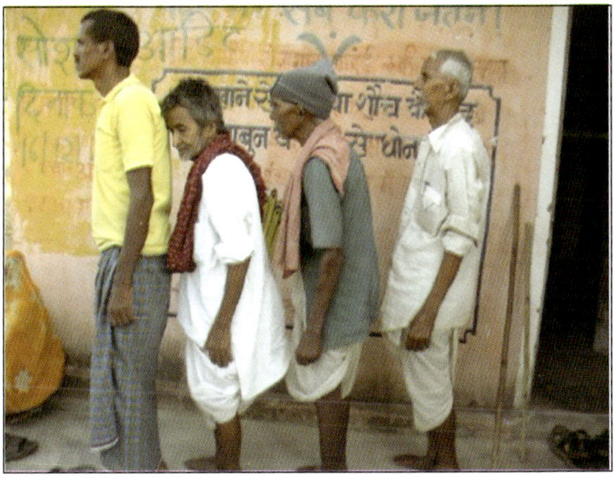

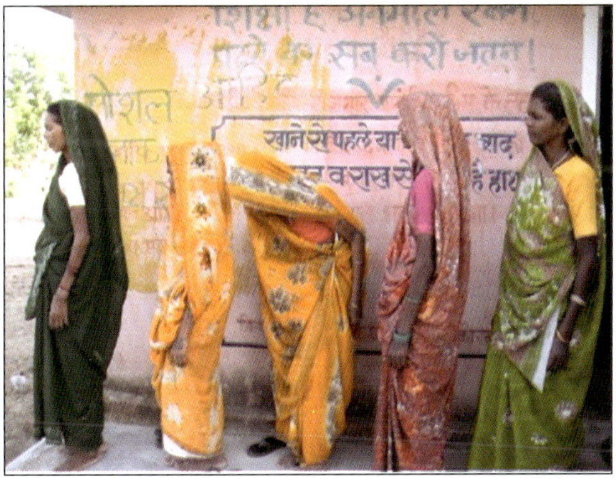

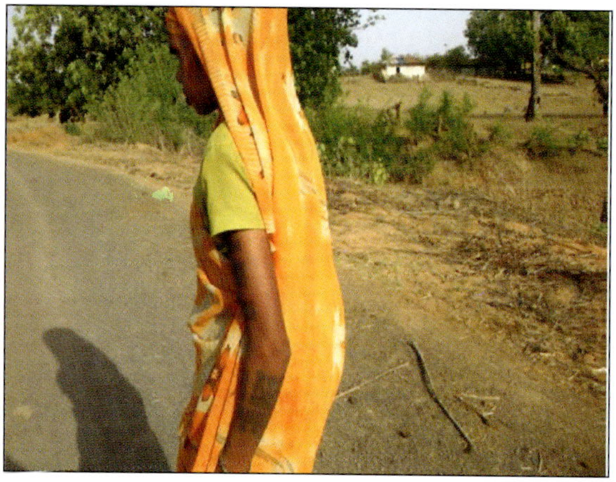 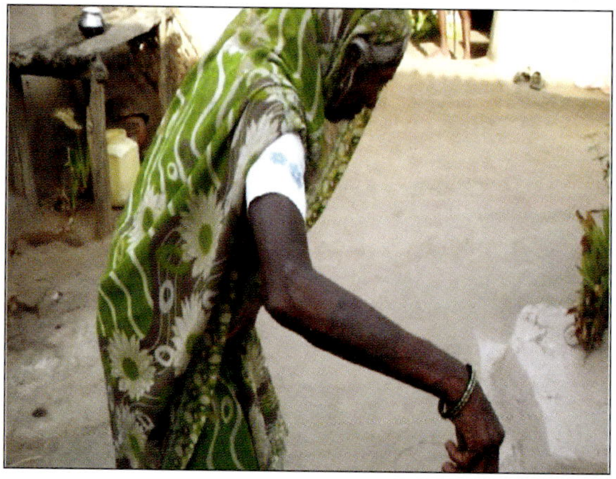

While Ved Prakash and Bhola Ram were started on calcium tablets, Vitamin C and D, JSS undertook an epidemiological survey of Amatikra village.

A house-to-house survey for symptoms of back pain and disability was done. And all the children in the anganwadis were examined for discolouration of teeth. A total of 15 adults, both men and women, were found to have back stiffness and/or disability. Their urine samples were taken for checking fluoride levels. Water samples from all water bodies in the village were taken to be checked for fluoride levels. The teeth of over 50% children were discoloured. It was clear that many people in this village suffered from skeletal or bony fluorosis, and most children were suffering from dental fluorosis.

The laboratory investigations done at the ICMR Regional Centre for research in tribals, now called National Institute for Research in Tribal Health (NIRTH), showed that:

1. The fluoride levels in all the wells was lower than 5 mg per litre, and thus well water was safe to drink with respect to fluoride.

2. Water in 15 out of the 25 hand-pumps had fluoride levels of more than 5 mg per litre, and thus was not safe for drinking.

3. Fluoride levels in urine samples of all 7 people with back pain and stiffness were more than 2 ppm, thus confirming the diagnosis of fluorosis.

After the reports came out, this information was shared with the residents of Amatikra village. Which wells and hand-pumps were safe and which were not was shared and also labelled as green and red respectively. The fact that domestic animals and livestock should also be given water from fluoride-safe water sources was stressed. The village communities were encouraged to demand a water defluoridation plant from the Public Health Engineering department. Information on fluorosis and our investigations were also shared with the district administration and health authorities for corrective action. We realised that many people in the surrounding villages were also affected, thus making a case for community action.

Fluorosis is one such illness in which the back can stiffen and become painful even in young age and may lead to disability. This happens due to deposits of fluoride in the bones and muscles. Since this happens due to excessive consumption of fluoride in drinking water in some areas, this problem is seen among many adults who may be using the same drinking water source. In children, this manifests as discoloured teeth called dental fluorosis.

Fluoride is a mineral found in the soil and rocks, and is necessary in very minute amounts for us to remain healthy. Usually, if the amount of fluoride in our drinking water and/or or food consumed increases beyond 1 ppm, the same fluoride becomes toxic and starts affecting the bones, muscles, teeth, genitals and eyes. One ppm means 1 g of fluoride in 1000 litres of water.

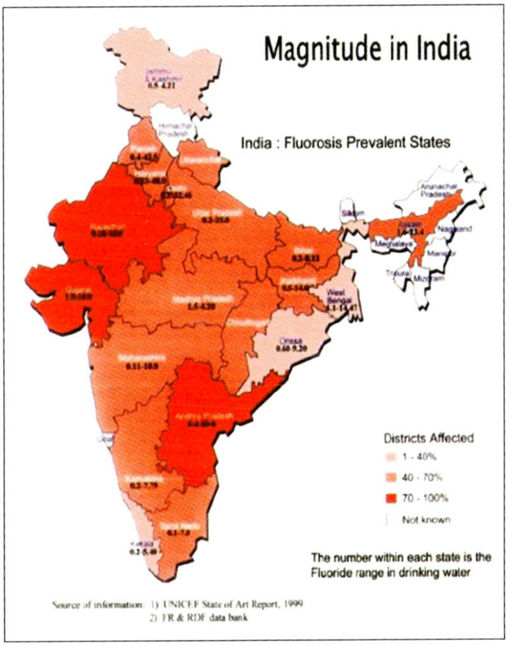

Fluoride content in the top soil and in superficial rocks is minimal. Any well that is less than 60 feet deep will never have excess fluoride. However, if we dig deeper than 300 feet, then fluoride rocks may be touched and thus water from these deep wells may have excess fluoride. But fluoride rocks are not found everywhere. In our country, fluoride-containing rocks are found in Rajasthan,

Gujarat, Uttar Pradesh, Andhra Pradesh, West Bengal, Bihar, Assam, Madhya Pradesh and Chhattisgarh, and in many sites in these states, the problem of fluorosis has been seen.

The teeth of children in these areas are the first to get spoilt and show discolouration, yellowing and chalky deposits. Then the bones and muscles stiffen due fluoride deposits. The blood vessels and reproductive organs, the testes and ovaries, also start malfunctioning due to excess fluoride.

Animals and livestock drinking this water also start having similar problems. Even crops grown in such high fluoride content water contain excess fluoride, and their consumption predisposes consumers to fluorosis.

Once this fluoride deposits in our bones and tissues, it cannot be removed and the damage caused is permanent. Medicines and drinking fluoride-free water in an already affected individual can only prevent further damage, not reverse the damage already caused.

Thus it is an important guideline that any new hand-pump that is set up should have its water quality tested for fluoride content before it is allowed for use by the community. This should be done by the Public Health Engineering department.

For symptomatic relief, one can give 1.5 grams of daily elemental calcium, vitamin C and diet rich in calcium plus some vitamin D. But the main thing is to change the drinking water source to one which is safe and checked for normal fluoride content.

vitamin b12 deficiency

Sanjana

Food choices, Nutrition and Severe Acute Combined Degeneration of the Spinal Cord

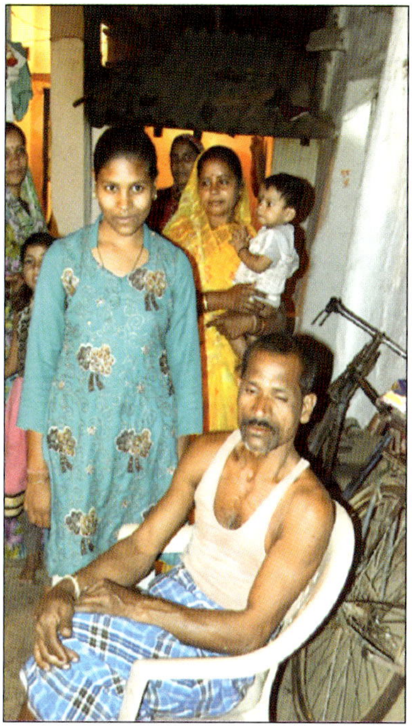

In Chhattisgarh, from the sprawling city of Bilaspur, 19 km towards Amarkantak offshoots a village road which takes you to the beautiful village of Beltukri. There is a small Hanuman temple in Beltukri, next to which are a bunch of huts where lives the family of Ashok Sahu. Ashok Sahu is a 46-year old peasant who owns two acres of land and grows rice during the kharif season. He has a buffalo which gives 6 litres of milk daily, which is shared among Ashok and his family—his four brothers and their wives and children, who together make up 22 members in all.

Back in the 1980s, as Ashok recalls, he and his brothers used to relish fish curry almost daily. 'Mostly during the period of June to November, when there wasn't much grain to eat, my late father Chhedi Lal Sahu used to catch fish from the local pond and my mother used to cook it in the evening. Sometimes, we brothers also caught some small rohu from the local ponds, or sometimes, brought foot-long fishes from a school friend of the Kewat caste, whose family used to catch fish in a big net and sell in the local market.

'We also had half a dozen hens, and that is how we used to get egg and chicken curry. My father was a huge fan of chicken curry cooked by my mother and we brothers, too, used to enjoy it. But once, on the suggestion of the village temple priest, my father had kept the fast of *Ekadashi*, during which you are not supposed to eat *maans-machchhi* (meat and fish). Since then, non-vegetarian food has never been cooked in our home. Although I would still eat chicken and fish at a friend's place sometimes and also at my in-laws', gradually that too stopped as father asked me to stop. Although he never said it forcefully, but I stopped eating non-veg. My in-laws still cook meat, but I don't eat it. My wife also stopped eating it along with me. Her brothers ask her to eat when we go there for a marriage or other functions, but she refuses. Our kids have never eaten it. Same is the story of my brothers and their families.'

On the morning of November 1, 2015, when Ashok went to his paddy fields nearby, Sanjana, the eldest of his three children, woke up and stretched. Sanjana, aged 16, was studying in the 10th standard at the Saraswati Shishu Mandir in nearby Ganiyari town, which was 2 km from Beltukri. Sanjana and the other children of the family walked to the school every day as there had never been any public transport to connect these poor farmer families to Ganiyari.

It was the day of her half-yearly maths exam. Thinking about her exam, Sanjana was going towards the kitchen, when she fell with a loud thud. Her mother came running and asked her to stand up and walk, but she quickly realised that Sanjana could not walk at all. Sanjana started crying and her mother too was anxious. The other children left for school for their half-yearly exams, but Sanjana could not go. Then Sanjana's uncle went to call her father from the fields. When Ashok Sahu reached home, Sanjana was still crying while her mother was massaging her legs with coconut oil, hoping she would soon recover. While the parents were worried about her legs, Sanjana was more worried about the exam she had prepared so well for and missed. She was the topper of her class and had got 92% in the 9th standard exams.

Ashok Sahu waited another day before deciding to bring his daughter to the Jan Swasthya Sahyog hospital in Ganiyari, hoping she would get better with bed-rest and massage. There was no health centre in their village, so people had to go to Ganiyari for their health needs. In Ganiyari, there were two hospitals—one was a government primary health centre and the other was the JSS hospital, which was quite popular in this area. 'This hospital was opened by some passionate AIIMS doctors back in 1999. People rely more on this people's hospital because of the availability of doctors and better quality of care. The treatment is even cheaper and better than that at the government hospital, where doctors always prescribe costly medicines,' said Ashok Sahu.

After reaching JSS Ganiyari with her father on a motorcycle early morning on November 2, Sanjana had to wait another three hours before she got to see the doctor. Her father took her on a hospital wheelchair to a crowded OPD room. During the examination, the doctor found her sense of vibration and position to be impaired, and there was no ankle jerk. Also, the Rhomberg's sign was positive. This neurological disability with the relevant history of little or no intake of eggs, milk or meat made the doctor suspect a vitamin B12 deficiency, which was further supported by an increased mean corpuscular volume (MCV) of red blood cells (RBCs) and macrocytic picture in the peripheral smear. As further confirmatory tests for vitamin B12 deficiency were not available, the diagnosis of Severe Acute Combined Degeneration (SACD) was made, and Sanjana was started on injectable intramuscular vitamin B12 on alternate days for 5 doses followed by oral vitamin B12 supplements, along with folic acid tablets.

On November 11, Friday, Sanjana walked into the JSS OPD after writing her social science exam. Exam was 'Okay' she said, but she looked happy. Although she has started walking again, her gait is still ataxic, and the Rhomberg sign was still found to be positive on examination. The doctor asked the nurse to give Sanjana a vitamin B12 injection and told her mother that Sanjana had improved significantly and that in a month, she would be completely fine.

Sounds like a happy ending? But wait, what is the connection between Sanjana's rare disease and her late grandfather Chhedilal Sahu's *Ekadashi vrat*? And above all, why is Sanjana's story even worth discussing?

Vitamin B12 and its deficiency

Vitamin B12 is one of the many micronutrients that our body needs in addition to calorigenic substances (carbohydrates, fats, proteins) for its proper functioning. Also known as cobalamin, B12 is a water soluble vitamin necessary for the proper development and functioning of the nervous system. It also plays an important role in the formation of blood cells. The recommended dietary allowance (RDA) of this vitamin is 2.4 micrograms daily for adults, 2.6 micrograms daily for pregnant women, and 2.8 micrograms daily for lactating mothers.

Vitamin B12 is produced by certain bacteria, not by plants or animals. But most animal foods are rich sources of vitamin B12 because of the symbiotic relationship of bacteria with animals. Rich sources of vitamin B12 include goat liver, shellfish, crabs, cheese, red meat and chicken eggs.

Vitamin B12 deficiency can have a range of manifestations, from simple fatigue and depression to oral ulcers and gastro-intestinal (GI) disturbances. It can show up as megaloblastic anaemia, or neurologically as in SACD. Deficiency of vitamin B12 can also lead to dementia and psychosis, and it has also been blamed for cerebral atrophy, autism-like features and low IQ according to various studies.

Vitamin B12 deficiency is rare in non-vegetarians as the liver can store it in huge amounts—the liver of a typical non-vegetarian adult can store up to 3000 micrograms of vitamin B12. The deficiency is more common in vegetarians and children born to vegetarian mothers. Pernicious anaemia is also a cause for this deficiency. In elderly populations, atrophic gastritis is a common reason for vitamin B12 deficiency.

Most vitamin B12 deficiency features are reversible and treatable with vitamin B12 supplements while some, like ill effects on cognitive development can only be prevented with a good non-vegetarian diet, milk and daily vitamin supplements in case of vegetarians.

India, B12 and Vegetarianism

According to a study published in the *American Journal of Clinical Nutrition* by Refsum, et al, 75% of a selected urban population from India (Pune, Maharashtra) was found to be vitamin B12 deficient. It also found that the deficiency was far more in vegetarians than non-vegetarians. A similar study done by Sri Ramachandran University Chennai in collaboration with Tufts University also indicates alarming prevalence of Vitamin B12 deficiency, clearly more in vegetarians.

The history of vegetarianism in India goes back to ancient times. The *Manusmriti* (an ancient book of Hindu codes) states: 'There is no sin in eating meat... but abstention brings great rewards'. A verse in the *Shrimad Bhagvad Gita* says: 'Those who are ignorant of real dharma and, though wicked and haughty, account themselves virtuous, kill animals without any feeling of remorse or fear of punishment. Further, in their next lives, such sinful persons will be eaten by the same creatures they have killed in this world'. The rise of Buddhism and Jainism further augmented vegetarian practices.

Country	Vegetarians (%)	Approx. No. of individuals	Source Year
India	31.0%	354,000,000	(2006)

According to the 2006 Hindu-CNN-IBN State of the Nation Survey, 31% of Indians are vegetarians, while another 9% consume eggs. Other surveys cited by FAO and USDA estimate

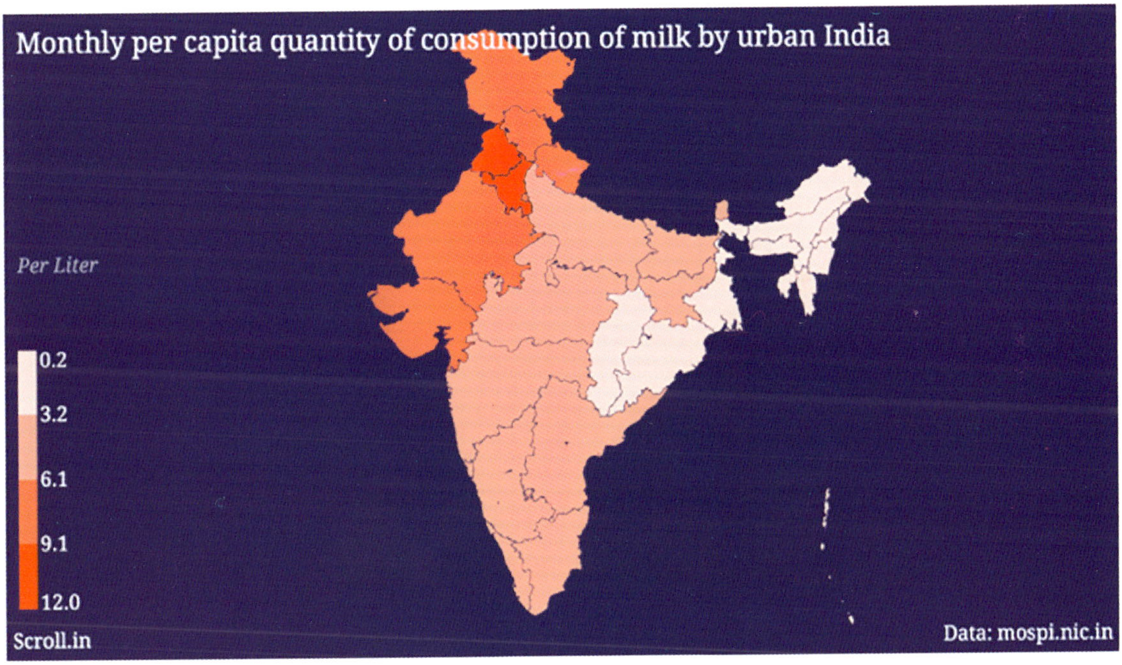

that 40% of the Indian population is vegetarian. These surveys indicate that even Indians who do eat meat do so infrequently, with less than 30% consuming it regularly, for reasons which are mainly socio-cultural and partly economic. Indian vegetarians are estimated to make up more than 70% of the world's vegetarians. But while being a vegetarian or vegan is a lifestyle choice in the West, it is predominantly culturally enforced in India.

To get the daily requirement of vitamin B12 equivalent to RDA, one needs 700-1000 ml of milk everyday, i.e., 21-30 litre per month per person, while 100 gm of red meat daily provides the same amount. For most Indians, per capita consumption of milk is much lower than this. Various religious/semi-religious organisations and animal advocacy groups have been pushing for adopting vegetarian diets, without considering that more than a quarter of the country lives on 32 rupees a day or less. This forced vegetarianism leaves this large population to rely solely on dairy products for their vitamin B12 requirements, which is not in everybody's capacity to procure, thus leaving them prone to cognitive and neurological underdevelopment in this competitive world and making them vulnerable to various other diseases besides.

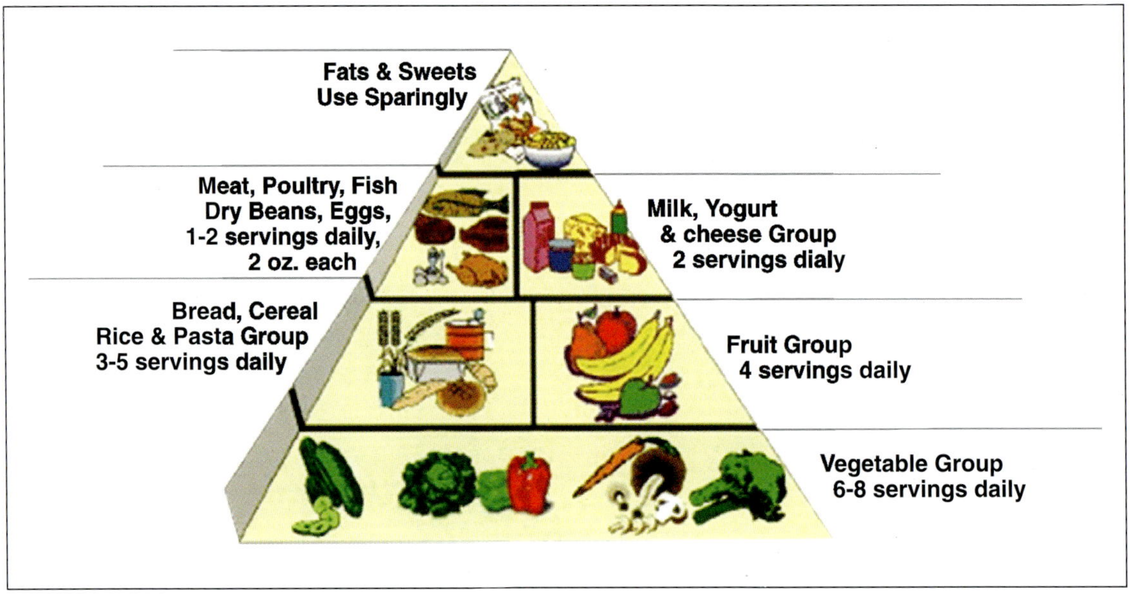

Those involved in health advocacy and policymaking should understand that it is not just calories but a balanced diet which is necessary to maintain good and complete health. Families should be made aware of the importance of a balanced diet for their own health and that of their children. Non-vegetarians should include meat, poultry, fish and eggs in their diet regularly as shown in the food pyramid above. Vegetarians should increase their consumption of dairy products and necessarily add daily vitamin B12 supplements in their diet. Along with this, the government should also take active measures to fight this key vitamin deficiency by including eggs and milk in its distribution system for the poor and in midday meals for school children, by fortifying cereals with vitamin B12 and supplying vitamin B12 supplements to vegetarians, especially to pregnant and lactating mothers. The state should actively encourage fisheries, poultry and the milk products industry and, alongside, promote their domestic consumption.

alcohol addiction

Mangal

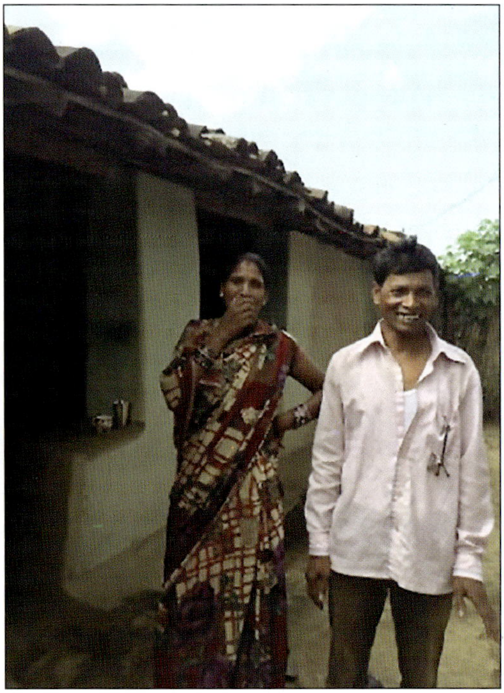

Mangal was twelve years old when he first had alcohol at his brother's wedding, and was struck by the ease and confidence it gave him to dance and engage socially with others. As he described it, his drinking started as a social activity, something to do with friends to pass the time. It boosted his morale as he enjoyed dancing and was generally more outgoing when under the influence of alcohol. This moderate drinking continued for many years, and looking back, Mangal felt that things were very much under control. However, he admitted that this may have been at least partly due to the fact that alcohol was relatively difficult to access in Katami and mostly had to be brought in from outside.

In 2000, Mangal got married to Sushila, a confident and outspoken woman from a village about 50 km from Katami. Yet not long after their marriage, Mangal's drinking habits started to change for the worse. Around the same time that Sushila moved in with Mangal, families in Katami were beginning to brew their own alcohol, encouraged by the potential business prospects. It so happened that Sushila was from a village where the brewing of alcohol was a big business, and her family was one of many that would sell their homemade liquor. Because she had experience in the trade, Sushila was encouraged to start up her own business in Katami. Mangal claimed that he was strongly opposed to the idea of brewing liquor in his own home, not wanting to support such an 'unhealthy practice'. However, the encouragement from others and the economic prospects overrode Mangal's hesitation, and he and Sushila began to brew their own liquor.

Over the years, with such easy access to alcohol and its high availability, Mangal started drinking more and more often. However, he had a steady job at Jan Swasthya Sahyog, which kept him occupied. When that job ended, he was briefly unemployed before landing a job with the Electricity Board in Bilaspur in 2010. That job lasted for 6-7 months, when a quarrel broke out between him and some other employees and Mangal was made to leave.

With no job and lots of idle time on his hands, Mangal turned to drinking. He had significant savings from his previous jobs, as well as from Sushila's alcohol business, with which he was able to support his drinking. Thereafter, things quickly spiraled out of control, to the point where he was drinking about 500 ml of liquor every day. His dependence was so great that not an hour would go by without a drink. Everything else in his life became meaningless. He lost appetite, sometimes eating only two to three times a week. The family's finances also worsened as Mangal had stopped tending to the farm, and their savings were being fast depleted. He even resorted to selling the family's monthly ration of rice to buy alcohol.

Alcohol also made him violent, and Mangal would beat his wife and sometimes his children. He was often irritable and angry. It reached the point that Sushila would run away to her relative's house for fifteen to thirty days at a stretch, before returning out of concern for her children. The whole family started avoiding him for fear of his uncontrollable rage. At the same time, Mangal grew weaker and weaker, eventually becoming confined to his cot. He would lie there all day, only getting up to find more liquor, and a couple friends with whom to drink. Over this period, he lost a lot of weight and would regularly experience bodily tremors. When asked if he thought about trying to stop drinking, he said that of course, he wanted to stop, but at that point things had gone so completely out of control that he didn't think it was possible for him to quit.

Then, in 2012, a few former colleagues from JSS approached Mangal to talk about some alcohol de-addiction groups that JSS was starting in some of their programme villages. They wanted to start one in Katami, and asked Mangal if he was willing to lead the group. Mangal agreed, and thus he became the head of a group of twelve men who joined under the agreement that they would all stop both the making and drinking of alcohol, and help and counsel other alcoholics to quit drinking as well.

Now, three years later, Mangal is completely sober, and his local de-addiction group has transitioned from holding weekly meetings to once a month. He and his wife are living happily together. Mangal is using a high-yield technique to farm an acre of his land, and is able to comfortably feed his family. He is in charge of overseeing six alcohol de-addiction groups in various neighbouring villages, and he hopes that such groups will help turn around the lives of other men addicted to alcohol, just as it had turned around his own.

Alcohol is probably the most commonly used drug worldwide. Alcohol or, more precisely, ethyl alcohol is made by fermenting the sugar available in fruits, flowers, grains etc. The concentration of alcohol after the fermentation processes can go up to 15%. Higher percentages are achieved through various distillation processes, done innovatively in villages using simple tools. Consuming small to moderate amounts of alcohol typically gives a pleasant feeling of relaxation and loss of inhibition initially, which is followed by unpleasant or unpredictable changes in mood as the concentration of alcohol in the blood falls and as the alcohol gets metabolized in the liver. On the other hand with the rising blood level of alcohol, a lack of physical and emotional control sets in. Alcohol is involved in about 50% of fatal accidents, an important factor in suicides and homicides, and a majority of domestic violence cases around the world, besides non-fatal hazards.

In tribal villages, locally brewed alcohol like *desi daru*, *mahua* and feni are commonly produced in households. Some experience and skill is needed to keep the concentration of methanol low as it is extremely toxic in higher concentrations. Serving alcohol to visitors and drinking during festivities is socially accepted among tribal communities. Thus, children often get exposed to alcohol quite early. Ten to 15% of people who drink alcohol regularly develop a dependency, and this is when a habit becomes a disease. On the one hand, there is physical dependence with tolerance, that is, more and more of alcohol is needed to get the same effect and withdrawal symptoms like tremors, agitation, sleep disturbance and even seizures and delirium can manifest when alcohol intake is suddenly stopped. On the other hand, the person increases the quantity and/or frequency of intake and continues drinking even though alcohol compromises his or her health, work and family life. At this stage it becomes extremely difficult for the individual to stop or cut down on alcohol. The first hurdle is to get over the withdrawal symptoms, which can be bad, and then to get over the craving. Many people consuming alcohol regularly in larger amounts, say more than 4 drinks daily, develop problems like liver and nerve damage, leading to numbness of feet and hands or memory difficulties. Furthermore, depressive symptoms are common. All this makes it extremely difficult for the person to reach a degree of sobriety, and to stay sober.

An alcoholic thus has good reasons to continue drinking. Therefore, in motivational therapy which forms the basis of change, it is important to recognize the reasons for continuing to drink and to discuss the pros and cons of both drinking and sobriety. This kind of discussion, particularly in a group setting, appears to work best in achieving de-addiction.

In JSS, we started the alcohol treatment programme in 2012, wherein we initially offer a detoxification regimen to patients in whom we expect withdrawal symptoms to occur. This comprises use of chlordiazepoxide, vitamin B1, multivitamins and carbamazepine to prevent seizures. Individual sessions with patients and relatives are offered to explain the de-addiction treatment and, if possible, patients are invited to one of the de-addiction groups now run primarily as self-help groups by former alcoholics. A recent meta-analysis of the results of past alcohol treatment estimates that more than 50 percent of treated patients relapse within the first three months after starting treatment. Relapses and relapse-management are a big challenge during alcohol treatment. It helps to have a strong support system evolve within the self-help groups to support the patient during a relapse and so keep the duration and severity of relapse as low as possible.

Alcohol is a major public health issue in rural settings but also in Chhattisgarh as a whole. Liquor consumption in Chhattisgarh is increasing at the rate of 30 percent every year. In 2013-14, Chhattisgarh has earned Rs. 1,900 crore from liquor sales, nearly Rs. 500 crore more than the revenue earned in the previous year. In the same period, revenue from alcohol in neighbouring states like Odisha or Madhya Pradesh has grown at half the pace or less—and this despite the fact that Chhattisgarh's population is half or one-third of these states. We have a long way to go in fighting this trend of growing alcohol use.

However secure and well-regulated civilised life may become, bacteria, protozoa, viruses, lice, ticks and mosquitoes will always lurk in the shadows ready to pounce when neglect, poverty, famine, or war lets down the defenses. And even in normal times they prey on the weak, the very young and the very old, living along with us, in mysterious obscurity waiting their opportunities.

- Hans Zinsser, 1934

Picture Stories

inaccessibility of healthcare and the need for caesarean section

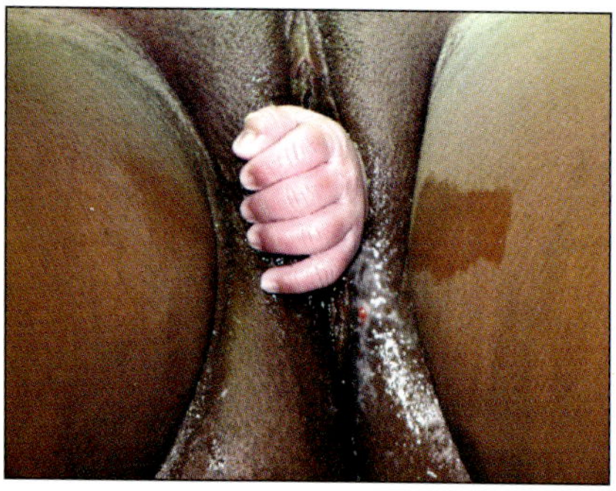

One of the biggest determinants of health in rural India is the physical and financial accessibility to health care. For this, you need a road that connects the house or village with an appropriate health facility, a vehicle on that road and money in hand to access that vehicle. These three determinants of access are poorly distributed in most rural areas compared to the cities and it is no wonder that health outcomes are worse in rural areas.

Two public health problems best epitomize this issue of inaccessibility. The first is the care of snake and rabid animal bites. A delay in accessing a vehicle at night and the consequent delay in reaching a health facility that can administer anti-venom to a person who has been bitten can decide if he or she dies or lives. The second example is of obstetric emergency of obstructed labour, where access to timely surgery like a caesarean section will decide if the mother and her newborn baby will survive.

In the district of Bilaspur, out of 1655 villages, 36% are not connected with an all-weather road to resources. Further, 55% of villages are not accessible by a bus or a similar four-wheeled vehicle. And there must be districts where inaccessibility to health facilities is even worse than in Bilaspur.

When a caesarean section (CS) is badly needed, like in the case of this child with a hand prolapse, a quick extraction is required in order to survive. This child is lying in the mother's uterus on the side and thus there is no way she can come out alive without a caesarean section.

CS rates vary hugely between the cities and villages of all states in this country. An expected CS rate is 15% of all deliveries, and in several rural areas of many states including Chhattisgarh, it is not even 5%. We feel this denial of appropriate health care for pregnant women is a structural denial and should be acted against.

cord prolapse

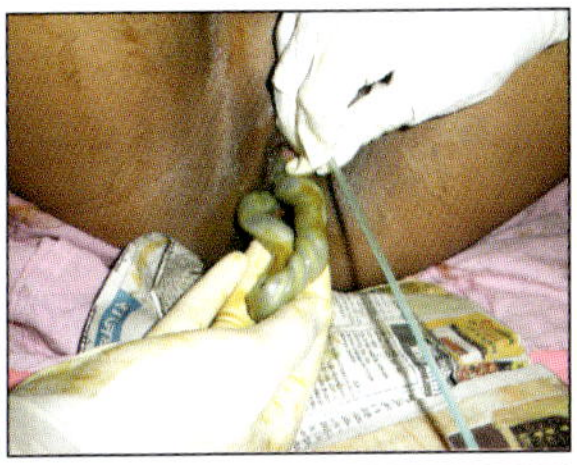

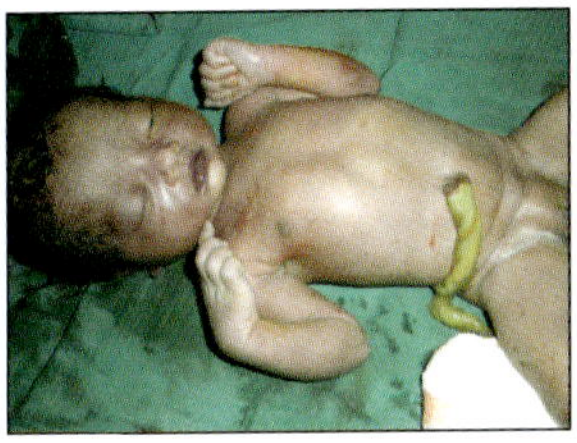

Cord prolapse is a frightful obstetric emergency which occurs when the cord comes out as the presenting part before or along with the head or the breech of the baby. The cord has a high chance of being compressed, compromising the blood supply to the unborn child. The risk of intrauterine death is very high. According to some studies, cord prolapse at home may result in over 40% perinatal mortality, but if it occurs at a hospital with facilities for emergency surgery, perinatal mortality can decline to 0-3%. The overall incidence of cord prolapse is 0.6% of all labour presentations.

Intrauterine growth restriction and prematurity are major causes for cord prolapse, and both are related to maternal malnutrition before and during pregnancy. Besides these, fetal malpresentation, polyhydramnios, multiple gestations, spontaneous rupture of the membrane as well as iatrogenic causes such as planned artificial rupture of the membrane and the use of oxytocics to speed up uterine contractions can result in cord prolapse.

One easy approach which can be tried to elevate the presenting fetal part is to introduce Foley's catheter, fill the bladder with 500-750 ml saline and clamp the catheter. It will cause some problems, but along with elevating the presenting fetal part, it will cause decompression of the cord and help in the relaxation of the uterus. This is called Vago's method.

Maintaining better nutrition in pregnancy and using dietary supplements may also help reduce the occurrence of cord prolapse. Carrying out a hospital delivery at centres with facilities to do cesarean sections on an urgent basis is an important step in helping preventing fetal mortality in cord prolapse, should it happen.

In this picture, the accompanying meconium stained liquor suggests coexisting fetal distress along with the cord prolapse. Despite doctors taking this woman for an urgent cesarean section, the baby was born dead.

neonatal intestinal obstruction

Neonatal intestinal obstruction is one of the most common emergencies in newborn children. Bilious vomiting, failure to pass meconium and abdominal distention are cardinal features of this condition, but they may be subtle and consequently overlooked. Any delay in diagnosis could lead to severe consequences, but if diagnosed in time and with the right intervention, there are good results.

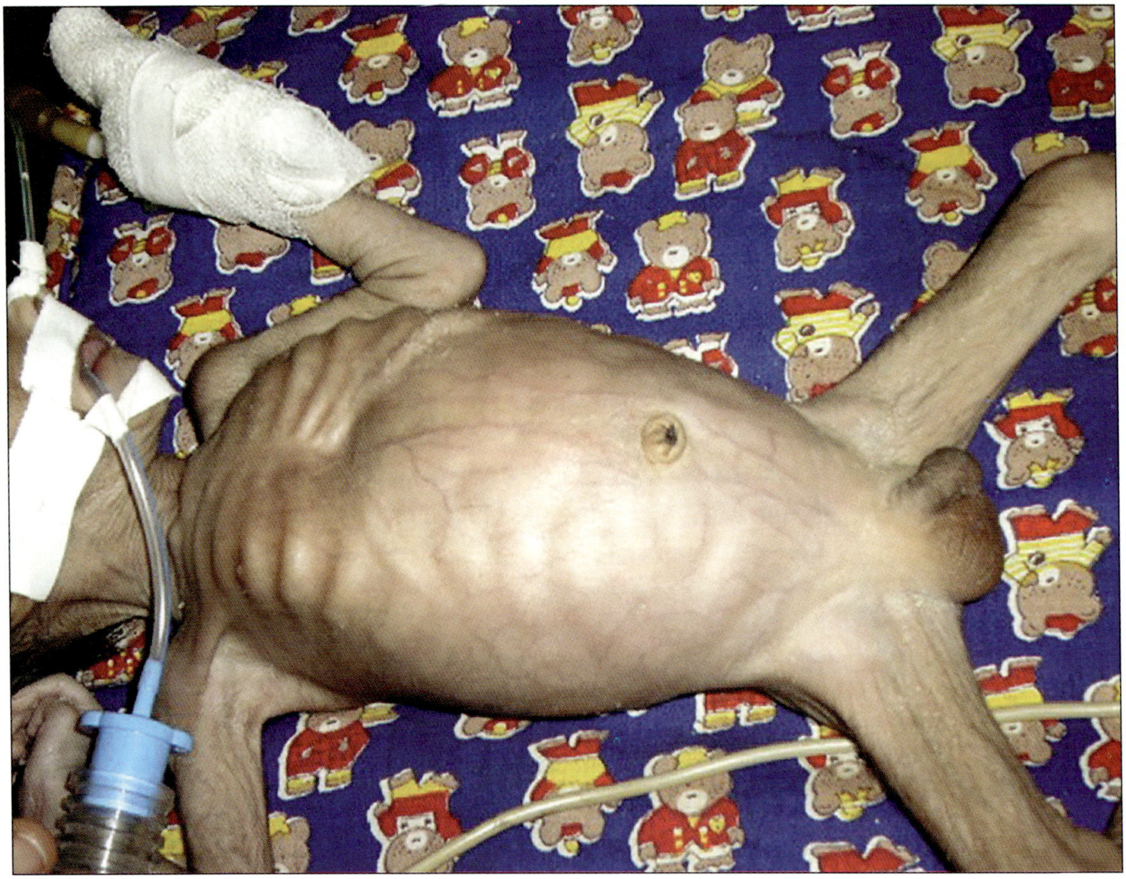

rheumatoid arthritis

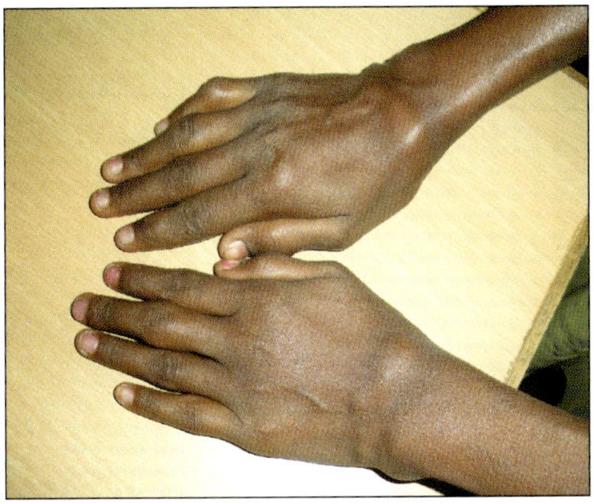

The description of crippling arthritis is encountered less frequently in Western textbooks, suggesting that there is an improper understanding of the burden of rheumatoid arthritis (RA) seen in rural areas of developing countries. If anyone would wish to see cases of the most crippling rheumatoid arthritis, they need to only attend one outpatient clinic at Jan Swasthya Sahyog's (JSS) rural health centre.

RA is a chronic progressive disease, causing inflammation in the joints. As the pathology progresses, the joint inflammatory (swelling) activity leads to tendon tethering, erosion and destruction of the joint surface, which impairs the range of movement and causes deformities.

The disease is seen disproportionately among women and is three times more common in females than in males. It occurs in young, middle-aged as well as elderly women. We have seen much harassment and depression on the faces of patients living with severe pain, fatigue and many other problems.

Most women present very late, after they are no longer productive and have been severely affected by the disease. They are often unable to walk even with a stick and cannot perform their own routine work, including their toilet needs. If there is no deformity yet, there is some hope that medicines may be able to work. Once deformities occur, proper treatment can relieve the pain.

The goals of treatment are to minimize symptoms, prevent bone deformities and maintain day-to-day functioning. It usually involves multi drug therapy along with physiotherapy. Medicines can also cause problems, so patients need careful monitoring and of course, empathy.

hyperthyroidism

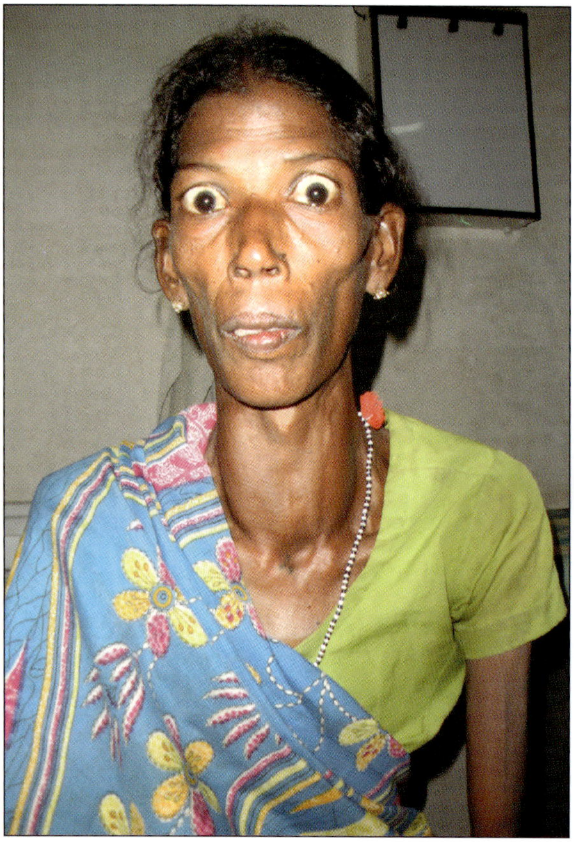

Hyperthyroidism is seen more among middle-aged and elderly women from rural areas, who present in a wasted state with swelling in the front of their necks, an affliction which often does not worry them enough.

An estimated 42 million Indians suffer from thyroid disorders, conditions which are largely prevalent in women. Most hyperthyroidism occurs in the form of either - Grave's disease, toxic nodular goiter or thyroiditis. This patient presented to us with marked weight loss despite a normal appetite, heat intolerance, sweating, palpitations, tremor, fatigue, irritability and lid lag. She also had an atrial fibrillation and congestive heart failure, presenting with an irregular pulse, severe edema, ascitis and effort intolerance.

A good symptomatic response happens with medical treatment in the form of anti-thyroid medicines, but there is a need for regular follow up over a long period, except in thyroiditis, where treatment may have to be stopped when thyroid function returns to normal. Radio iodine is also required sometimes, for which a referral is needed to a tertiary care facility.

Screening for thyroid disorders and having treatment facilities can decrease the burden of this problem in rural India.

hypothyroidism, hyponutrition and hypodevelopment

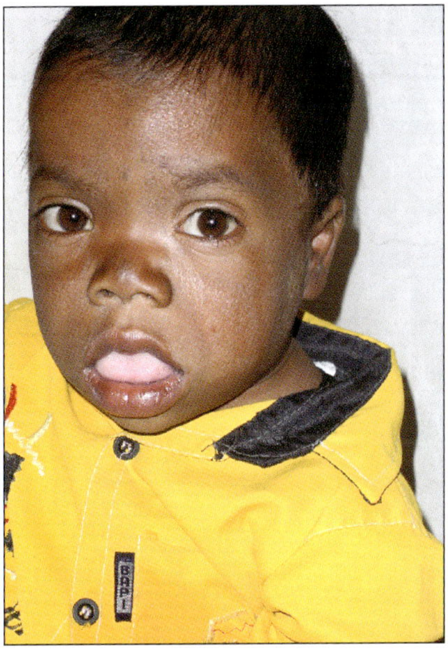

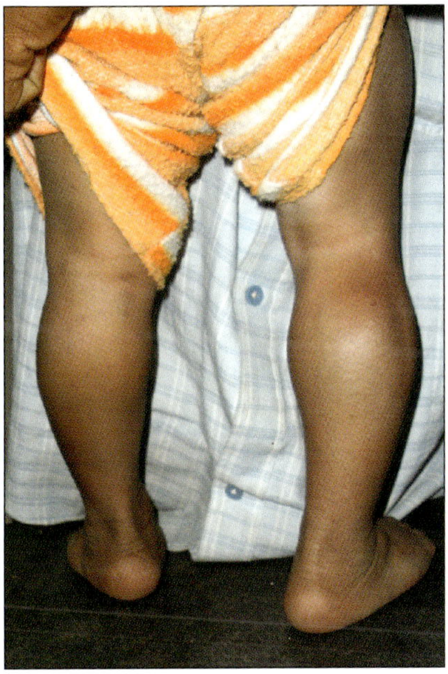

This picture shows a stunted childhood which could lead to poor adulthood as a consequence of poor thyroid development. The role of iodine deficiency is disputed, but what is not disputed is that every one of us should be screened at birth for hypothryroidism, something which is not done in India. Screening has been recently recommended in the Rashtriya Bal Suraksha Karyakram under the National Rural Health Mission, but has yet to take off. The fact that one still regularly sees such problems as in the case of this child, who will remain permanently stunted and mentally challenged is proof of the structural neglect of poor people.

The best outcome of therapy is when we start it by the age of 2 weeks. When treatment initiation is delayed until 3-6 months, the child's mean IQ will be only partially improved, which according to some studies is seen to be an average of 71. When treatment is delayed beyond 6 months, the final mean IQ drops to 54, and if left untreated, then there is life long suffering.

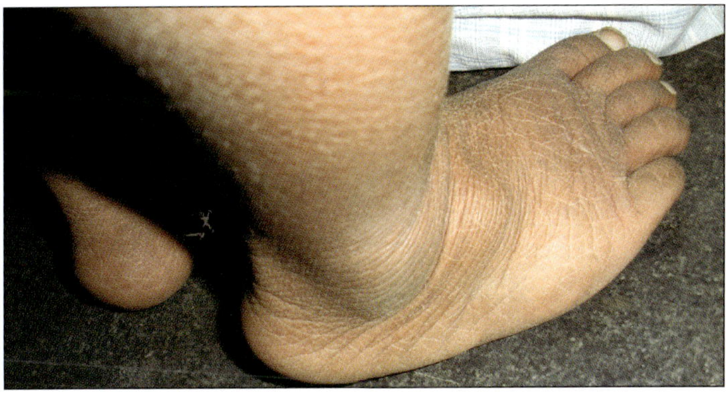

gas gangrene

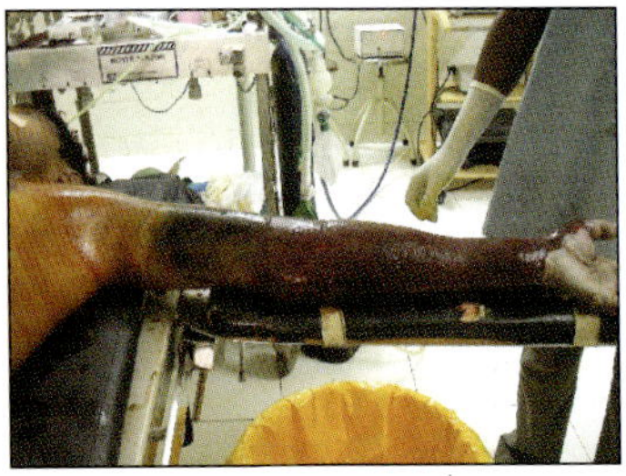

Gas gangrene is a miserable condition and those who suffer are the ones who live off the land. We have seen young adults coming in with severe pain and tense bluish skin, usually involving their extremities. Sometimes we see very small lesions, but within no time they become a very large patch of blackish discoloration if left untreated.

Gas gangrene, also known as muscle necrosis, is often seen in people with infections by clostridium perfringens or any of a number of soil borne anaerobic bacteria. Soil borne bacteria are well adapted to surviving very harsh conditions and produce toxins for their existence in order to compete with other bacteria of the environment. They are not easily killed by disinfectants and show their venomous nature when they get an opportunity.

In anaerobic or oxygen-poor conditions, the bacteria causes a tissue infection in the devitalised tissues following a wound and then forms a gas that spreads locally and extends along tissue planes, causing excruciating pain and progresses rapidly over 18 to 24 hours. The skin color changes from pale to bronze or purple and the tissue becomes tense and swollen. The gas is very obvious and we can easily feel crepitus (a Velcro- like feeling) on local clinical examination. This condition is easily visible on x-rays, CT or ultrasound scans and is usually fatal.

The signs of systemic toxicity also develop fast due to the release of toxins by the bacteria. Multi-organ dysfunction rapidly ensues.

Poverty is one of the big triggers for any disaster relating to human health and those who work in fields far away from health facilities often don't realize the severity of day-to-day injuries. They often start working again after the application of some local herbs. If people don't recognize the problems of deep wounds, they can be life threatening. If toxemia occurs, aggressive surgical debridement and antibiotics in the form of high-dose intravenous penicillin, clindamycin and metronidazole are needed urgently. Any delay may lead to the loss of limb and further delays may result in death.

bacterial pneumonia

The picture shows three children between 5 and 6 years old who were undernourished and had fallen prey to bacterial pneumonia. They received treatment very late and when they did, it was inadequate. The infection from their lungs leaked into their pleural cavities, causing large volume of pus to accumulate, a condition called empyema. After futile attempts to drain the fluid at different healthcare facilities and having exhausted their meager financial resources, the family arrived at Jan Swasthya Sahyog. The children required a surgical removal of the fibrous peel to allow their lungs to expand.

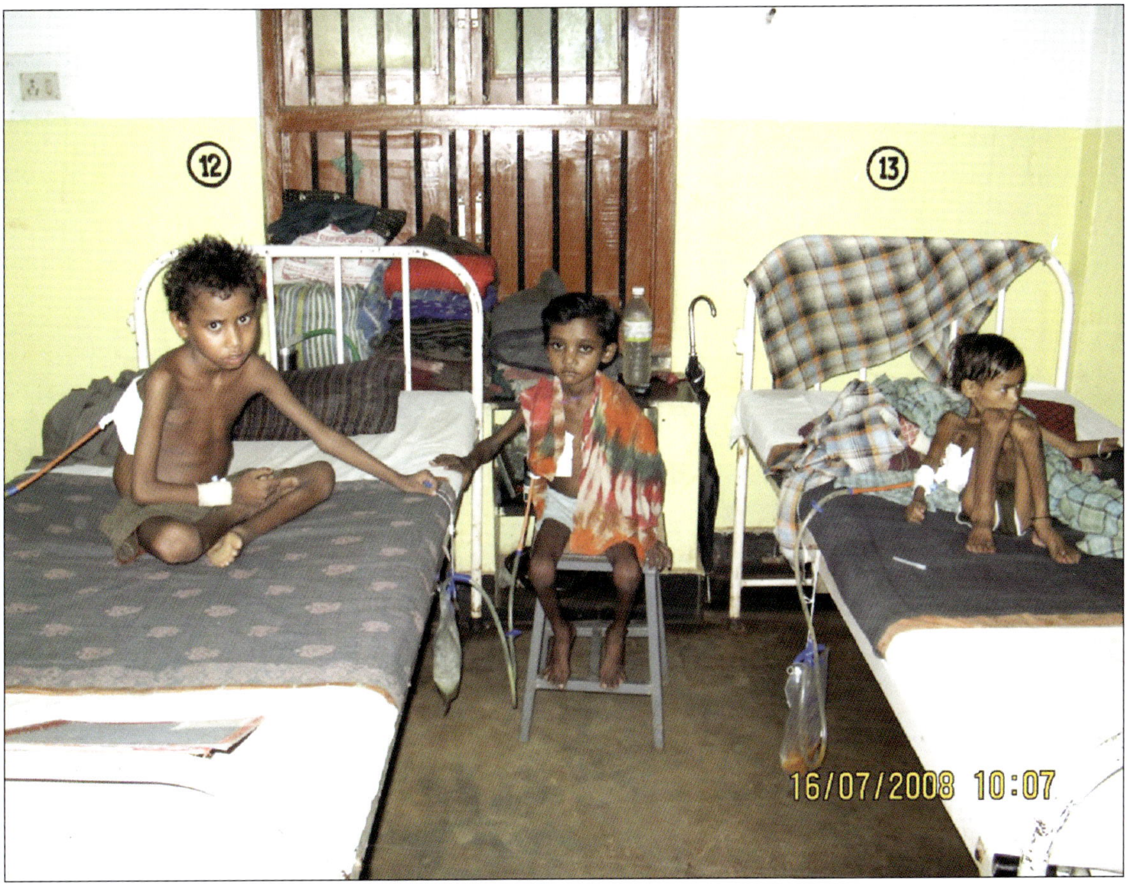

lymph node tuberculosis

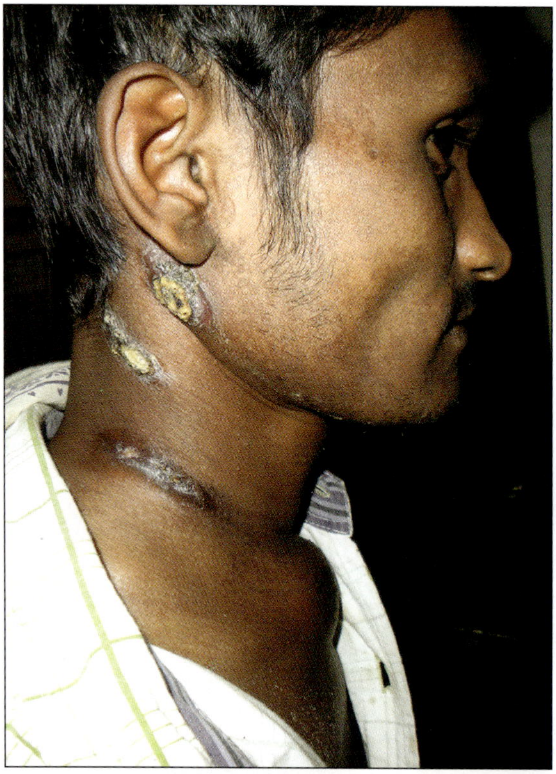

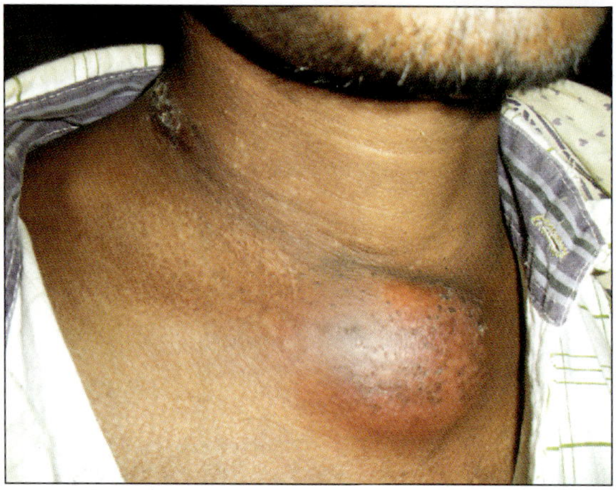

This picture is of a patient with lymph node tuberculosis who came too late to the Jan Swasthya Sahyog (JSS) health facility for treatment. He had multiple lesions which were only partially healed, one of which was inflamed and ready to burst. These lesions may be misdiagnosed by an unwary physician as common abscesses.

In the past, tubercular lymphadenitis was considered as a disease of childhood. However, the peak age has now shifted from childhood to the age group of 20 to 40 years. In developing countries where tuberculosis is endemic, extrapulmonary disease is common and lymphadenitis is the most frequent presentation of it. When it occurs in the neck area and involves the surrounding skin, it is known as Scrofula.

Extrapulmonary tuberculosis is caused by decreased immunity. In most developed countries, it is mainly associated with HIV. However, in central India, this association is not so common and undernutrition is the most common causative factor.

bone tuberculosis

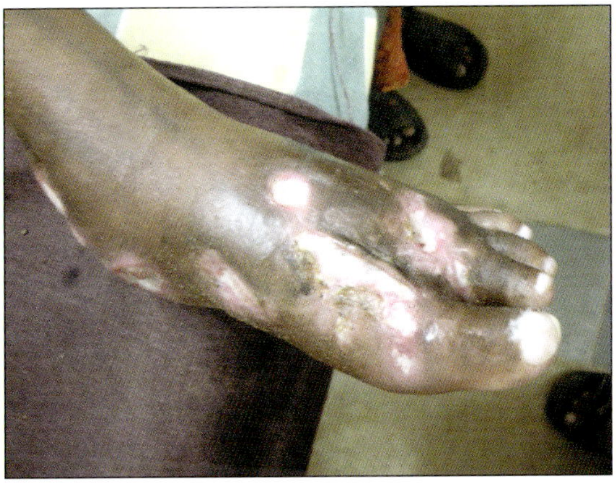

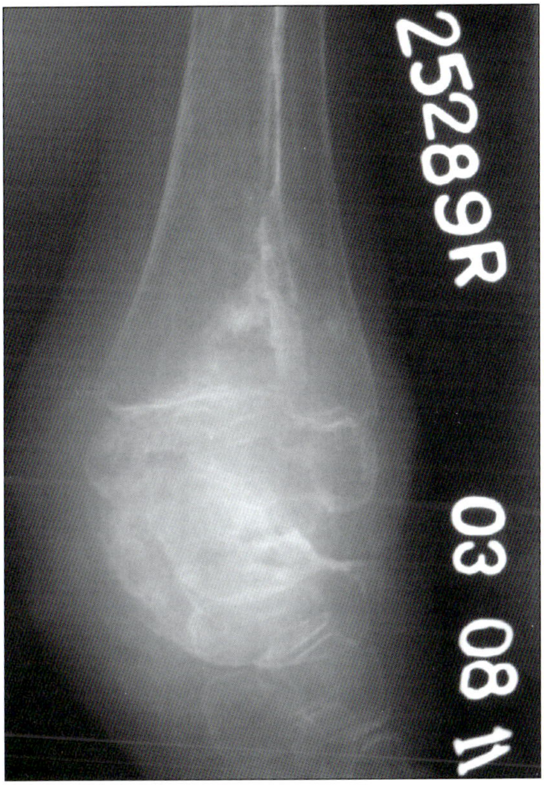

Bone tuberculosis is a chronic manifestation of tuberculosis, which occurs more frequently in those who are exposed to physical trauma and under nutrition.

In rural India we have observed many patients with bone tuberculosis, mainly involving a single joint, but in some cases with more than one joint affected. Occasionally we see the occurrence of polyarthritis due to an immune reaction - a form of tubercular rheumatism called Poncet's disease. Spinal tuberculosis, also known as Pott's disease, is most commonly seen in children and young adults. If not treated in time, it may result in paralysis. Lack of awareness may lead to a diagnostic delay and increased morbidity. Sometimes, bone tuberculosis presents with multiple discharging sinuses.

The course of treatment for bone tuberculosis is slightly longer for 12 months, than for other types of TB although the same drugs are used.

tuberculosis and wasting

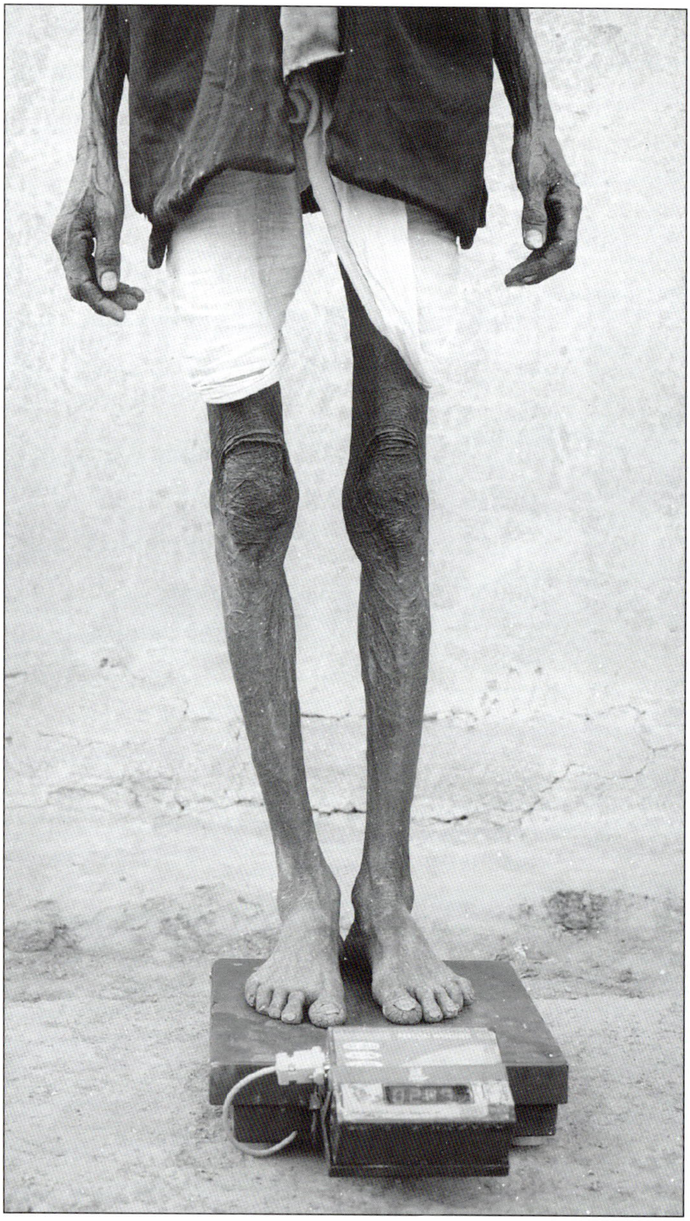

This picture shows the wasting of a 55 year old man with tuberculosis. He weighed only 28 km, with a Body Mass Index of 11.4. Such levels of wasting are seen in only a few illnesses such as tuberculosis (better known as consumption), thin diabetes, HIV, hyperthyroidism and often, as a result of starvation.

crippled due to sickle cell disease in young adulthood

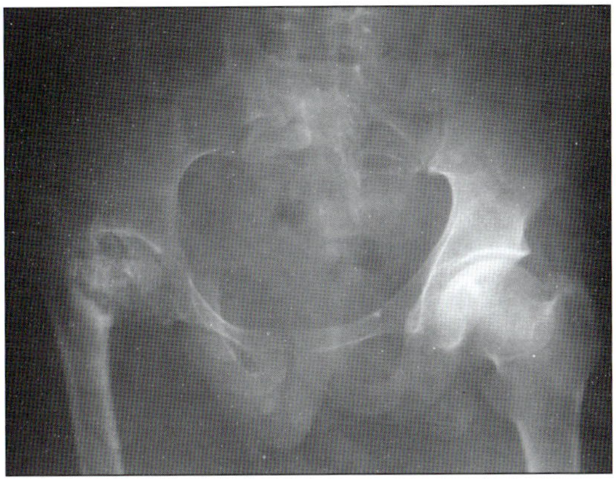

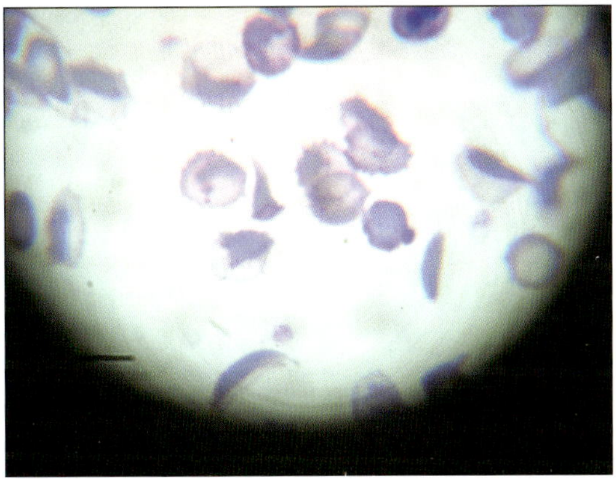

Sickle cell disease (SCD) is a primary genetic defect making a rounded red blood cell (RBC) sickle shaped. This makes the RBCs rigid and they tend to block circulation and become sticky enough to form a plug.

The distribution of this illness parallels that of falciparum malaria and it is most prevalent in the tribal population, which is settled mainly in forested and in rural areas. People with SCD do not always have access to good healthcare.

SCD patients usually come to the hospital as children, suffering from unbearably severe pain in either the whole body, multiple joints or in the chest or abdomen, a condition known as vaso-occlusive crisis. Severe chest pain is one of the most life-threatening condition in SCD. Plugs in the pulmonary blood vessels put the patient at risk for pulmonary arterial hypertension and further cardiac complications. These are emergencies and must be treated aggressively.

Chronic complications of SCD includes avascular necrosis (AVN) of the hip joints, in which the head of the femur collapses due to a blockage in the blood vessel of the femur and immobilizes the patients permanently. Along with suffering severe pain, patients stand to lose their daily wages and self-confidence.

About 50% of people affected by this condition would have developed some AVN by the age of 33. Those who have associated alpha thalassemia have a much higher prevalence of AVN.

AVN of the hip joint causes chronic pain and disability. The pain is usually worse when walking, relieved by rest, and may be accompanied by a moderate to severe limitation of motion when the patient bears weight on the affected extremity. Almost half of the AVNs are bilateral.

If a young man or woman walks into the Jan Swasthya Sahyog (JSS) outpatient department with a painful hip or a limp and is also a little anemic, the doctor's first suspicion is of an avascular necrosis of the hip.

This is a cause of significant disability in adults with sickle cell disease, even if they have escaped childhood without many infections and a painful vaso-occlusive crisis.

With the advent of science, we can treat SCD with Hydroxyurea, a type of chemotherapy drug which increases fetal hemoglobin in the blood and makes oxygen delivery in body sustainable.

For this genetic disease of tribals and others who live in malarious areas, hip replacement surgery or any other surgery like core decompression for AVN seems difficult to provide, but it is the right of every one with this disease to have access to treatment and we should try hard to get this done for all who need it .

dactylitis

This image shows a case of dactylitis or painful bilateral finger swelling. This form of vaso-occlusive crisis can happen in very young children with sickle cell disease below two years of age. There are hardly any other illnesses that cause such painful bilateral hand swelling. The treatment for dactylitis includes pain relief using opiates and blood transfusion, after which hydroxyurea can be started.

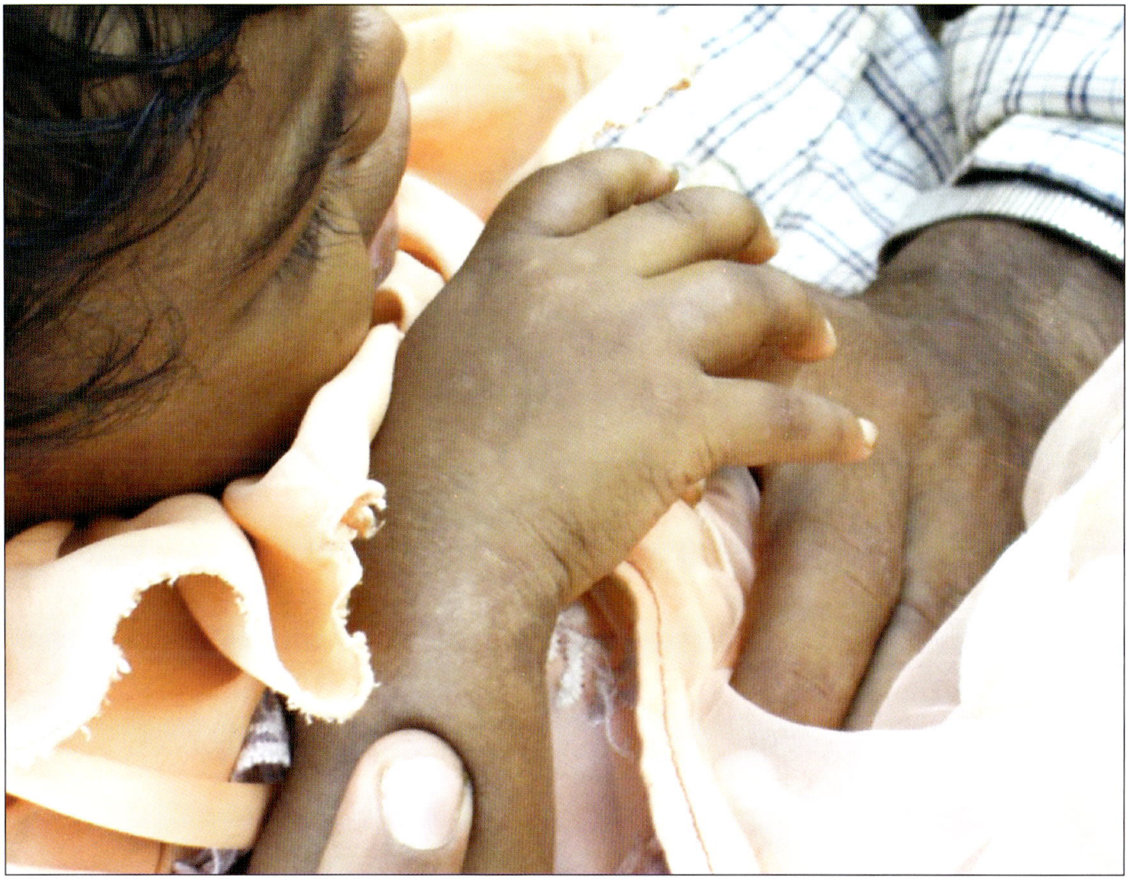

Marjolin's ulcer

The picture shows a 30 year old woman who had fallen into a fire 12 years previously, burning her back. There was repeated ulceration after the wound had apparently healed, until she developed this foul-smelling malignancy at the site over a period of nine months, a malignancy known as Marjolin's ulcer. The patient required extensive resection and large skin grafts.

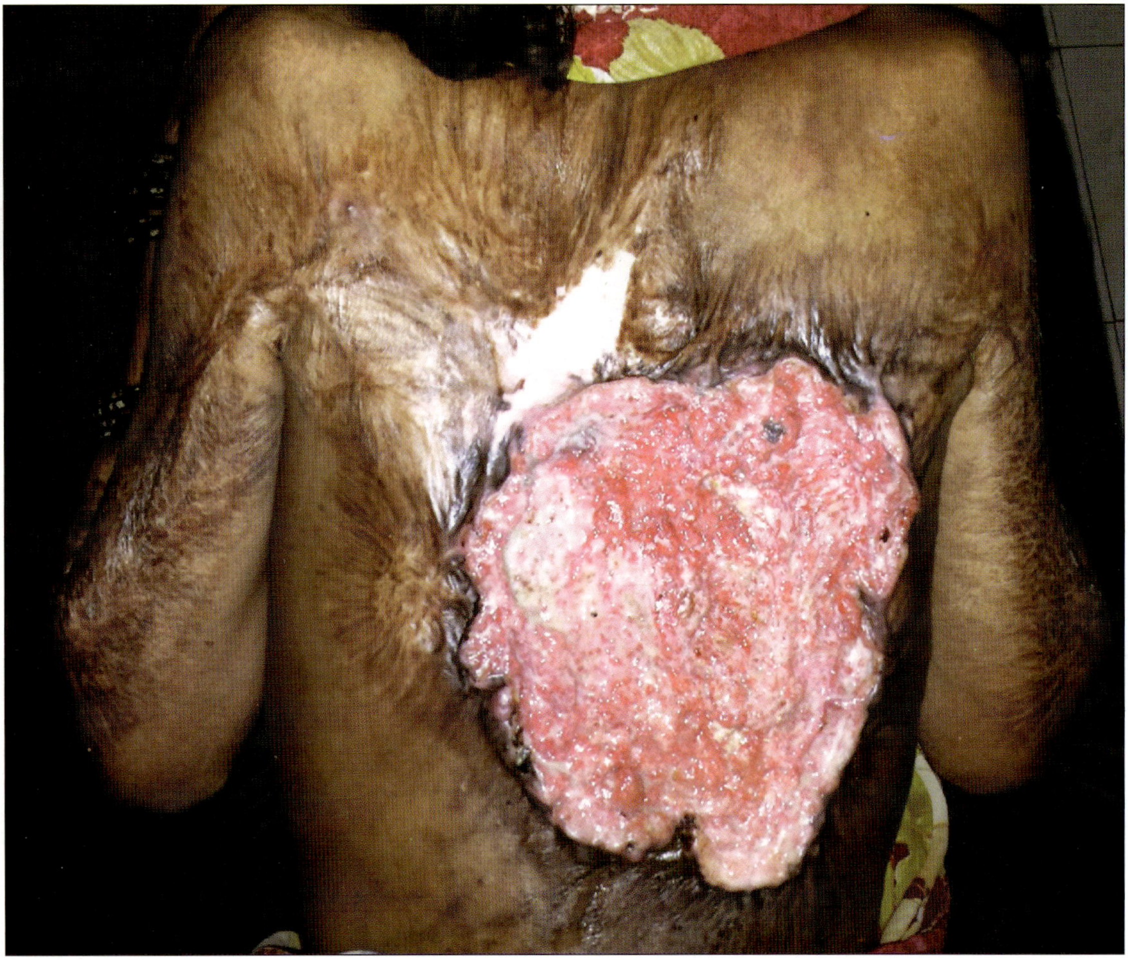

necrotizing fasciitis

A one year old girl had an infection in her right leg that spread behind her knee. Local practitioners treated her with intravenous antibiotics but she got no relief. Four days later she was brought to Jan Swasthya Sahyog in a critical condition, with the infection along with gangrene (Necrotizing Fasciitis) having spread to her abdomen. Despite extensive surgery and heroic attempts to save her, she died the same night.

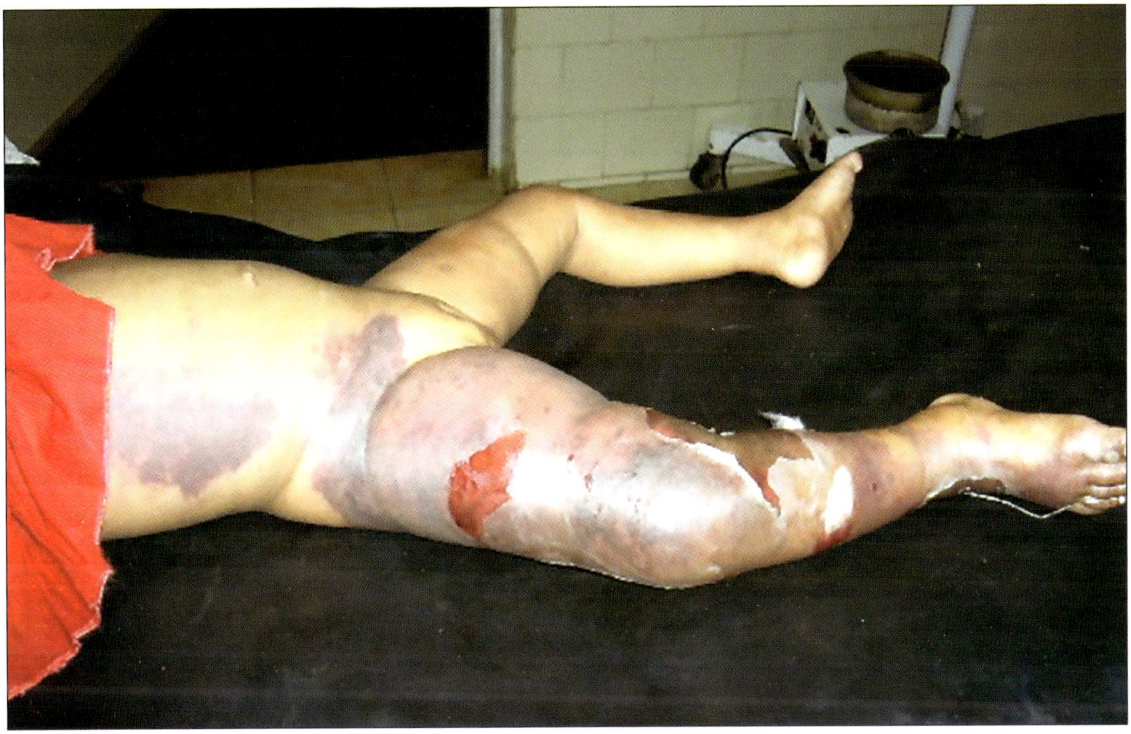

osteomyelitis

This image shows the osteomyelitis of the lower end of the femur, a chronic pyogenic infection of the bone, in adults. It usually has a subacute to chronic presentation and needs a minimum of six weeks of treatment with proper antibiotics, debridement and stabilization of the joint.

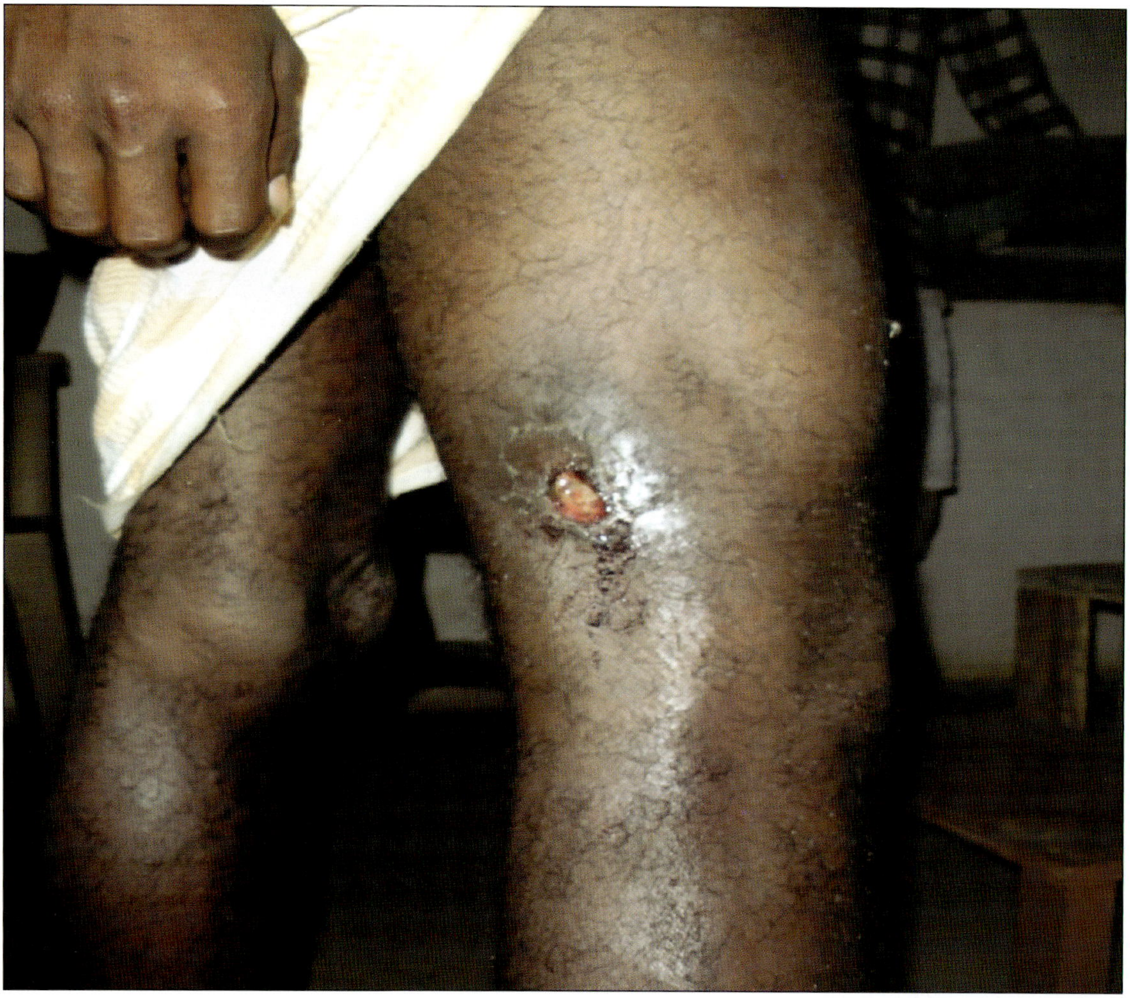

nerve abscess

Nerve abscess is a severe complication of leprosy. Patients with various forms of leprosy and particularly those with the borderline tuberculoid form may develop nerve abscesses with a surrounding cellulitic appearance of the skin. The affected nerve will be swollen and usually very tender.

Although prednisolone in doses of 1-1.5 mg per kilo of body weight may reduce signs of inflammation, rapid surgical decompression is necessary many a time to prevent irreversible nerve damage, which can result in claw hand and other motor weakness.

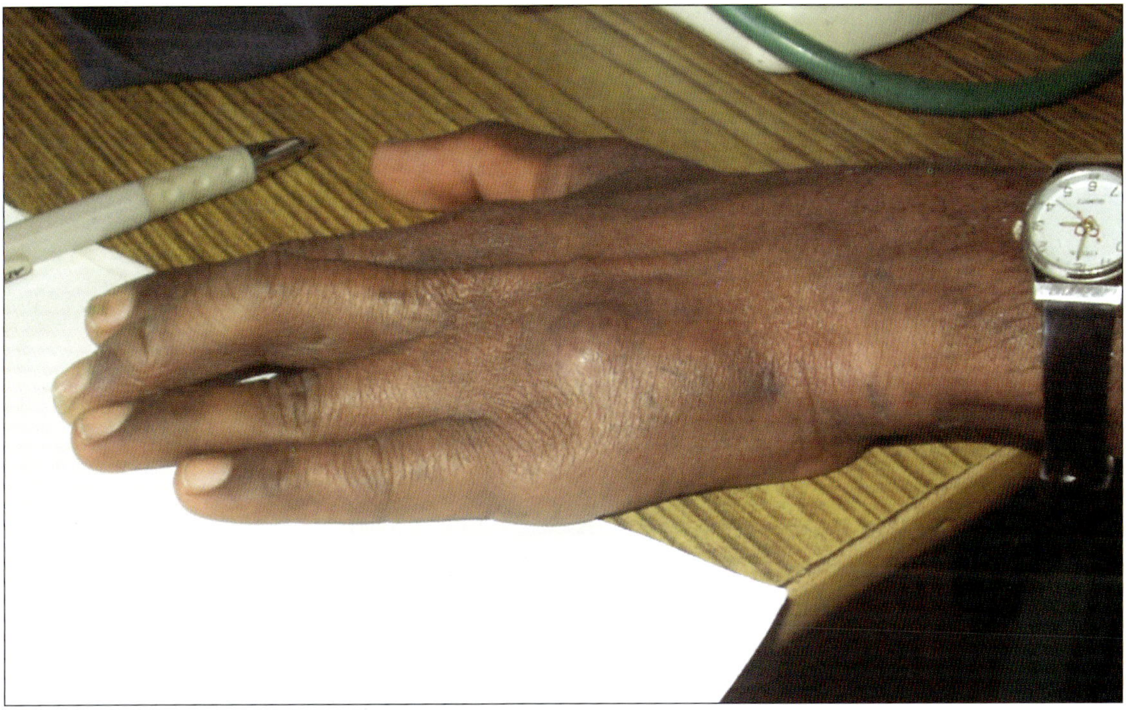

iron deficiency anaemia

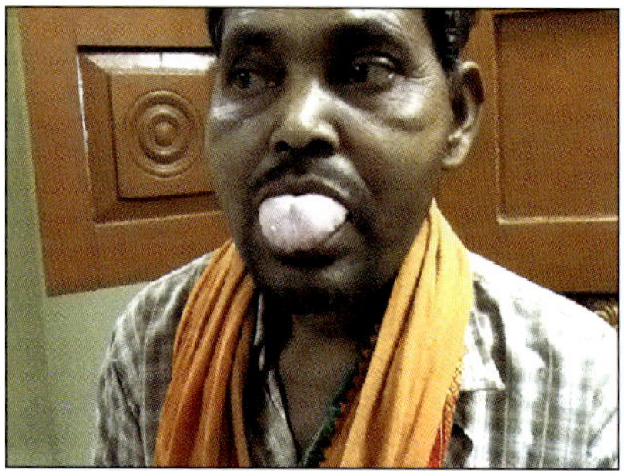

This is a picture of a young man of 35 who presented with exertional breathlessness and the inability to work in the previous three months. On examination, he was very pale and had a high resting pulse rate. His nails showed a spoon-like deformity called platynychia. His haemoglobin level was at a life threatening value of 1.1 grams per decilitre. He had to be admitted and investigated for the cause of his severe anaemia that seemed to be due to iron deficiency. The red cells on microscopic examination were much smaller than normal and had much less haemoglobin. His diet was predominantly rice, some chutneys and occasional green leafy vegetables. He was a vegetarian and consumed almost no fruits. Investigation for a possible bleed from the gastrointestinal tract did not show any site of bleeding.

He was treated with two units of cross-matched blood and was started on a six-month course of therapeutic iron tablets given on an empty stomach. He was also advised to eat dried amla (Indian gooseberry) every day and was given antihelminths. One month after starting treatment, his haemoglobin was 8 grams per dl and he felt much better.

Iron deficiency anaemia (IDA) in men and post-menopausal women is most commonly caused by gastrointestinal blood loss or malabsorption. In the premenopausal period in women, menstrual blood loss is the main reason for such severe iron deficiency. Dietary deficiency of iron causing severe anaemia is common in infants who were born with a low birth weight, or were born premature. We still see a few adults with severe anaemia due to dietary deficiency in extreme poverty.

Patients with asymptomatic colonic and gastric carcinoma may present with IDA and the exclusion of these conditions is of prime concern. Malabsorption, poor dietary intake, previous gastrectomy and Nonsteroidal anti-inflammatory drug (NSAID) use are not unusual but there are many other possible causes. The management of IDA is often suboptimal, with most patients being incompletely investigated, if at all.

tetany in a young lactating mother

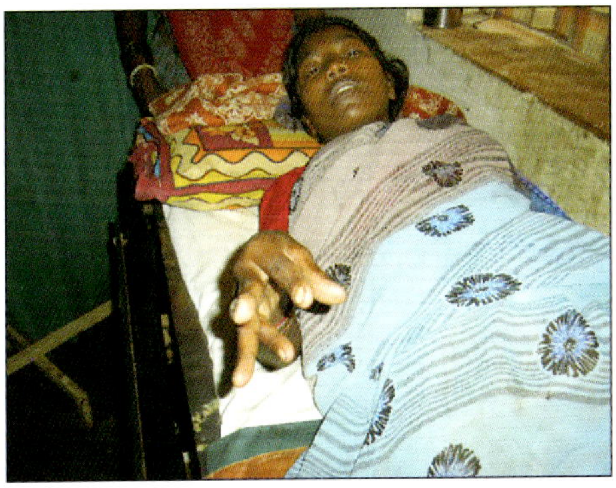

Hypocalcemia (tetany) may be associated with a variety of clinical manifestations, ranging from few, if any, symptoms if the hypocalcemia is mild and/or chronic, to severe life-threatening symptoms if it is severe and/or acute.

The major factors that influence the serum calcium concentration are parathyroid hormone (PTH), vitamin D, the calcium ion itself and phosphate. Low serum calcium concentrations are most often caused by disorders of parathyroid hormone (PTH) or vitamin D, or decreased calcium in the diet.

While sodium and chloride are more ubiquitous, minerals like potassium, calcium and magnesium are usually present in fewer foods and most of these foods are more expensive. Thus, with food deprivation, there is a higher likelihood of a deficiency of these minerals. The deficiency of calcium and magnesium, if severe, manifests as the horrific and scary neuromuscular symptom of tetanic spasms of the hands, and sometimes of the feet.

This dietary deficiency of calcium may occur when the increased need in certain situations such as pregnancy and lactation are not met with increased dietary intake. This picture is of a lactating mother, whose 4th pregnancy had culminated in the birth of a child weighing 2.1 kgs.

The other major causes of hypocalcemia include inadequate vitamin D intake or inadequate sunlight exposure, decreased parathyroid hormone secretion and chronic kidney disease.

The diagnosis of hypocalcemia is made by measuring serum levels of calcium, both total and ionised, observing clinical symptoms and by checking an electrocardiogram (ECG).

The management of the disease depends upon the severity of symptoms. In patients with acute symptomatic hypocalcemia, intravenous calcium gluconate is the preferred therapy, whereas chronic hypocalcemia is treated with oral calcium and vitamin D supplements.

rickets

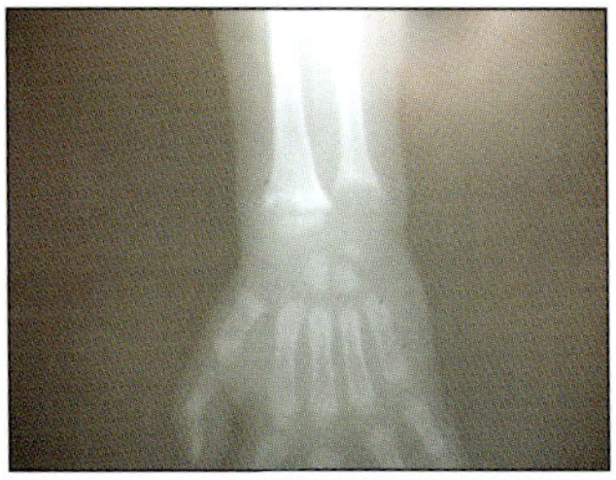

Rickets in children and osteomalacia in adults are the commonest manifestations of vitamin D deficiency prevalent in the rural population of India. These disorders are largely responsible for morbidity in the young and are characterized by defective mineralization of the bone. The lack of exposure to sunlight and a poor diet are predisposing factors. The x-ray shows frayed and flayed epiphysis with expanded metaphysis and some epiphyseal dysgenesis. If not treated early in childhood, then deformities will persist in adulthood.

Cases of rickets are found in larger families of a lower socioeconomic status due to a lower almost non-existent intake of dairy products. Rickets develop when a low dietary calcium intake coexists with a low or borderline vitamin D nutritional status. Malnutrition and intestinal infections aggravate each other and this causes malabsorption of both vitamin D and of calcium. Dark skin is also one of the causative factors for vitamin D deficiency because the absorption of ultra violet rays is low as compared to fair skin.

The majority of cases occur in children who suffer from severe malnutrition in the early stages of childhood, usually resulting from famine or starvation. Osteomalacia is a similar condition occurring in adults, generally due to the deficiency of vitamin D, but it also occurs after epiphyseal closure.

During the Industrial Revolution rickets appeared in the temperate zone, where pollution from factories blocked the sun's ultraviolet rays.

Rickets can cause many skeletal deformities in toddlers, including bowed legs or knocked knees and double malleoli (genu varum/valgum), skull bossing, spinal deformities such as kyphoscoliosis or lumber lordosis, rachitic rosary in the chest wall or widened wrists and short stature. Deficiency of vitamin D also increases the predisposition to infections including tuberculosis.

Prevention can only be achieved with the supplementation of calcium and vitamin D in the proper amount to all women before and during pregnancy and after delivery. Adequate sun exposure and the consumption of dairy products and eggs are highly desirable.

vitamin a deficiency

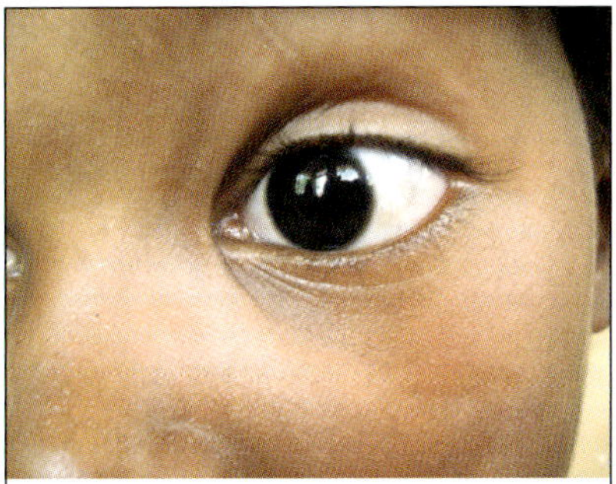
Bitot

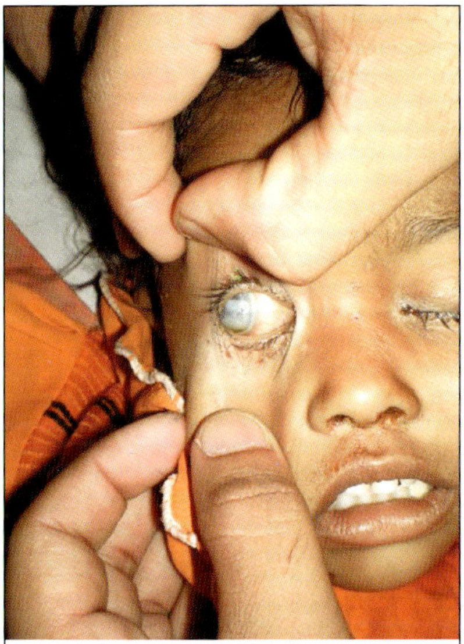
Keratomalacia

Chronic dietary deficiency of vitamin A is caused by the inadequate intake of animal food sources and edible oil, both of which are expensive. This, coupled with seasonal unavailability of vegetables and fruits and concurrent zinc deficiency are leading factors in avitaminosis A. The depletion in the body, along with recurrent infections, aggravates vitamin A deficiency.

Vitamin A is responsible for the production of the eye pigment which allows vision in low light situations, as well as for the functioning of goblet cells in the conjunctiva which secrete mucus to keep the eyes moist. If deficient, xerophthalmiaor dry eyes develop, resulting in corneal damage and Bitot's spots on the sclera. If the cornea gets damaged, then blindness may result due to keratomalacia.

India has the highest prevalence of clinical and sub clinical vitamin A deficiency among other South Asian countries : 31-57 % of preschool children and 5% of pregnant women manifest signs and symptoms. Among these women, 12% are severely affected by this condition, which has a higher prevalence in the rural population.

Vitamin A is essential for the normal maintenance and functioning of body tissues, and for growth and development, including during pregnancy, when the fetus makes demands of the mother's vitamin A stores and during the postpartum period, when the newborn is growing rapidly. In most cultures, young infants depend on breast milk. If the mother is deficient then both will suffer.

alcoholic cardiomyopathy

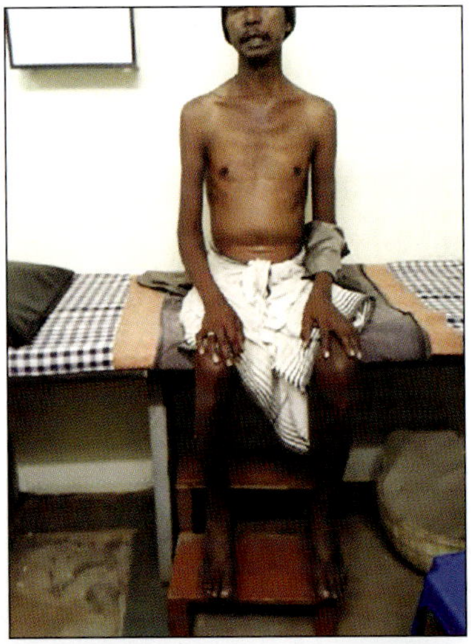

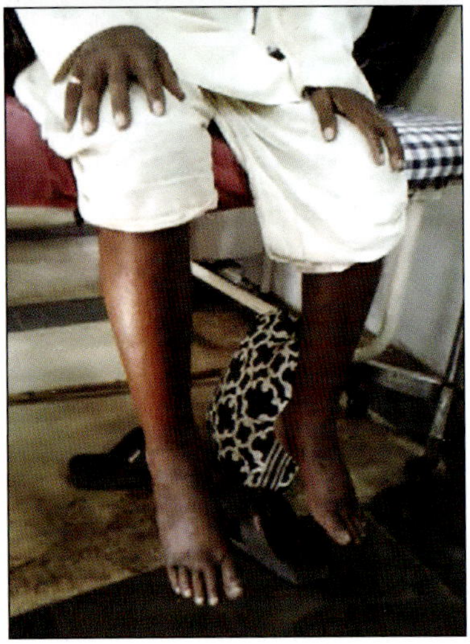

This man was unable to take even a few steps without feeling tired and his exercise tolerance had been decreasing. He could not sleep lying down because of a shortness of breath and would wake up in the middle of the night with a feeling of uneasiness. His weight was increasing, not because of muscle or fatty mass, but due to excessive salt and water retention in his body. In contrast, his appetite was failing because the slight fullness in his abdomen was making it difficult for him to draw breath.

The man had consumed more than three pegs of alcohol every day for 10 years and the stress on his myocardium had caused his heart pump to stop working properly. He developed dilated cardiomyopathy a year before this photo was taken.

Modern science has repeatedly emphasized that alcohol affects various organs and systems of the human body. Alcoholic cardiomyopathy in turn affects human life and longevity. The recovery of cardiac functions can occur if the disease is diagnosed early and alcohol consumption is halted. Patients also need treatment for congestive heart failure and the vitamin B1, B6 and B12, supplements along with folic acid.

This patient recovered well. There are, however, numerous others at the risk for disease, bearing in mind that the state government of Chhattisgarh earns Rs. 3,000 crore a year from the license fees on alcohol sellers.

elephantiasis

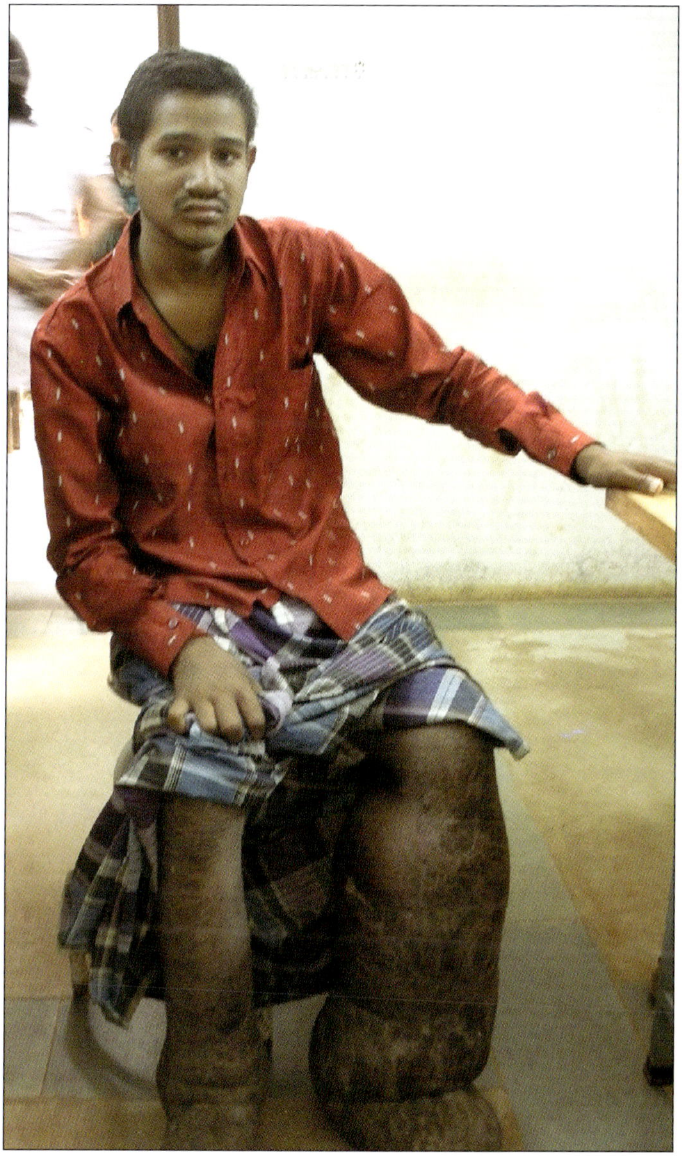

Elephantiasis, also called *pheelpaon* or *hathipaon* in Arabic and Hindi is the end result of neglected filariasis and secondary infections of the skin and subcutaneous tissues.

It is a relic of the past, and several people are still affected by it, many of whom take to begging because they are unable to earn a livelihood. This problem can be prevented by timely treatment. Treating elephantiasis is difficult despite doctors' best attempts at surgery, although at a moderate level of infection, it can be treated with pressure bandages and antibiotic use.

We still see about half a dozen such patients every year with elephantiasis.

airborne contact dermatitis

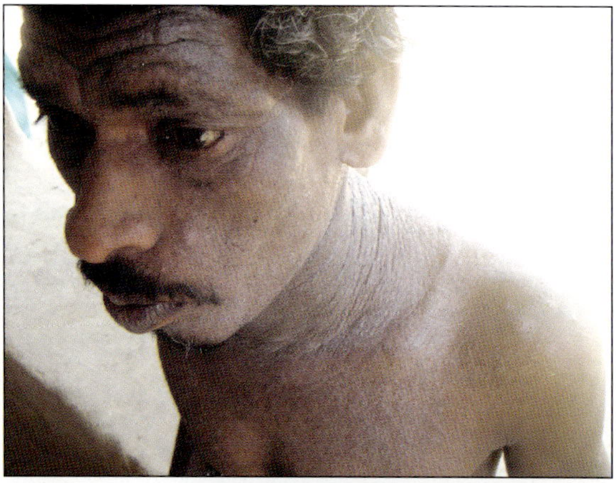

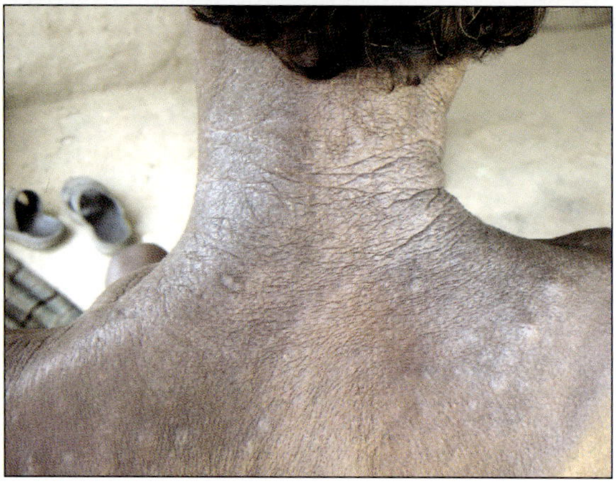

In the forest villages of Chhattisgarh, a troublesome air borne contact dermatitis due to the plant Parthenium is common. We have seen at least 15 such people in one village cluster made miserable due to this chronic and persistent illness. Contact dermatitis, caused by the airborne pollen of the Parthenium (also called Congress grass), is an allergic skin condition that results in itchy papules and plaques on the exposed areas of the body, especially the face, hands and feet.

The itching is very severe and is naturally most common in the months of the year when this weed plant is flowering. Parthenium weed came to India along with the PL487 wheat donated by the United States in 1967 and is now ubiquitous in Indian forests, villages and cities. However, we see this problem maximally in the forest dwellers and in forest fringe villages. This condition is seen mostly among adults. It is rare to see it in those below the age of 25. There is associated depression with this disabling skin illness.

Airborne contact dermatitis is treated with anti-inflammatory drugs, including oral and topical steroids and anti-itching drugs. But the mainstay of management is to prevent recurrences by avoiding exposure to the plant, covering exposed areas of the body, and washing the pollen off when entering the house after an outdoor visit.

chronic atopic dermatitis or bemchee

This chronic skin condition, seen in wide patches on both legs and occasionally elsewhere, is a common problem with which young adolescents and children are brought to Jan Swasthya Sahyog (JSS). They have often tried many different types of treatment and failed to get relief, necessitating a hospital visit.

This condition is primarily an allergic condition of the skin and may be precipitated by exposure to pollens. The skin frequently gets infected and becomes thicker, and sometimes oozes pus and becomes painful.

Treatment includes topical cleaning, an oral antibiotic to take care of the infection and then anti-itching medicines and topical steroid ointment for four weeks. There may be a few recurrences, but usually people recover fully.

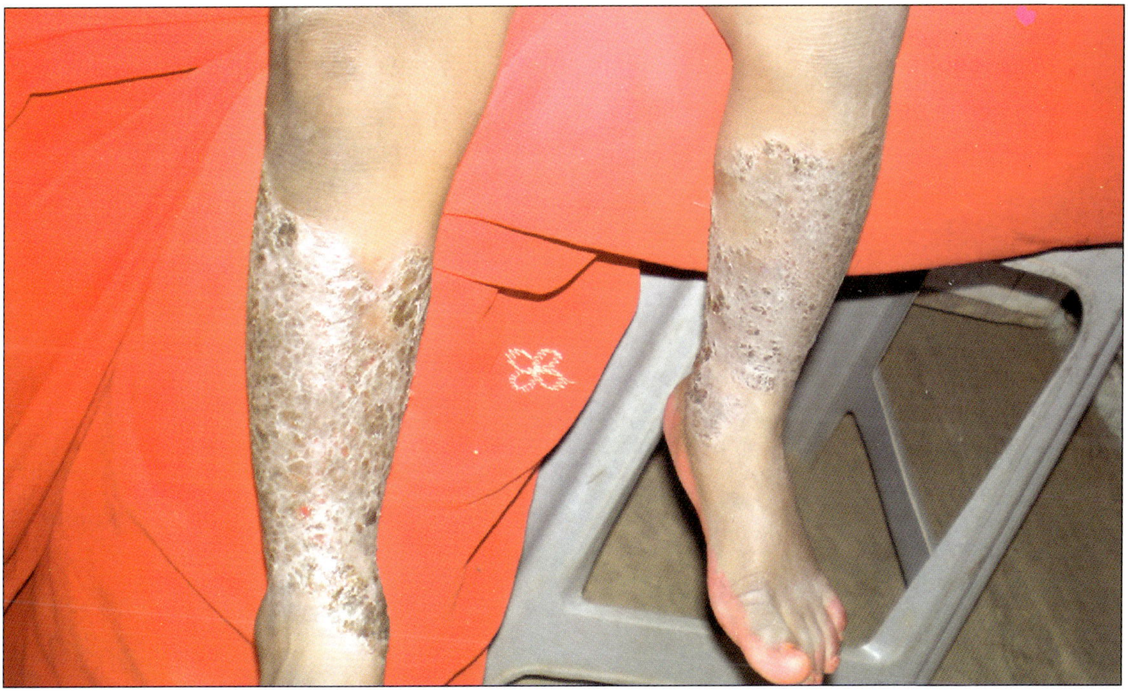

scabies

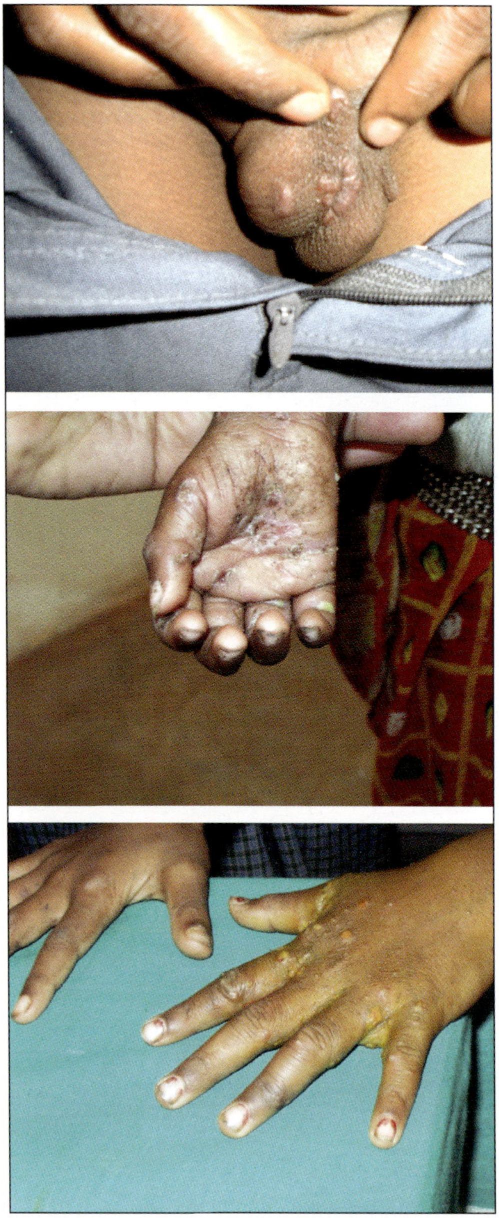

In tribal and rural areas of India, where residential schools or hostels exist for children from remote interiors, children often return home for summer or winter vacations with lesions on their bodies. These lesions, which are horrible, very itchy and infect their hands, feet and genital areas, are all due to a parasitic infection called scabies. These children soon infect their family members and co-dwellers as well.

Just like many other diseases, the prevalence and burden of scabies is high in the poorest communities of the world. Some of the highest prevalence is seen in the vulnerable tribal groups of India as well as in the aboriginal tribes of Australia. This infection is caused by a mite called Sarcoptes scabiei which burrows into the top layer of the skin. Scabies in endemic areas is characterized by skin lesions - burrows (classic), papules and vesicles with itching which worsens at night. Neglect by the healthcare and hostel system, poor availability of water for washing linen, late diagnosis, reduced access to appropriate treatment and subsequent re-infestations leads to a persistence of this problem.

Secondary infections by Group-A streptococci and staphylococcus are very common and can lead to pyoderma and lymphadenitis. Acute post streptococcal glomerulonephritis, a kidney problem, is a complication found particularly in children. An association with acute rheumatic fever has been well documented and is a major cause for rheumatic heart disease (RHD). We witness many cases of RHD from rural communities.

The treatment of scabies includes a variety of topical compounds such as permethrin, benzylebenzoate, malathionandoral ivermectin. It should be given at the same time to all householders and to other close contacts such as inmates of hostels and prisons, to avoid re-infestations of those already treated. Bed linen and towels should also be treated.

Control of scabies at the community level is not an easy task. Integrating mass therapy, community involvement, health education, training of health professionals and ongoing surveillance can reduce disease prevalence.

post-burn contracture

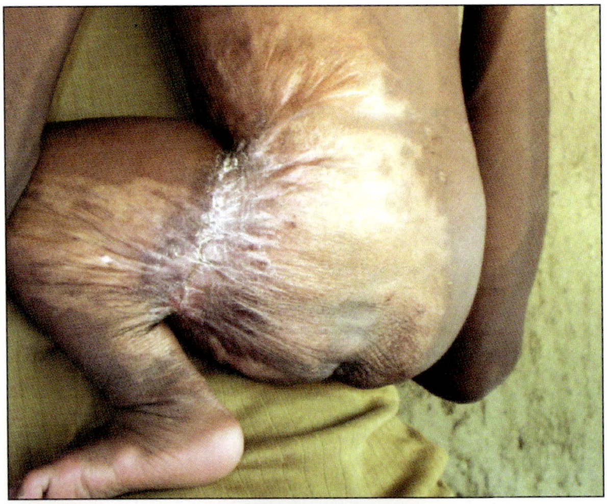

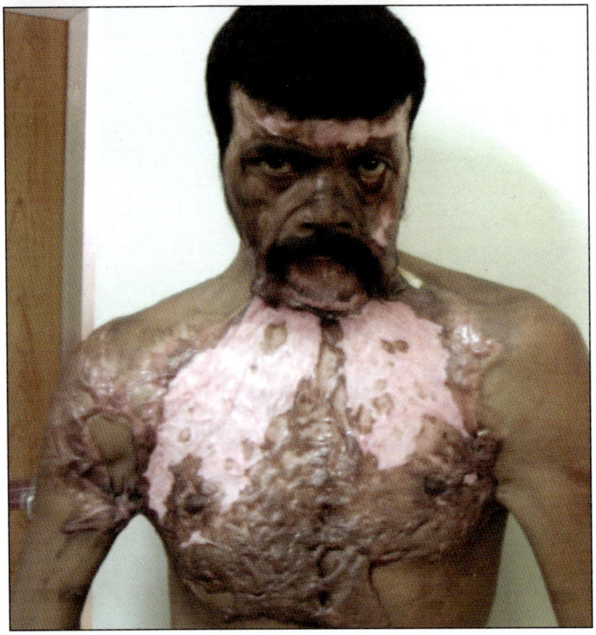

The picture of a baby with post burn contracture overlies a tragic story. Her elder sister, a 10 year old, suffered from untreated epilepsy. She was holding her sibling in her lap near a stove when she had one of her frequent seizures, and they both fell into the fire. The older girl sustained severe burns and succumbed to her injuries.

This infant survived with a large contracture which was operated upon by a plastic surgeon. Untreated epilepsy is quite common in rural areas, and it is estimated that the half the cases go untreated. We need awareness of possible treatments, to be spread as well as an efficient public health system to handle the large number of people who need medicines, counselling and other support.

The second case of severe post-burn contracture is of a man with self-inflicted burns contracted during an episode of psychosis and inebriation. He required expert surgical care and with the aid of anti-psychotic medication, was integrated back into society.

gingival hyperplasia or gum overgrowth

One of the complications of taking Phenytoin, an anti-seizure drug, is gum overgrowth which is seen in varying degrees of severity in 30-50% of patients. However, Phenytoin is one of the most commonly prescribed drugs in India because it can be given for tonic clonic seizures and complex partial seizures. If a doctor is unsure of the type of seizure, this would be the drug to prescribe. Neurologists call this a "fire-and-forget" drug. If it works with no adverse effects at a moderate dose, it is continued for at least two years.

This drug is easily available in rural India and its low price makes it easily affordable for the poor. The doctors have to weigh the cost of developing gum overgrowth against the risk to life and limb if a person with epilepsy is left untreated.

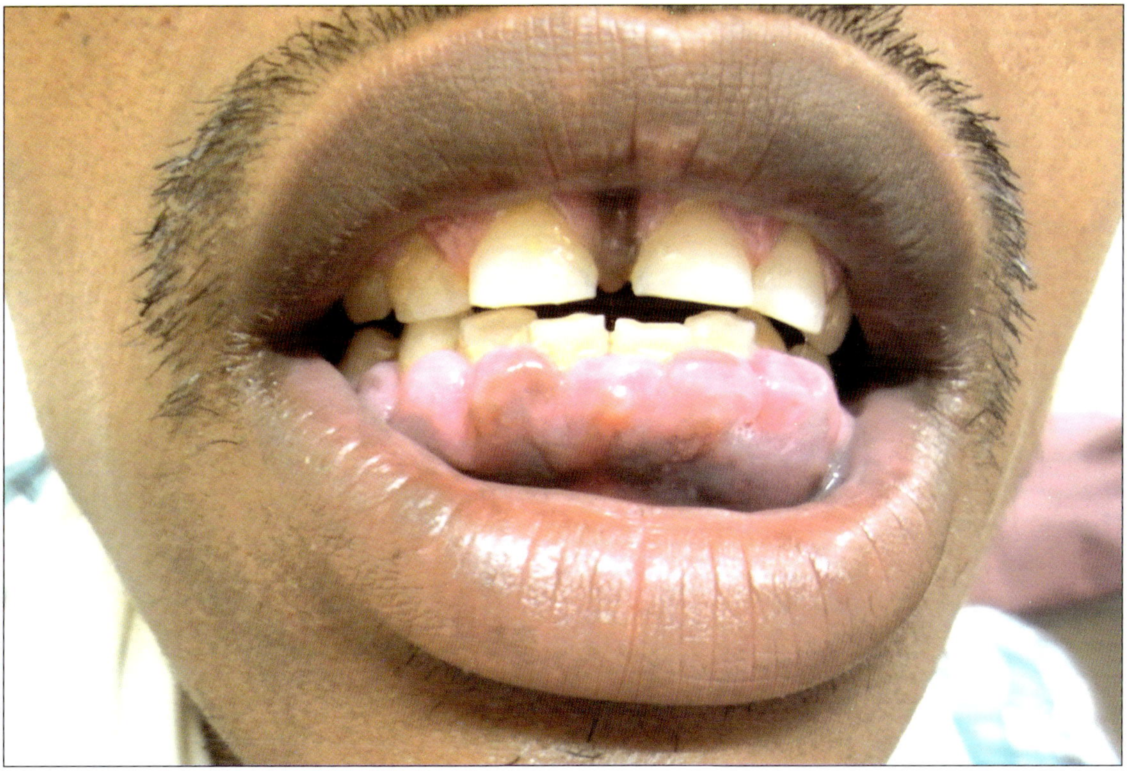

Bell's palsy

Bell's Palsy is a condition caused by a viral infection that affects the facial nerve. The facial nerve stops functioning, as a result of which the person is not able to use one side of the face. The person may not be able to close one eye or masticate food. One side of the face may droop. There is of course a problem of asymmetry of the face, but the major suffering is due to inability to close one eye or to chew and swallow food.

If affected people come in within a day or two of the onset of symptoms, they can be treated with oral steroids which can reverse the facial weakness.

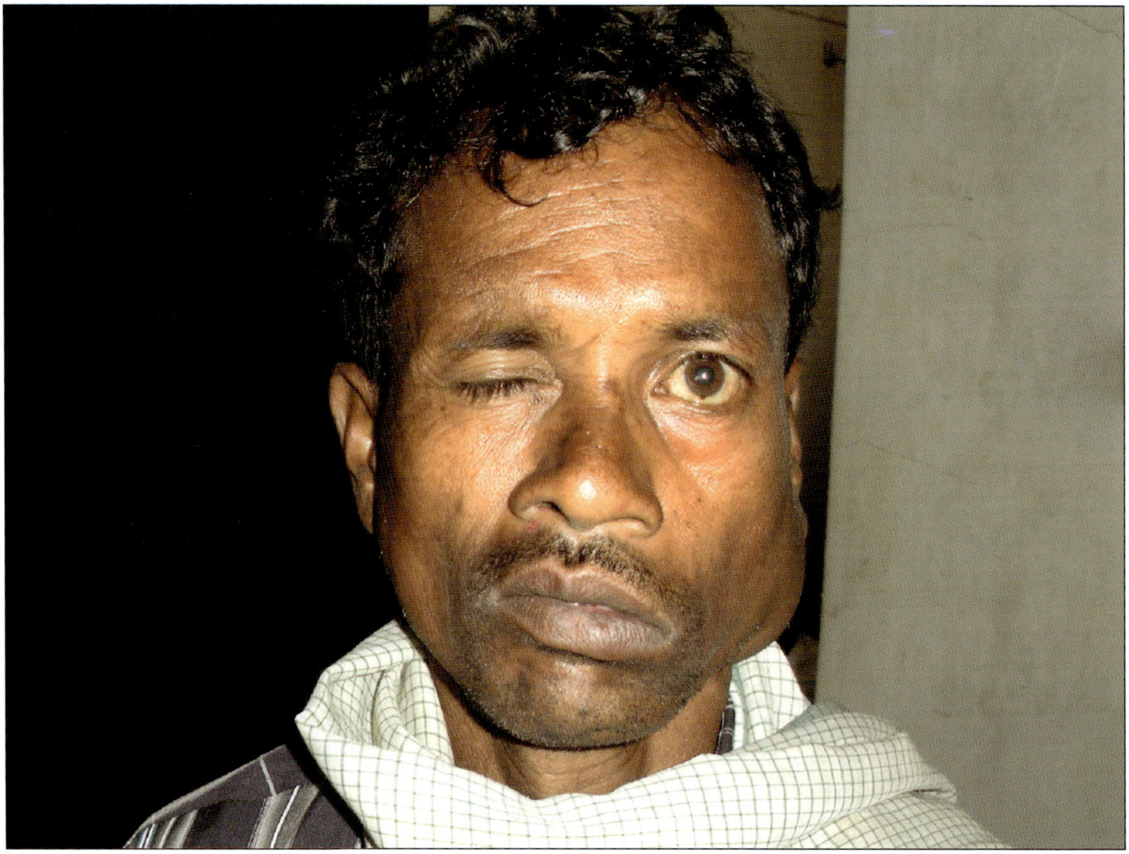

down syndrome

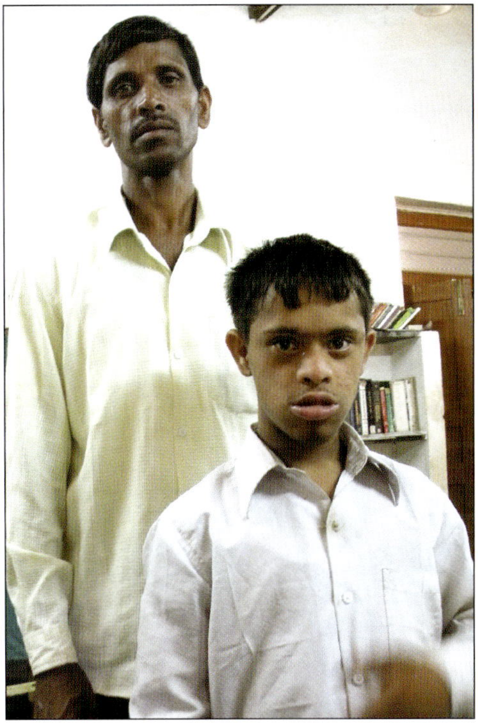

Down syndrome, also known as trisomy 21, is a genetic disorder caused by the presence of all or part of a third copy of chromosome 21. It is one of the most common chromosome abnormalities in humans, occurring in about one per 1000 babies born each year. It is typically associated with physical growth delays, characteristic facial features, and mild to moderate intellectual disability. The average IQ of a young adult with Down syndrome is 50, equivalent to the mental age of an 8 or 9-year-old child, but this varies widely.

It is a genetic abnormality that happens spontaneously, and parents are typically genetically normal. Down syndrome cannot be prevented and there is no cure. The mother's diet or activities before and during pregnancy have no bearing on it. Although a woman of any age can have a baby with Down syndrome, there is a link between the probability of having a child with Down syndrome and the age of the mother. As a woman gets older, her odds of having a baby with Down syndrome, becomes greater. Down syndrome can be identified during pregnancy by prenatal screening followed by diagnostic testing, or after birth by direct observation and genetic testing.

Education and proper care have been shown to improve the quality of life of a child with Down syndrome. However, it is a challenge for the parents to bring up a differently abled child up over the course of their lives. The child's life expectancy is around 50 to 60 years in the developed world with proper health care, but is much poorer in our part of the world because of infections and heart diseases.

rhinosporiodosis

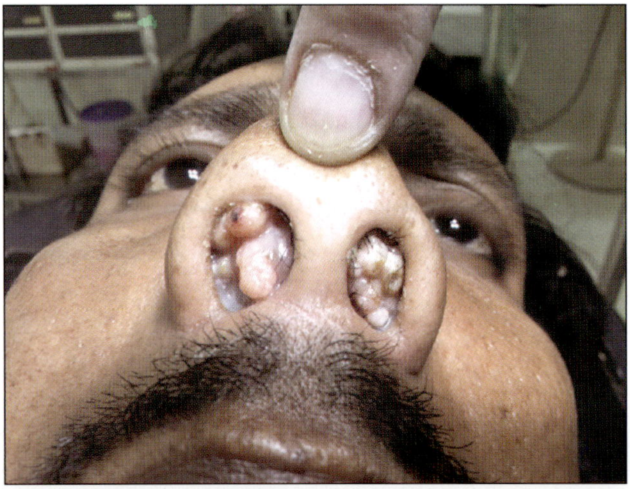

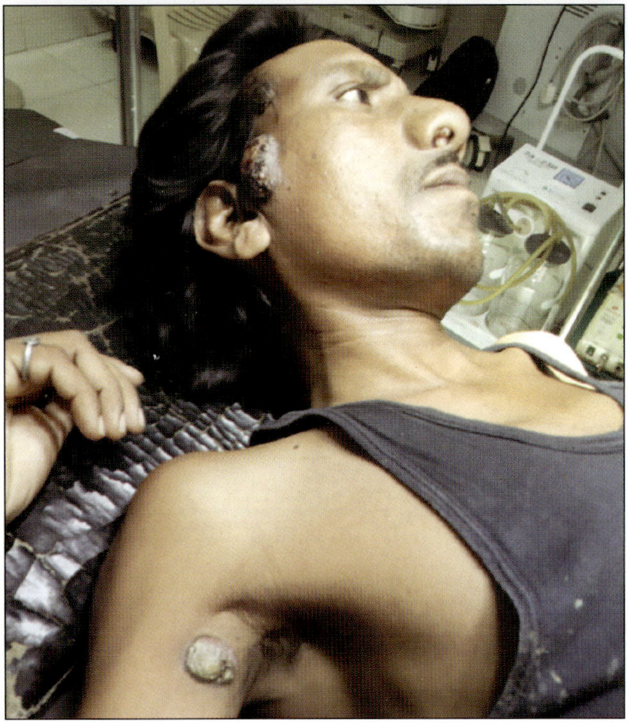

Rhinosporiodosis is caused by a common pathogen present in the ponds where village people bathe and source their drinking water. Sometimes it can take on a 'Rudraroop', causing widespread devastation in the body such as in this young man who had his nasal passages choked, his skin and bone and joints involved, necessitating besides other surgical procedures, an amputation of his upper limb above the elbow.

Bone and joint get involved if there is a spread to remote sites through the blood. This spread is rare.

oral cancer

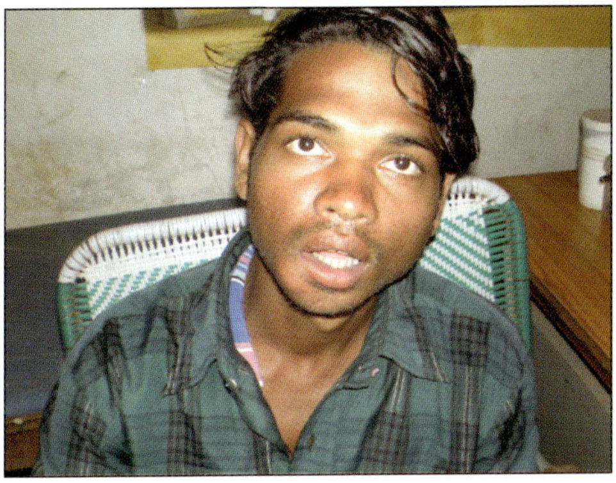

This young man came to the hospital just to get an opinion on the lesion in his mouth. He had been ignoring it for some time, but someone suggested that he go for a medical check-up at a time when oral cancer awareness campaigns were reaching out to rural areas. Oral cancer is the most common cancer among men in India, which accounts for about 40% of the world's oral cancer cases.

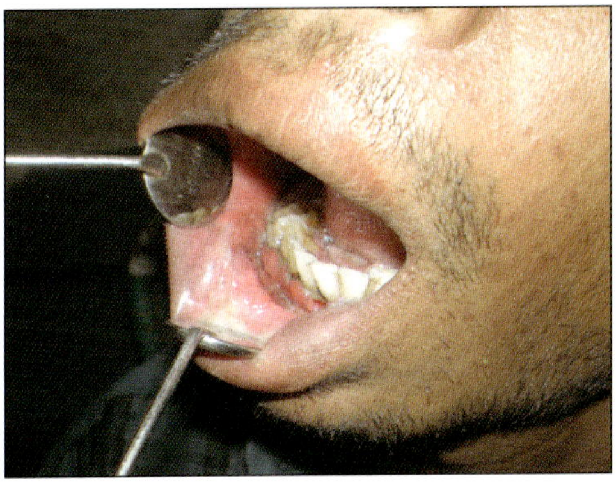

The practice of consuming paan containing betel leaf with betel nut (areca), lime, kattha and tobacco is very common in India. There are numerous paan and tobacco shops in every hamlet, road, village and town. Even in the Jan Swasthya Sahyog (JSS) campus, where tobacco consumption is banned, scores of empty gutka pouches litter the ground every evening.

The other risk factors for oral cancer include poor oral hygiene, poor nutrition and infection with the Human Papilloma Virus16.

The disease may be preceded by pre-malignant lesions which look benign, morphologically altered tissue, leukoplakia, erythroplakia or a mix of both. Submucous fibrosis is very common, manifesting as the inability to open the mouth wide. If there is no response to treatment in 15 days, a biopsy will be required for early detection of cancer.

In established cases we can see a visible or palpable growth, which many times bleed on touch. It is more commonly found on the lateral and ventral side of the tongue, lips and the buccal mucosa.

a nursery for cancer - paan shops or mukh shudhi kendra

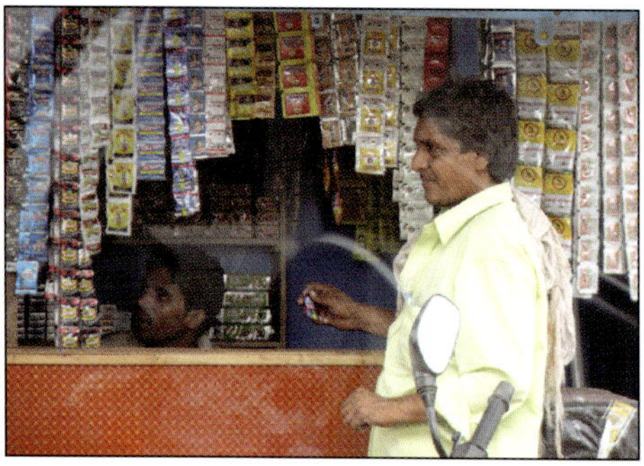

It is common to have paan shops at cross roads, where gutka pouches, rather than paan is available now. Gutka, under the brand names of -Paan Parag, Sitar, Rajshree, Khazana, Paan Bahar, Rocket, Chutki, Paas Paasand Deepak are consumed by almost every section of society in significant amounts. The shiny long hanging strings of pouches and the fragrance of agarbattis in these shops have attracted not only men, but even children and women.

Gutka is of two kinds. The plain gutka is a masala mixed with some fragrance to freshen up the mouth (fennel mixed with fragrance). The second is mixed with zarda or tobacco which provides some heat to the body after eating. People who start eating plain gutka don't take much time to switch to gutka with tobacco because the sweetness and fragrance of plain gutka soon gets dull.

Gutka is easily available everywhere, in villages and in cities, because it is cheapest for consumers and most profitable for sellers, priced between Rs.1 and Rs.10 per pouch.

Consumers of gutka say it is stimulating, helps in reducing fatigue and allows them to pass time. Some say it is necessary to digest their food. People who eat gutka find it to be hassle free, compared to preparing gudakhu or tobacco paste using water. Beedi and cigarette smoke could cause objections if taken in public, but gutka doesn't have these problems and can be kept and eaten wherever and whenever wanted.

Some states in India have banned the sale of gutka, but the manufacturers haven't been wholly banned. Its advertising hasn't been regulated either. It is sold illegally even in places where it is banned. It is found being sold close to schools, colleges and hospitals, whereas the law bans its sale within a 100-metre radius of such institutions.

There is thus no wonder that the list of tobacco related illnesses and the numbers of those affected by them are large.

the frightful spectre of antibiotic drug resistance

This is a culture report with an antibiogram of multi drug resistant coliform bacteria that grew in a urine sample of a cancer patient from a village about 30 km from Ganiyari. We don't know whether he will die due to his cancer or because of infection with this highly resistant bacteria.

New Delhi Metallo-Beta Lactamase-1 (NDM-1) is an enzyme produced by highly resistant bacteria that enables them to break down broad-spectrum antibiotics called carbapenems. Bacteria that break down carbapenems can be very difficult to treat and only at a cost that few Indians can afford.

The enzyme is encoded on a circular piece of DNA which has a penchant for jumping between bacteria. The bacteria can travel across continents in the wounds and intestines of travellers. In August 2010, the worrisome emergence of this extremely drug-resistant bacteria was published in 'The Lancet Infectious Diseases' journal.

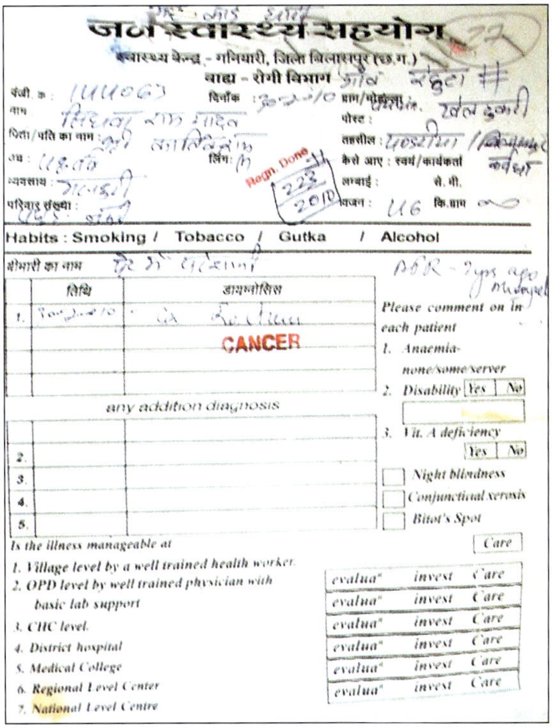

जन स्वास्थ्य सहयोग

स्वास्थ्य केन्द्र - गनियारी, जिला बिलासपुर (छ.ग.)

वाह्य - रोगी विभाग

Habits : Smoking / Tobacco / Gutka / Alcohol

CANCER

any addition diagnosis

Please comment on each patient

1. Anaemia- none/some/sever
2. Disability Yes | No
3. Vit. A deficiency Yes | No

Night blindness

Conjunctival xerosis

Bitot's Spot

Is the illness manageable at

1. Village level by a well trained health worker
2. OPD level by well trained physician with basic lab support
3. CHC level
4. District hospital
5. Medical College
6. Regional Level Center
7. National Level Centre

Care

evalua° invest Care

Extended-spectrum beta-lactamase (ESBL) enzymes, which enable Gram-negative bacteria to hydrolyse third-generation cephalosporin antibiotics, were first detected in Germany in 1983. The first report of ESBLs in India was from the Christian Medical College, Vellore, in 1995. By the turn of the century ESBLs had stepped out into the countryside.

Many ESBL-producing bacteria carry genes

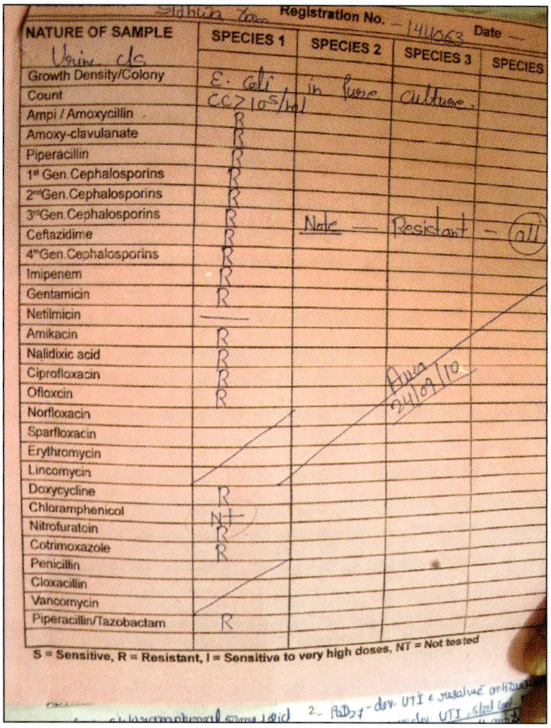
Registration No. 141063 Date

NATURE OF SAMPLE	SPECIES 1	SPECIES 2	SPECIES 3	SPECIES
Urine c/s				
Growth Density/Colony	E. coli	in pure	culture.	
Count	CC>10^5/ml			
Ampi / Amoxycillin	R			
Amoxy-clavulanate	R			
Piperacillin	R			
1st Gen.Cephalosporins	R			
2nd Gen.Cephalosporins	R			
3rd Gen.Cephalosporins	R	Note —	Resistant	— all
Ceftazidime	R			
4th Gen.Cephalosporins	R			
Imipenem	R			
Gentamicin	R			
Netilmicin	—			
Amikacin	R			
Nalidixic acid	R			
Ciprofloxacin	R			
Ofloxcin	R			
Norfloxacin				
Sparfloxacin				
Erythromycin				
Lincomycin				
Doxycycline	R			
Chloramphenicol	NT			
Nitrofuratoin	R			
Cotrimoxazole	R			
Penicillin				
Cloxacillin				
Vancomycin				
Piperacillin/Tazobactam	R			

Anu 24/09/10

S = Sensitive, R = Resistant, I = Sensitive to very high doses, NT = Not tested

for resistance to other antibiotics and the only antibiotics that were consistently effective against them were Amikacin and the carbapenems. Now, the logical thing to do in this kind of a situation would have been to reserve these two drugs for patients who were dangerously ill and treat the other patients on the basis of their culture and sensitivity test reports. Unfortunately, most chose the easy way out and started using carbapenems as drugs of first choice. These precious and expensive reserve drugs quickly became routine drugs, not only in tertiary care hospitals and intensive care units but also in community practice, provided the patient could afford it. A single course of Meropenem could wipe out the resources of a poor family. Once that happened, it was only a matter of time before resistance appeared. In the absence of a national resistance surveillance system, it spread right under our noses from hospitals into the community.

It seems that we have been foolishly squandering away the benefits of one of the most important discoveries of the 20th century - the antibiotic - and we may have to go back to pre-antibiotic era therapeutic methods in managing infections.

an attempt at suicide

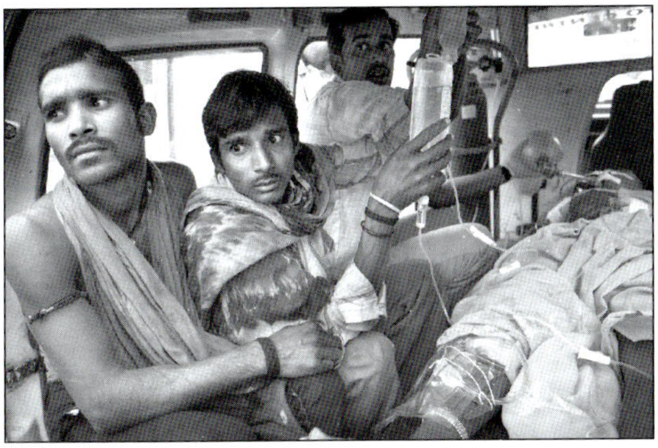

Every 40 seconds, a life is lost due to suicide, according to the World Health Organization. The most preferred method for killing oneself is by consumption of toxins, most commonly pesticides or rodenticides. In India, suicide by poisoning has been found to be the main cause for 40% of reported suicides. In Chhattisgarh, the rate of suicides was 21 per 1 lakh population as against the national average of 11, according to a 2013 report of the National Crime Records Bureau.

The picture shows one such woman in her 30's being brought to Jan Swasthya Sahyog (JSS). She had consumed pesticide of the organochlorine variety, which is commonly used for agricultural purposes. The menace of this poisoning induced recurrent seizures which could not be controlled. A situation like this requires intubation to support the patient's breathing as drugs cannot help. She had to be referred to the regional medical college for intensive care and ventilator support, from which she was weaned off in four days.

She was fortunate to reach JSS for primary care, after a journey of 45 minutes . Several lives are lost due to the delay in reaching health facilities, while others who are saved receive no further care or counseling. Mental illness and alcohol abuse are risk factors for suicide attempts, apart from cultural, social and economic factors. Not all depressed people commit suicide but most suicidal individuals have one or more psychiatric problems.

This highlights the need for a comprehensive package for primary care that has a socio-cultural dimension to help face a public health epidemic of suicides. It will require a multipronged effort, including developing mental health care services, availability of suicide support services and a strict regulation on pesticides and other toxins.

urinary passage injury becoming complex due to neglect

This image is of a 16 year old boy who was buried under a collapsed wall and had sustained a pelvic fracture a year previously. After repeated attempts at catheterisation and attempted urethral bouginage, he was left with this urethral catheter. For three months the family had no money to take him to any doctor even for a change of the dirty catheter. The scarred segment of his urethra was excised and an end-to-end anastomosis was done at Jan Swasthya Sahyog, allowing the boy to urinate normally. This is a case of a simple illness becoming complex because of neglect.

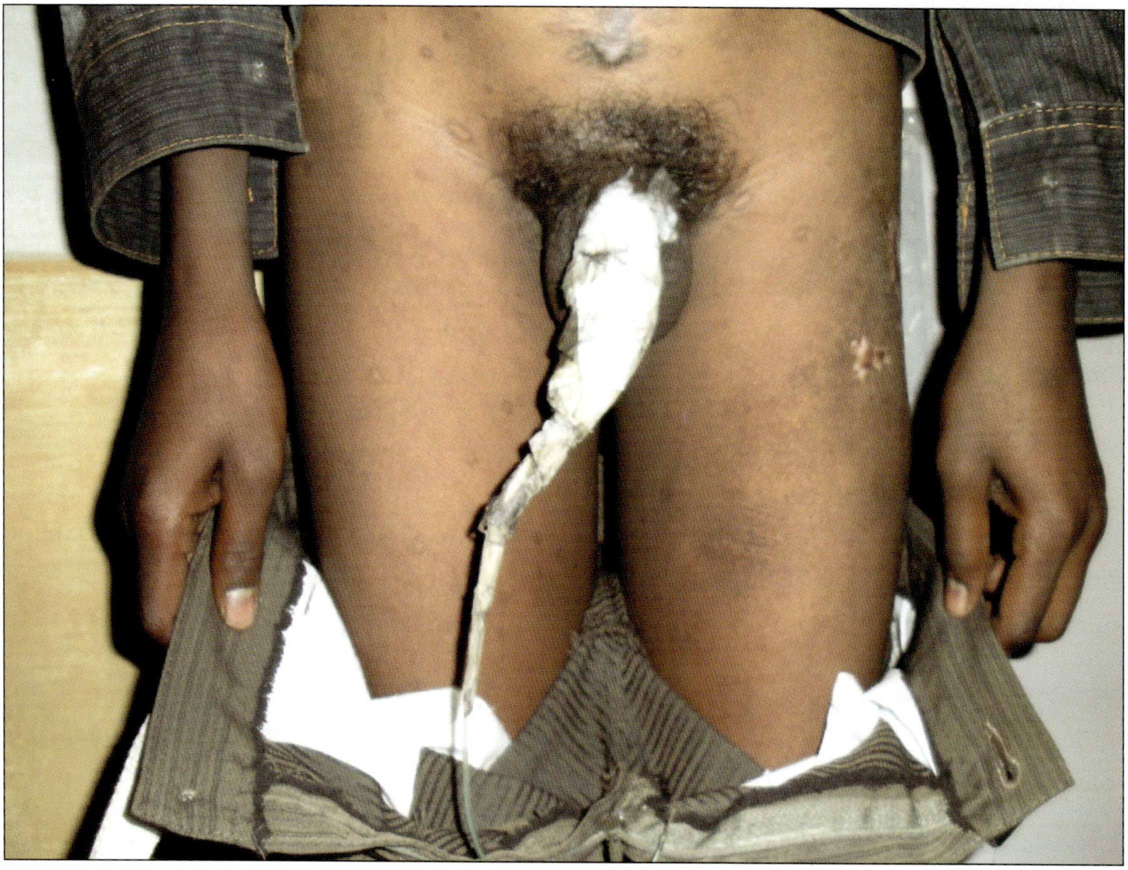

broken bones from a tree fall

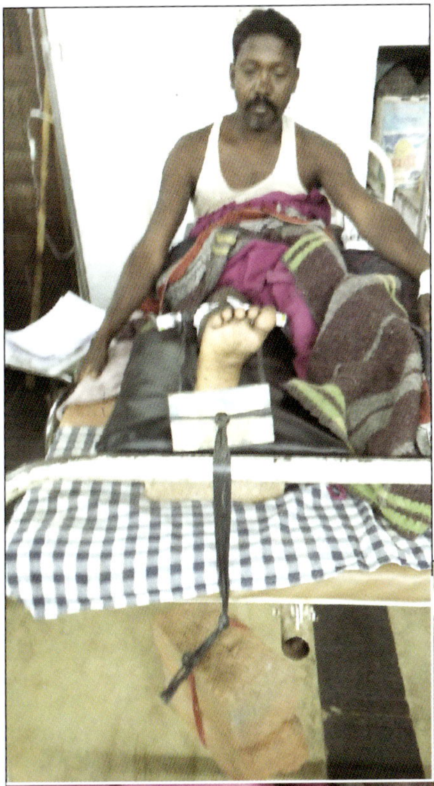

This 35 year old man fell from a tree while collecting forest produce close to his village at the fringe of the forest, 30 km from Jan Swasthya Sahyog's (JSS) sub-centre in Bamhani. He was bedridden and in much pain for the first month, when it was raining too heavily to make a journey to the clinic possible. He had broken a major lower extremity bone, the femur, which - by the time of his presentation was dangling loose and had gone into non-union. He was brought to the referral hospital at Ganiyari, where an operative internal fixation was carried out.

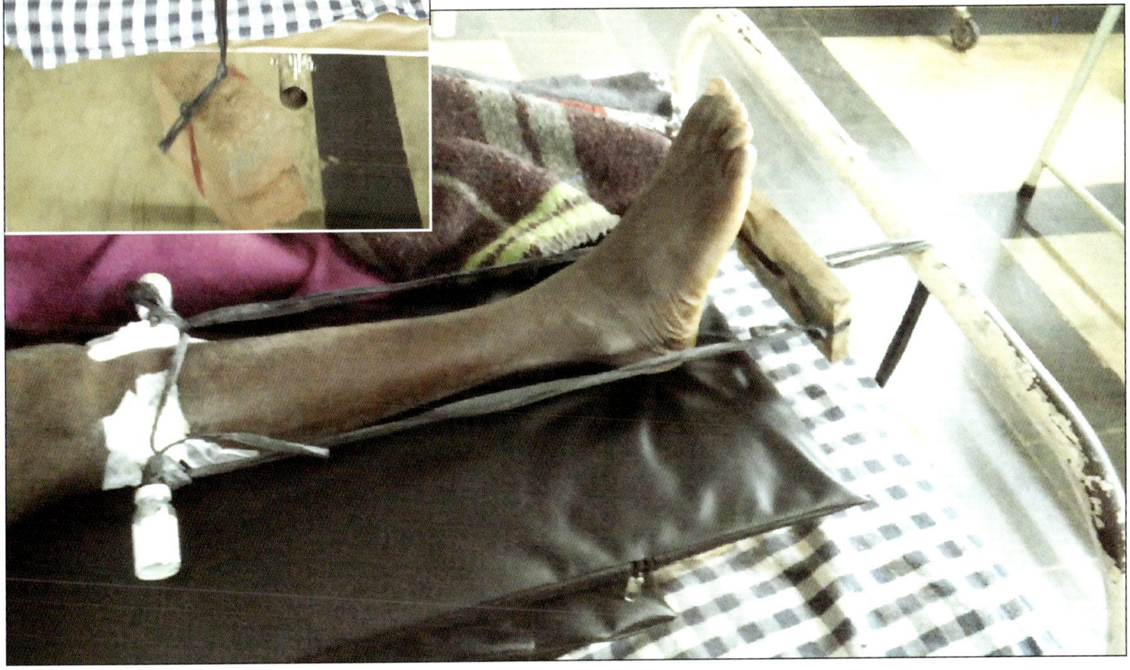

shoulder fat pads

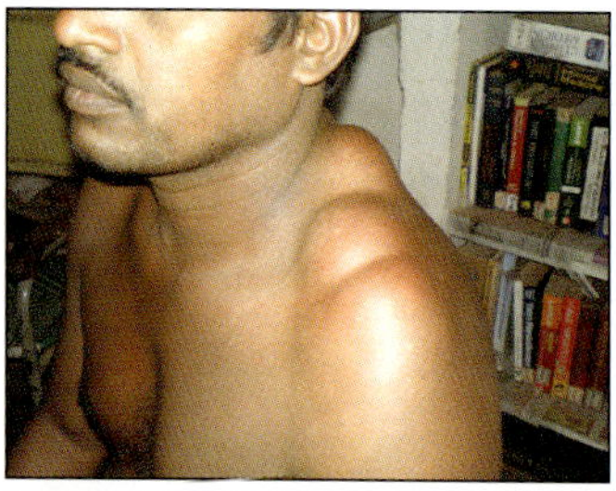

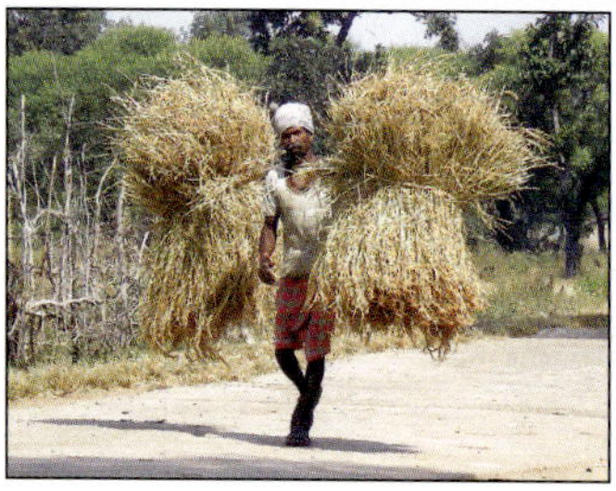

The humps on this man's shoulders are a reminder of the weight that people have to carry to earn a livelihood. These are the Atlases who ferry around the weight of the world on their backs and shoulders.

These fat pads fulfil the function of providing some cushioning to the shoulders which are forced to lift loads sometimes heavier than the labourer's entire body and carry them over long distances. For example, carrying firewood from the forest or countryside to one's home on either the head or shoulders is a daily burden for most families in rural India. The transportation of the harvested crop to home stores is done by both men and women. It is not uncommon to see people lift loads of 50 kgs on their heads or shoulders to carry over long distances.

A weight of 25 kg is heavy to lift for most people and should thus be the maximal load that anyone should be carrying manually. If heavier weights have to be lifted, it is advisable to divide the load and restrict one time lifting to less than 25 kgs.

Lifting heavy weights on one's shoulders and head can have many adverse health consequences. Besides muscular strain, back ache, early cervical spine osteoarthritis and the risk of cervical disc prolapse, it can cause inguinal hernias, which in turn can get obstructed and become very painful.

At Jan Swasthya Sahyog (JSS), we see a large number of people presenting with hernias in the inguinal area. While they may have been triggered by many reasons such as congenital muscular weakness and increased abdominal pressure caused by a number of factors, lifting heavy loads is a definite cause for increased hernias.

Pregnant women who lift heavy weights are at risk for miscarriages or uterine prolapses.

copper-t (intrauterine contraceptive device)

This x-ray was taken for a patient having pain in the lower abdomen. What it shows is a copper-T, which is an interval method of contraception that should be encouraged. An intrauterine device (IUD) is a piece of plastic usually with copper wire wound around it. An IUD prevents fertilization when placed in utero.

The advantages of an IUD are its suitability for mothers who cannot attend clinics regularly to take pills, its low cost, reversibility, its immediate action and a low failure rate of 0.3%. The disadvantages include a fall out rate of 3-5%, bleeding difficulties - like spotting and heavy cycles which diminish with time, and pelvic inflammatory disease.

IUD scan be inserted anytime when a woman is not pregnant or within 72 hours of having unprotected sex, after an abortion or immediately after delivery of placenta (Postpartum IUD), 4-6 weeks after delivery when involution is complete and immediately after a caesarean section.

It is indicated as an interval contraceptive if a woman has no pelvic infection, in breast feeding mothers and someone who can't take pills regularly. But it is contraindicated if there is a known or suspected pregnancy, a pelvic infection, or abnormal bleeding per vaginum or a history of previous ectopic pregnancy.

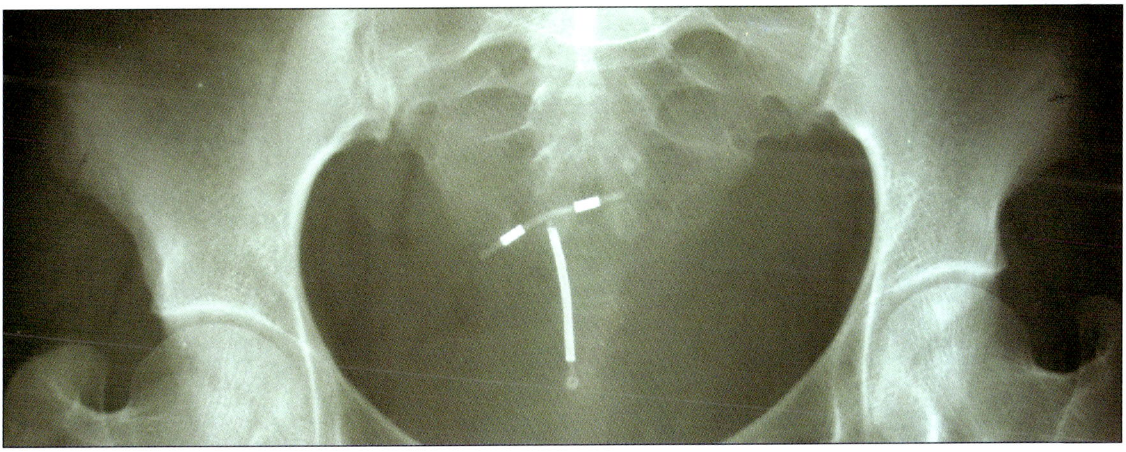

sanvaahan

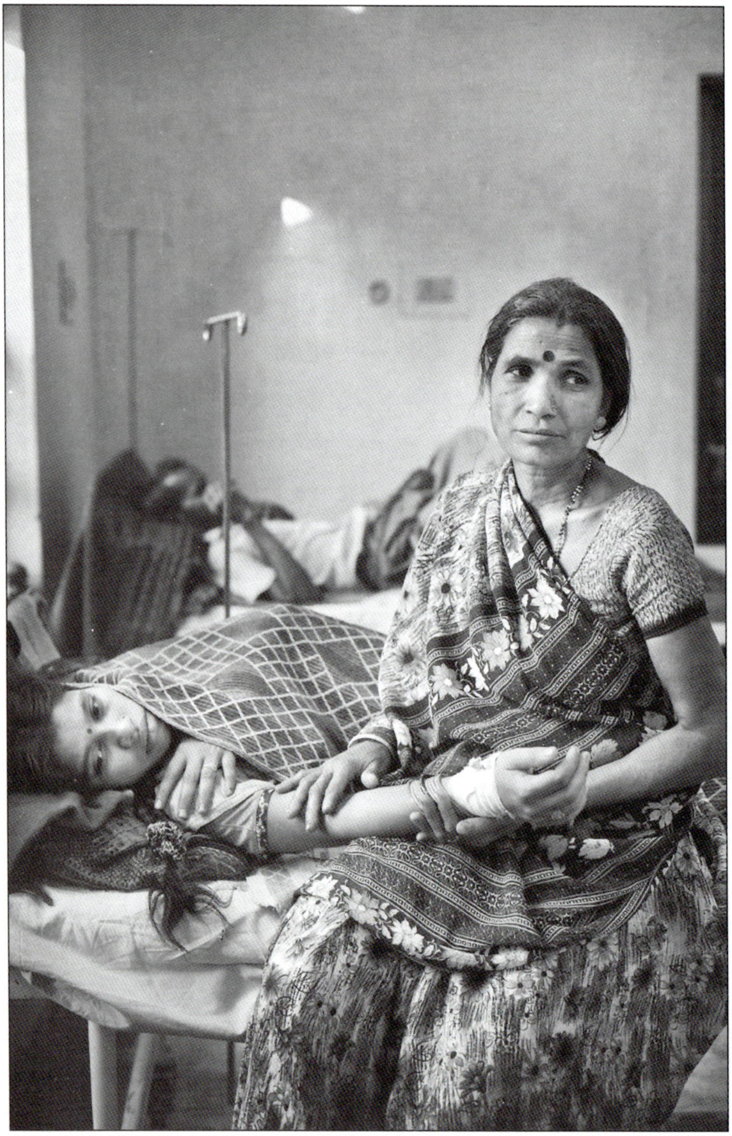

This is an image of caring; caring for the daughter or daughter-in-law by a mother or mother- in-law, and sharing the wisdom of age. Is there any evidence of the benefit from pressing the legs in improving disease outcomes? Ayurvedic physicians call it "sanvaahan" and claim it helps to decrease pain in affected patients and reduces the "vaat", besides giving a feel-good sensation.

Vaat is one of the three tattva's (others being pitta and coff) or principles in Ayurveda, whose imbalance causes illness.

construction labourers packed in an auto

This is the way humans are carted off to aid in the construction of buildings. Over 20 people have been packed into a small vehicle to be taken to a construction site. Their wages have always been low. These labourers are likely to have migrated from the villages to the cities in search of jobs and more. However, this comes with the risk of poor hygiene and lack of access to clean drinking water, the lack of personal safety and poor availability of health systems even for minor illnesses. Several times, their efforts to attain a better standard of life by migrating to the cities may backfire if they lose a lot of money in undue expenditure on treating their illnesses. In the cities, these people from villages are like medical refugees in their own country.

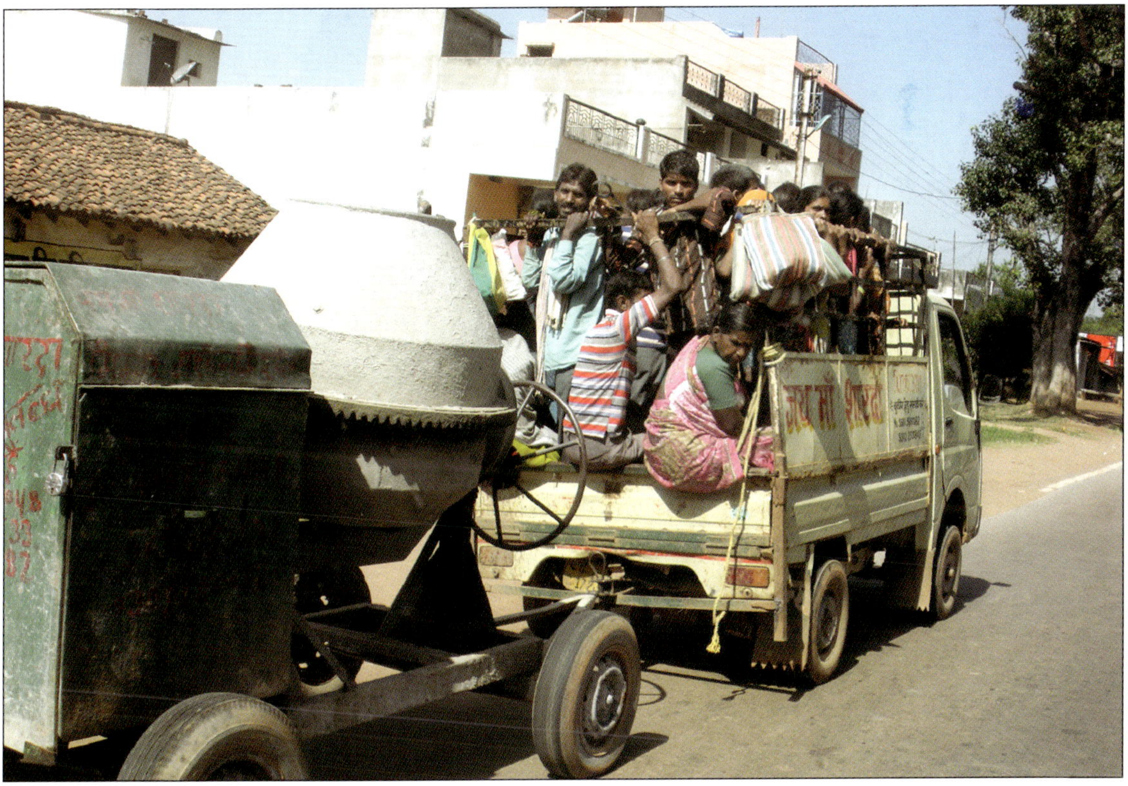

the marketing of fear

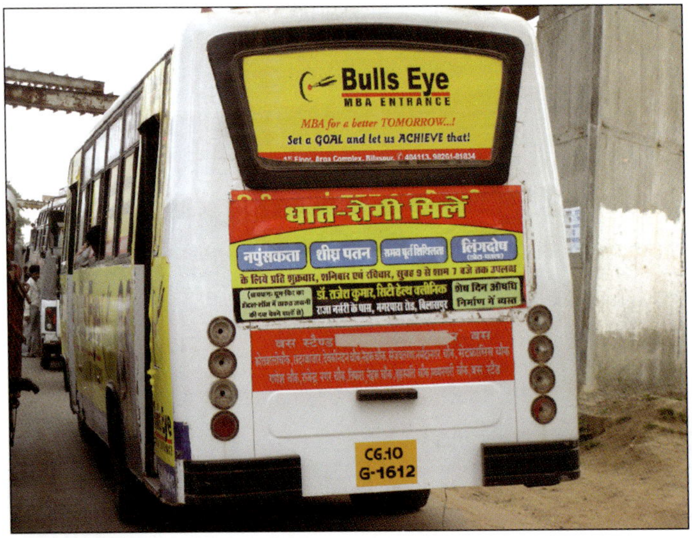

There are some innate fears like the fear of loss, failure, disease and death, which may be exploited for profit particularly if they get potentiated by cultural factors or taboos.

How the capitalist world takes advantage of this phenomenon is well illustrated in this example. One of the two advertisements on this bus is titled "धात रोगी मिलें", welcoming patients with "Dhat-Syndrome", a condition in which some penile discharge is passed at night, no evidence of which is usually found during medical examination. We meet men in real distress, sometimes to the extent of getting depressed by the constant worry of losing their strength and virility. It is extremely difficult for the patient to get rid of this irrational thought as it does sound plausible and corresponds to the belief system of society. "Dhat-Syndrome" is endemic and often occurs with anxiety and/or depressive disorders. Receptivity to any suggestions in advertisements which claim to help is likely to be high, particularly if the person involved does not have much self-confidence or is misinformed.

The lack of information and distorted information on a subject like sex leads to misconceptions. One can be misinformed about masturbation and think that it makes people weak, is a sinful act or can lead to premature ejaculation. Another common misconception is about the size of the penis, about which many young men have an inferiority complex. Advertisers often target people with the fear of a small and thin penis and is ready to help them solve a problem that does not exist. This is the marketing of (irrational) fear.

voluntary blood donation

The annual blood requirement of India would be met if 1% of our total population donated blood each year, amounting to 14 million units. Voluntary blood donors are not remunerated with any inducements in cash or kind. Such donations are very useful to society, because they are the best source of safe blood. However, in India only 55% of the total blood donations are voluntary and non-remunerated.

It has been difficult to convince healthy individuals to voluntarily donate blood due to the false notion that blood donation makes one weak and incapable of hard work. People are keener to buy blood from paid donors than to donate for their kin.

If we want to ensure availability of safe blood for our rural population, there is no other way than to ensure 100% voluntary donation and phase out replacement donation. Of course, paid donations are unacceptable.

Jan Swasthya Sahyog (JSS) has tried to create a movement amongst the youth in our program villages, where we encourage groups of blood donors to regularly donate voluntarily.

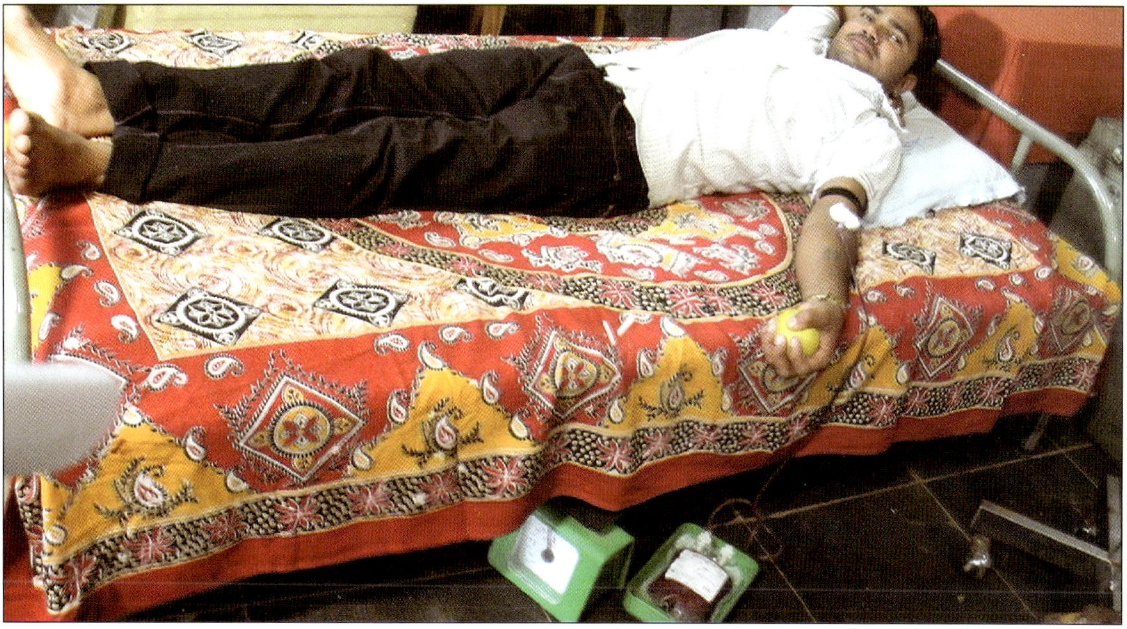

training village health workers

This photo shows Dr. Yogesh Jain teaching village health workers the jaundice and joint examination of a young girl who had both sickle cell anemia and rheumatoid arthritis. The pedagogy for the training of village health workers, most of whom are neo-literate, has to be through doing and by demonstrating and not so much by seeing and listening, and that is what we try to practice in Jan Swasthya Sahyog's training programmes.

It is more important to train workers at the periphery so that they can provide first contact care, pick up chronic and significant illnesses and refer them in time, rather than to focus all one's efforts in training doctors in medical colleges.

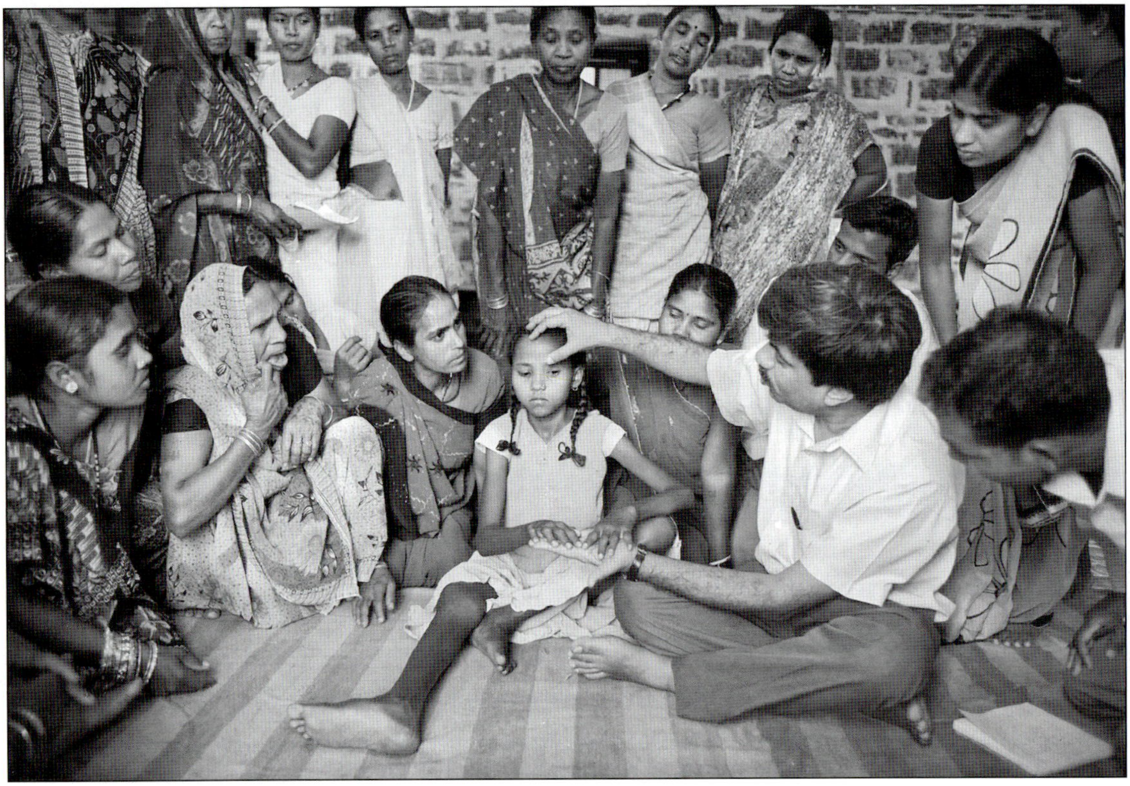

pictorial drug slips

Pictorial drug dispensing slips are used by Jan Swasthya Sahyog to dispense medicines, among other therapeutic aids. These allow the patient to remember which medicine to take at what time of the day and how frequently. Drug intake errors are rather frequent and their prevention includes avoiding polypharmacy as much as possible and then developing patient friendly dispensing aids that take into account poor levels of literacy.

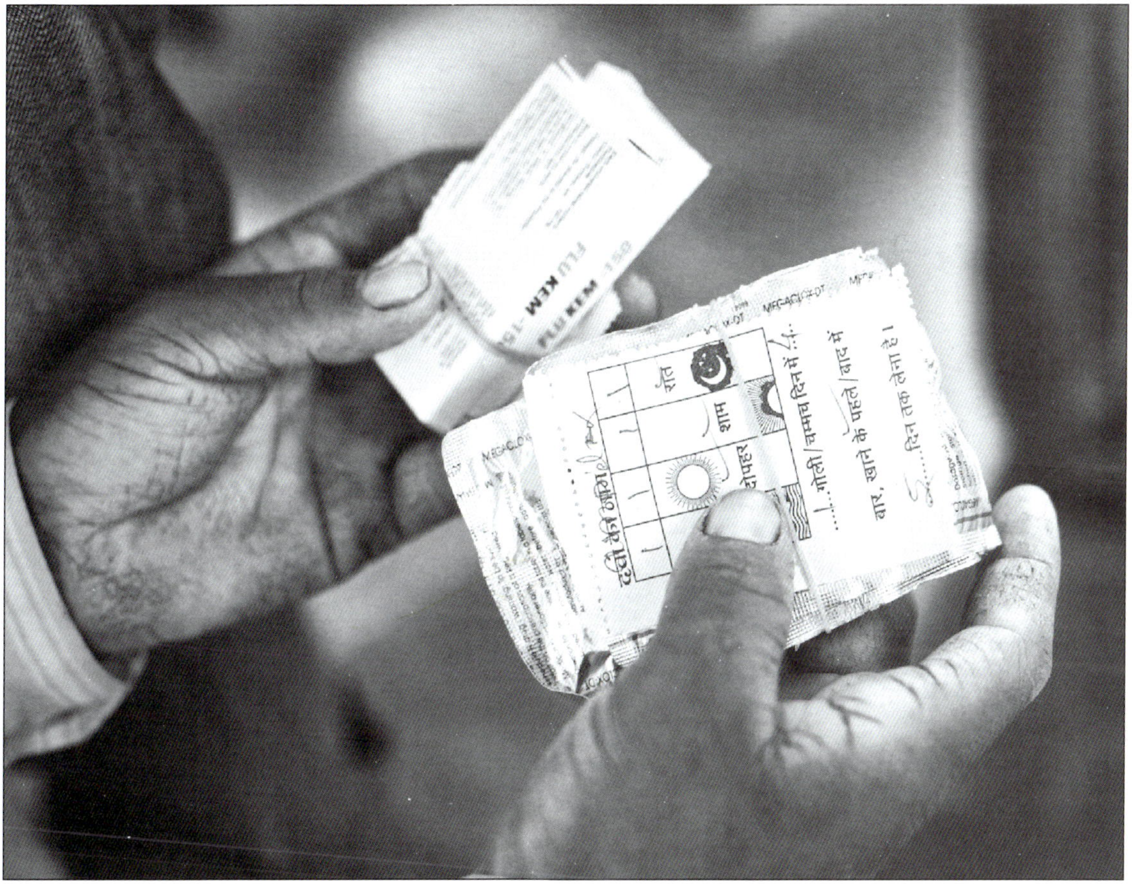

the healing touch

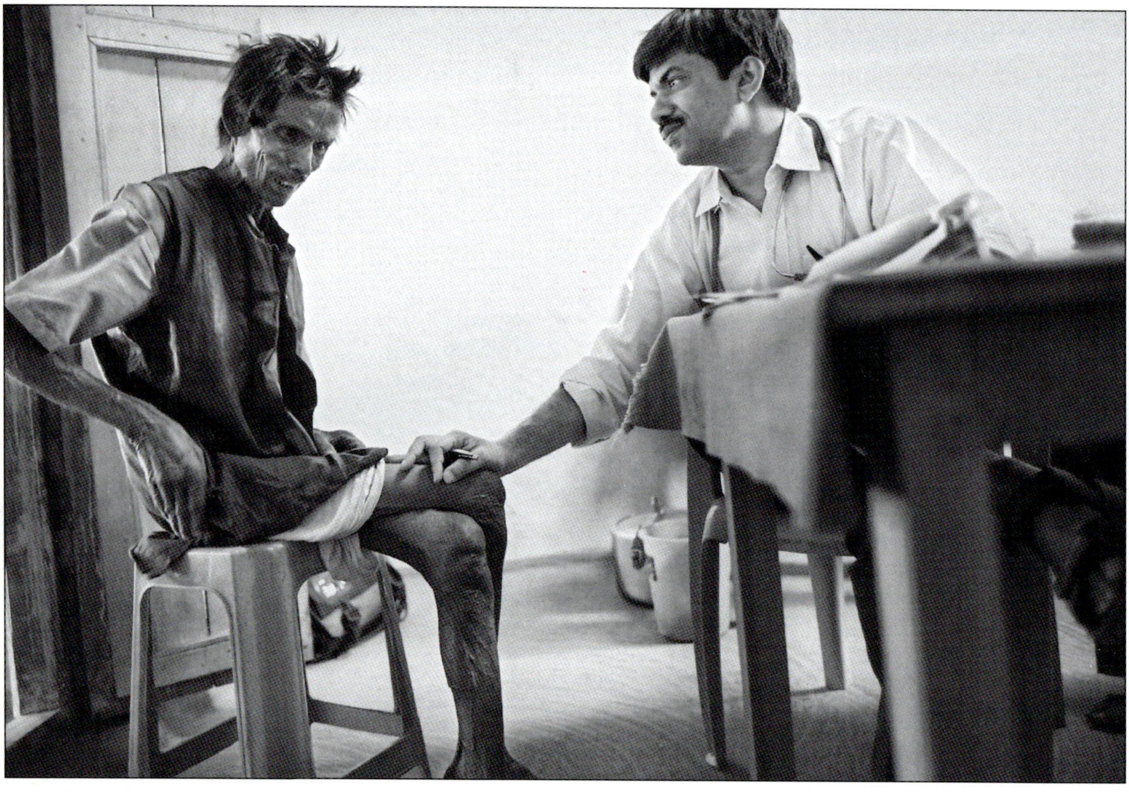

"Our lives begin to end the day we become silent about things that matter."

- Martin Luther King, Jr.

The Blogs

other voices from the hinterland

the walking stick sign

They come, literally by the hundreds, to the small examination room where I work in rural Chhattisgarh, India. Usually a friend supports them on their weak side, often a younger male family member. They resolutely hold a thin piece of wood worn smooth by the hand on the side of the body that has not betrayed them.

Our patients and their loved ones sit on small blue stools in front of the exam table that abuts the wall where a lithe green gecko lives behind the clock. Each of these patients performa a carefully choreographed dance as they attempt to find a seat. The safer ones make the long, slow trek around the blue stool, stoic or apologetic as they go. The more daring attempt to step over with their good leg, precariously balancing on a failed extremity, their loved one, and that same thin piece of well-worn wood.

My resident looks at me and says, "They have a walking stick. I promise I won't forget the aspirin and atorvastatin if I think it was a thrombotic stroke. I promise I will get an ECG if I suspect atrial fibrillation. I will enroll them in physiotherapy." These patients come so often I have drilled this workup and treatment plan into them, like the rhythms of the drums during the Festival of Ganesh.

I have come to call it "the walking stick sign." With the exception of one older man with a superior gluteal nerve injury and Trendelenburg gait, it has been almost 100 percent sensitive for stroke in my time in rural India. I'm proud that my residents are everyday becoming more competent and confident. I am happy they are imbuing a systematic approach to each patient, including stroke patients like these.

These interventions, though, are worth only so much weeks and months after a devastating cerebrovascular catastrophe. They are part of a larger system that is only worth so much when a poor person in the Global South abruptly loses the ability to move one side of her body one morning out in the fields.

With the gentle clack of each walking stick, it is impossible not to notice how the medical professionals of high resource, urban settings have forgotten or failed the residents of the rural, poor regions of the Global South.

We have a medicine (tissue plasminogen activator) that can greatly improve outcomes in the first hours of an acute stroke. This medicine is a recombinant technology, a truly impressive modern research marvel that can literally melt clots that are cutting off blood flow to the brain. Recombinant technology is a complicated technology, and it cannot be made available generically. Its complexity and cost make it impossible to manufacture or acquire in the Global South. From the time this medicine was conceived of, to the first successful animal tests through to the Clinical Trials in humans, we must recognize that poor residents of the Global South were never intended for inclusion as beneficiaries of this wonder drug.

One stick gently clacks.

We have other medicines (streptokinase) that are used for heart attacks in the Global South. They could perhaps deliver some of the benefit of these aforementioned recombinant technologies. They were previously studied with mixed results in stroke and certainly warrant further investigation. No researchers have taken up the mantle of these medicines (though some are calling for these studies to be done. Our research agenda is driven by the new and the innovative. We must admit our research agenda often excludes the concerns of the poor residents of the Global South. They are often already systematically excluded when the very research question is hatched.

Two sticks gently clack.

We make important medical devices like head CT's available through kind hearted but often poorly planned donations or the capitalistic system of wealth. Neither of the latter has even been shown to consistently do right or minimize harm for the residents of the Global South. If and when these machines arrive, they struggle with the load sharing, power surges and rolling outages that are part and parcel of life in the Global South. It is as if these machines were only ever intended to function at their best in the parts of the world that produce the lion's share of the world's carbon dioxide.

A dozen sticks firmly clack.

We have spent too little time building up systems, and paid too little attention to the silent chronic diseases that cannot make a galling poster or a galvanizing fund raising campaign. We know that strokes occur a full decade earlier in many parts of the Global South, and we know that much of this phenomenon can be attributed to the poor, chronic control of major stroke risk factors like diabetes and hypertension. But we have not yet found a way to consistently get insulin, the best and final medicine for poorly controlled diabetics, safely into the hands of those without refrigeration. We are letting the wildfires of tobacco abuse and processed foods spread throughout the Global South even as we restrict or ban them from our own shores.

A hundred sticks loudly clack.

In the Global North, we have divided medicine into small fiefdoms and led the medical institutions in the Global South into believing this is a behavior worth copying. In the major urban centers of this world, doctors and trainees become more and more test and imaging and technology dependent, until a stroke patient is hard pressed to find a Neurologist more than a few kilometres from an MRI. We have even made Global Health into its own "specialty" of sorts, with its own lingo and peer reviewed journals and conferences. In so doing, we have confirmed our collective suspicions that, while this is one planet, it really is made up of three separate worlds. We, the medical professionals of the Global North, are often only interested in providing health care to those living in the first of those three worlds.

A million sticks clack like thunder.

Timothy Laux

the freedom to dream

Three 19 year olds presented themselves at the hospital at Jan Swasthya Sahyog (JSS), Ganiyari.

The first, a male who was apparently alright one year back when he started complaining of increased frequency of micturition, especially nocturnal urinary frequency due to which he couldn't sleep in the night. He had weighed 48 kgs some seven months ago and now was 28 kgs. He had developed cataract in both eyes due to which he lost his vision and was unable to give his HSC exam. He could no longer draw pictures which was his favourite hobby before his vision was affected. Due to these health issues, he gave up all the hopes about his dreams of studying Arts or drawing beautiful pictures. His body was alive but his hopes were dead.

My Impression : Loss of Freedom to Dream.

The second patient, a 19 year old was a girl who was apparently alright, playful and cheerful 20 days back. Then she fell from a jamun tree, had a fracture of T12 vertebra and also a resultant spinal nerve injury. She then consulted with a private doctor but he ignored her swollen right hand completely. After 7-8 days, she noticed that her right hand was turning blue and subsequently black. She was experiencing the worst pain of her life. And then she had to undergo the even worse pain of amputation of her right hand: her working hand. She also noticed that her legs had no power below the waist. Even for her day to day activities like bathing, she had to depend on her father (her mother had died in her childhood due to some illness).

She was now crying continuously, not due to the fact that she had to have her right hand amputated nor because of her useless painful legs, but due to a feeling that she could not do anything in her life.

My Impression : Loss of Freedom to Dream.

The third 19 year old who came to the hospital was a medical student who was alright when he first went to a Modern, Urban 'International' school which was famous for its success rate in academics. There however he was bombarded with some artificial concepts and dreams about 'life' and 'success' and he then had been thrown in the ruthless river of extreme competition. His eyes were covered by green coloured glasses that allowed him to see only in a straight direction and along a fixed path. Every time, he achieved a milestone, he was told that this was not a real achievement and that the real achievement was at the next milestone. Finally, he got admission at a medical college after clearing the tough entrance exam with flying colours. But from the very first day of college life, hypothetical dreams about success and the 'Real Meaning of Life' for a Medico to get a good PG seat were imposed upon him.

Running behind some hypothetical dreams set by society, many a times, he was frustrated but could not express this to anyone. The hypothetical dreams didn't even allow the newly minted Medico to ask his own self about his own health.

My Impression : Loss of Freedom to Dream.

After thinking about these three cases, I think most of us have lost their freedom - due to poverty and hunger in some cases; due to diseases and ill health for some; violent injustice for others ; and some people willfully lost their freedom - the Freedom to Dream. Unfortunately, most people don't know that they have lost their freedom for the sake of some things and some people act like they have nothing to worry about.

Sagar Kabra

the art of letting go

In rural India, there are a lot of ways to get to the hospital. People come via public transport, hitchhiking, foot, taxis, rickshaws, bicycle and rarely the ambulance. People are helped by family, friends, compassionate lorry drivers and empathetic complete strangers. I've seen family members sandwich a very sick loved one between two healthy individuals on a motorcycle. I've met a father who walked through the night with his suddenly paralyzed son in his arms, stopping only inside the Emergency Department's doors.

While there are many ways to get to the hospital in rural India, there is only one group of people who can take you home: your family. This reality is a mixture of legal precedent and cultural tradition. If you're alive, the diversity of options listed above - some expensive, some reasonably priced, some free - are available. But, if and when you should die, there is only one option. Gone is the train or the bus or the friendly lorry driver. Where I work in India, your family must arrange a ride in a private vehicle capable of transporting a dead body. Such vehicles and the rides they provide are few and far between.

And they are bankruptingly expensive. In a bad monsoon year, they can consume the entirety of an extended family's savings. When this happens, it threatens food stability, malnutrition and further illness in a brutal cycle.

We are presented with a challenge previously unknown to me, as I trained in a tertiary care hospital in the United States, but which is not uncommon in Ganiyari. In a non-palliative, acutely sick individual with a treatable condition, when and how do you decide when "enough is enough"? We can treat lymphomas and pulmonary tuberculosis and severe sepsis, but we are not successful 100% of the time. This fact is frustrating, horrifying and horrifyingly undeniable. When does one gather a patient's loved ones and say, "It's time to rush to the train station (or the bus station). You have no more business being here."

You can die on the train if you boarded alive, no extra fee.

Such thought processes run completely counter to the intrinsically aggressive narrative of medical training no matter where one trains on this planet – London or Boston or Ganiyari. There is a code of ethics, perhaps even a code of honor, in all medical specialties which states "Never abandon the patient." One strives and struggles (provided that is the patient's or their loved ones' wishes) until the patient dies. In high resource settings, we have the ability to provide substitutionary therapy for multiple organ systems with more under development. Neurology research has shown us that meaningful commentary about the state of a person's cerebral function cannot be made until 48 hours after a cataclysmic event. In some sense, high resource settings have a built-in two day waiting period for miracles (which is frequently extended based upon a family's wishes).

In Ganiyari, these possibilities do not exist. One does not get a second more in a hospital bed than one is entitled to. One's family may not be able to afford that extra second anyway.

You might counter by saying, "Does this really happen? Is this really a decision tree you navigate? Would you really tell the family of a 15 year old with an APACHE score of 70, 'Time to go home'?"

I will probably never get to a place where I will be willing to do anything other than rage against the dying of the light for a child or adolescent or parent who has young children at home. But one would be amazed at the number of highly functional middle aged and elderly adults who come to the hospital in rural India with treatable conditions who, despite our best and ongoing efforts, creep ever closer towards death. Individuals who fit exactly into this category.

In the process of creeping towards death, the patient is usually exposed to more treatment modalities and is generally started on more powerful and more expensive medicines. In most cases, the bill for these treatments and medicines will be partially or completely covered by the family. In coming to the hospital, doctors and patients / patients' families enter into a tacit agreement where the doctor promises to do what is necessary and prudent but not more while the patients trusts the expenses of care were justifiable.

There is probably a tacit agreement that also says, "Tell me when it's hopeless." This same tacit agreement existed as I trained in the United States. However, there is a huge difference between "Tell me when it's hopeless" and "Tell me when it's hopeless and the bus is leaving soon."

It's so hard. It's awful watching someone leave the hospital hours from death with a problem you believe you can still intervene upon. But it's equally awful imagining a grieving family having to face the music of paying for a body's transport home.

As a fourth year doctor, I do not have enough experience to accurately predict death hours or days in the future. I am using my gut and when there is no evidence my gut feelings are useful.

Yet of all the clinical decisions I make in rural India, there is none that inspires a faster response. I've seen many things happen rapidly in a US hospital, but I have never seen a rapid discharge. That was until rural India. I've seen two generations of a family bundle up and move Grandpa to the hospital's front gate in 600 seconds.

As a US resident, I was familiar with CPR, grieving loved ones and death certificates. But I never had to greet death until it was already fully present. Death was a sworn enemy to at times acknowledge but always combat. When I took the Hippocratic Oath, I never imagined I would one day be letting the ultimate harm (death) happen to an individual so as to avoid another harm for the living who remain.

Timothy Laux

the distance to healing

The late afternoon sun filtered through the broad, yellow-tinged leaves of teak and Sal, creating kaleidoscopic patterns as we drove in second gear through the Achanakmar Tiger Reserve, in northwestern Chhattisgarh. Ajay was driving us to the remote village of Boiraha, where 55-year-old Matwarin and her husband Chherturam Baiga, along with their daughter seated in the back seat, were to be safely dropped off at their home. It had been a gruelling few weeks for the family, with two members having taken seriously ill and a lone daughter tending to them. Matwarin remained silent throughout the journey, pensively looking out of the window with a mix of homecoming relief and the residual anxiety that had shaken her up in the preceding days.

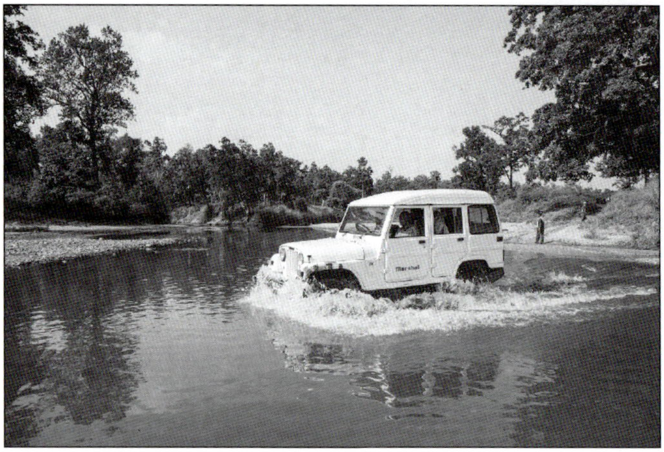

Before our vehicle left Jan Swasthya Sahyog's (JSS) Hospital in Ganiyari where the couple was treated, driver Ajay was doubtful we would get past the village of Katami. The Maniyari River had to be negotiated and even though this was the tail end of the monsoons he anticipated an unfathomable level of water. The rest of the journey, the last 22 km of the 76 km long journey, was to be made by cautiously wading across the river on foot and then ride pillion on motorcycles to Boiraha.

However, nature's frugality turned out in Matwarin's favour; the scanty rainfall this season combined with consecutive dry days enabled our Mahindra Marshal to gingerly ford the river. We then navigated delicately along a 100-foot-wide rift in the forest - it was dark and beautiful, the kind where Kipling's Mowgli would be spotted.

In 1999 a group of doctors pursuing their masters at the All India Institute of Medical Sciences (AIIMS) in New Delhi decided to do something unexpected. Instead of plotting their way into plush air-conditioned clinics in metros, they decided to put their heads together to set up a healthcare system in a much-neglected tribal region of Bilaspur district in Chhattisgarh. The need for primary and secondary medical care was of course apparent and well acknowledged, but the doctors were also keen on laying the edifice for an effective community-based health system that had preventive medicine at its core.

The Jan Swasthya Sahyog thus began slowly, gathering a holistic view of the lives of the people they intended to work among – the social structure of various tribal groups, their customs and rituals, agricultural practices and their implications on diet, areas of disengagement with the system and of course a clear mapping of prevalent ailments. A set of abandoned buildings close to the village of Ganiyari (23 km from the town of Bilaspur) originally built for an irrigation project was reclaimed and redesigned into a referral hospital with a current capacity of 70 beds, a fully-functional lab and two sufficiently large operation theatres.

News soon spread of the 'good' doctors and the outpatient department (OPD) clinics were soon brimming; they now see up to 400 patients a day, three days a week. In addition, JSS has set up sub-centres in three far-flung areas to dispense basic medical care to people living on fringes of the forests.

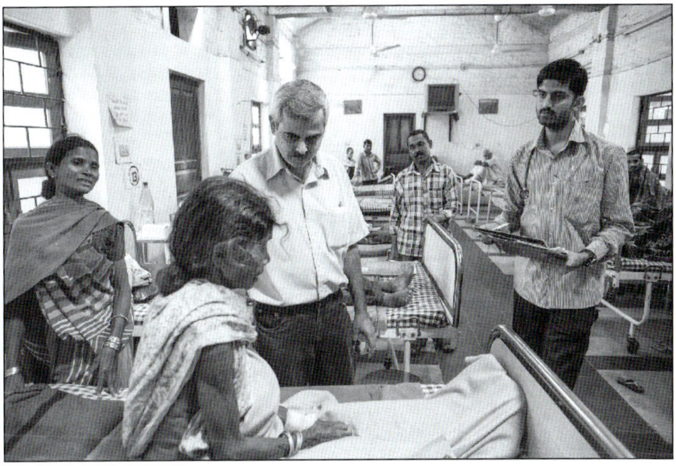

It was at one such sub-centre in Bamhani village that the Baiga couple of Matwarin and Chherturam first presented themselves. Matwarin looked frail and distressed, weighing a mere 35 kgs and had a swelling in the abdomen coupled with recently worsened pain. Chherturam looked no better, and complained of

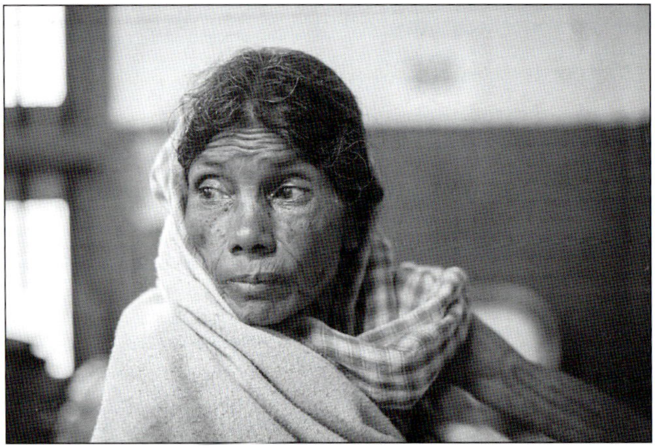

persistent cough with occasionally bloodstained sputum. The senior health worker at the sub-centre, Kamlabai, eventually directed the couple to the JSS Hospital in Ganiyari.

Dr. Rachana Jain, the gynaecologist at the JSS hospital ran the necessary investigations on Matwarin and elected to perform a panhysterectomy (removal of the uterus along with ovaries and cervix). A piece of the tumour was sent for histopathological analysis, a microscopic examination to study the nature of the tissue. Meanwhile, Chherturam was deduced to have had tuberculosis in the past that probably went improperly diagnosed or treated, and that the current episode might be a relapse. However, the tests proved inconclusive and he was put on palliative treatment.

Boiraha is among the many remote villages in the Anchanakmar Tiger Reserve that is served by JSS. The nearest hospital is a good 76 km away, but distance isn't the only predicament. Roads are simply non-existent and there are no bridges over rivers. The village is hence cut off from the rest of the world during monsoons, for about two months.

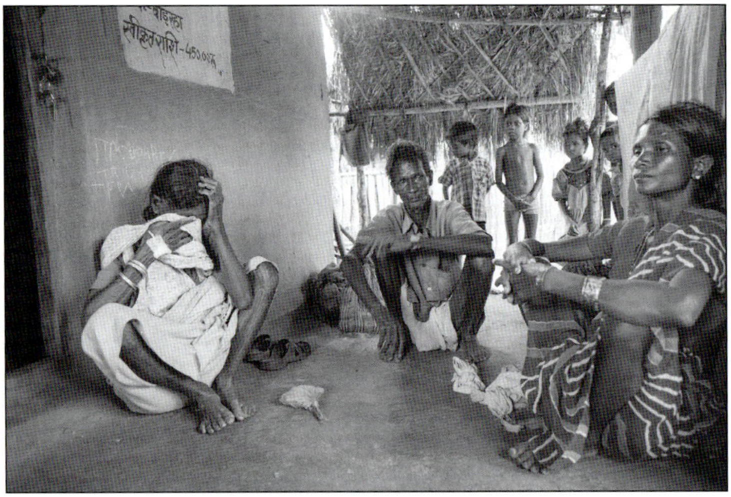

After a bum-numbing three and half hours of travel, we made it to Matwarin's home in Boiraha. On entering her house, Matwarin sat down on the earthen floor and broke down. Then, fishing out a much-crinkled plastic pouch hidden deep in her bag, she pulled out two hundred-rupee notes to thrust into Ajay's hands. She only had five more notes left in the pouch. Ajay of course refused to take it, and we left wishing them well.

It is difficult to imagine Matwarin's ordeal in the absence of JSS, and I shudder to think of the many Matwarins across India who are in need of help, every single day. Matwarin was fortunate to have had warm and caring hands tending to her during her two-week stay at the JSS hospital. As we left her to enjoy the familiar confines of her house I could tell from that her eyes that she was indeed grateful.

A week later, after returning to Bangalore, I emailed to enquire about Matwarin's histopathological report. Dr. Sushil Patil, the program coordinator at JSS and a general handyman who does everything from fixing plumbing woes at the hospital to overseeing the organization's annual report, wrote back with bad news. Matwarin's tumour turned out to be cancerous, and she was being asked to report to the hospital for chemotherapy. Dr. Yogesh added one line to the email thread: "Mucinous adenocarcinoma is a cancer of the ovary. Bad disease."

Vivek Muthuramalingam

how do we treat the poor?

Rajkunwar's Gond's slender frame looked taller than the actual 5 feet 4 inches she measured. This is because she was light : exactly 31kg and 700 gm. Ten days earlier, she weighed only 31 kg. Noticing her condition, the Jan Swasthya Sahyog (JSS) village level health worker at Katami, a forest village, immediately took Rajkunwar to the nearby JSS sub-center at Bamhani where she was diagnosed with tuberculosis but she was sent to the JSS rural hospital in Ganiyari, a 2 hour ride over some rough roads for confirmatory tests and treatment.

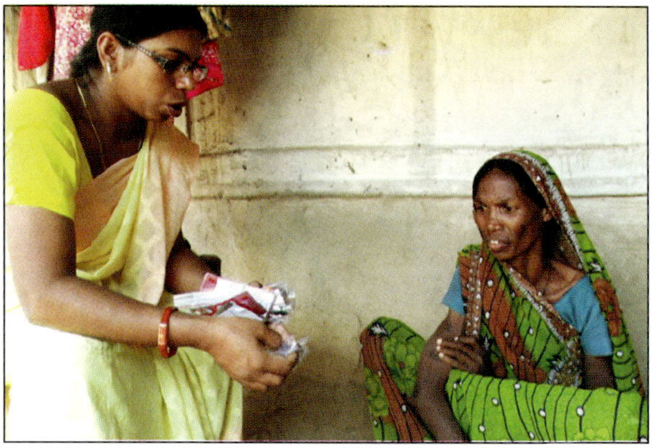

Rajkunwar and her husband were landless and earned their living through agricultural labour and the few days of work available through MGNREGA. I followed Reena, a social worker with JSS, who was visiting Rajkunwar in her home to follow up. Had it not been JSS's explicit aim to reach out to the most marginalised, about 55 forest villages in this area would not have expected any access to healthcare, much less a home visit. In the early days of the sickness, Rajkunwar had gone to a jholachhap (quack) who treated her for malaria and gave her a bottle of saline intravenously. Five hundred rupees of their hard earned money was wasted!

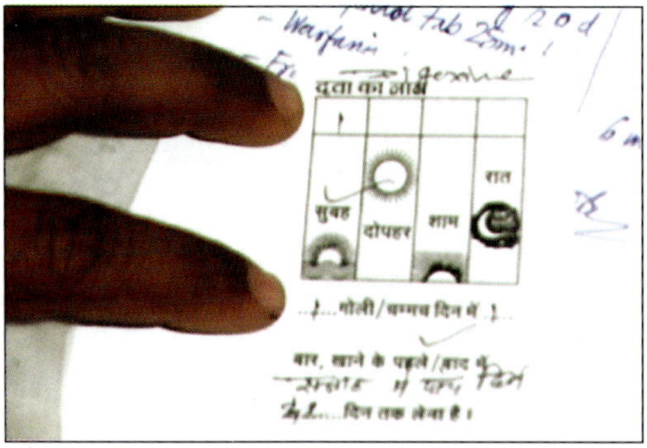

Reena located the home at the edge of the village overlooking a valley where the river was reduced to a trickle in the winter month. Bright yellow fields of mustard swayed in the gentle breeze in the small valley. It was hard to imagine such beauty could coexist with the cruel deprivation that Rajkunwar's family lived with – 1.5 kg of rice and 500 gm of potatoes was the average daily diet of this family of five adults. The death of two grandchildren in the recent past added to the heaviness inside their home.

As we settled in the courtyard, Rajkunwar briefly disappeared into a room and brought out a plastic bag with substantial number of medicines in them. At Reena's urging, she began explaining which medications she has been taking and at what time of the day. The slips on the drug pouches were aptly colour-coded with a sheet of paper illustrating the time of day they were to be taken. Could modern healthcare be made so poor-friendly, I wondered? Could socio-economic status and the cultural context play such an important role in taking healthcare to the marginalised people of India?

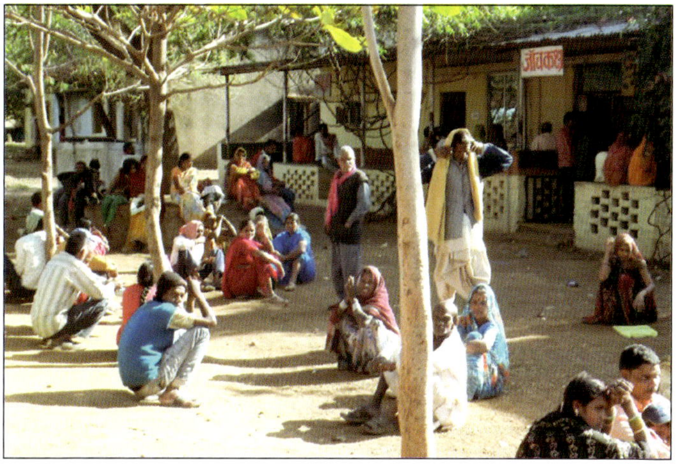

The first thing that strikes a visitor to JSS is the respect and compassion with which a poor person (or any person for that matter) is treated – for human dignity should not have to calibrate itself to appearances, economic backgrounds, and the ability to read. What makes the efforts of JSS unique is not its medical expertise alone, but its ability to read the pulse of a society. At JSS, modern science has not been able to induce contempt for a people living with a different world view. JSS puts significant effort in improving agriculture, in developing technology appropriate for the region and people, in understanding social processes that lead to illnesses. JSS operates with about 100 village level health workers centered around 3 remote sub-centres that are finally backed by the rural hospital in Ganiyari with the capacity to perform complex surgeries and an in-patient facility of 60 beds. Ambulances travel daily to the sub-centres and one is stationed in Bamhani, the furthest sub-centre, at night for any emergency.

"Your urine might turn red due to the medication," Reena patiently explained to Rajkunwar sitting on her haunches, "But do not be alarmed. Don't stop taking the medicines. You have to continue them for 9 months to get well completely".

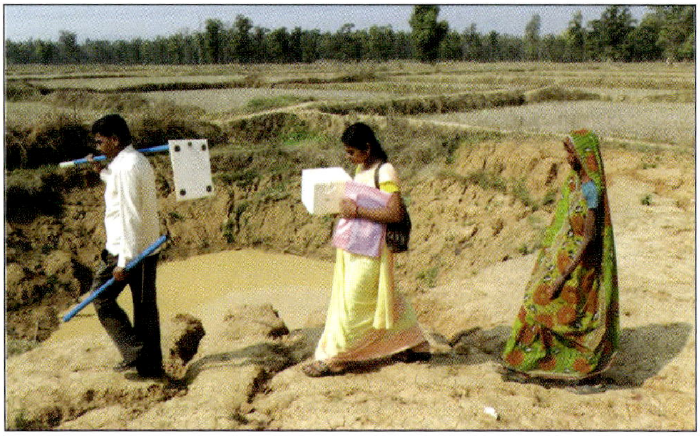

Rajkunwar reported a slightly improved appetite which was corroborated by the marginal increase in her weight; marginal yet trend-reversing. Her BMI was a precarious 11.8 (<18.5 is considered to be a state of chronic undernourishment). Reena wanted to see the bag of 2 kg Kala Chana (Black Gram) that was given to TB patients on a monthly basis as a protein supplement. Barely 100 gms were left – it had just been 7 days. Reena understood that even in her condition it was not possible for Rajkunwar to eat the Chana by herself.

"How do you feel?"

"Not too well. I am still very weak to do any work at home," Rajkunwar says.

Ill-health steals the most precious belonging of the poor – their capacity to labour.

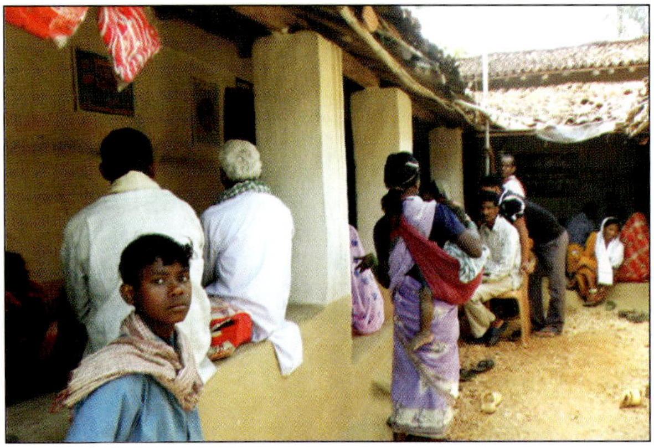

"Come with us to the Bamhani sub-centre, the doctor is here today. We will bring you back to the road in a vehicle," Reena tried to persuade Rajkunwar.

The Bamhani sub-centre is a miracle of appropriate technology that defies all limitations of remoteness from urban centres. It is completely powered by solar energy including a refrigerator to store anti-venom and other emergency medicines, UV purified drinking water, WLL phone, and is staffed round the clock by a senior health worker. On Tuesdays a doctor from Ganiyari is here and so is a mobile diagnostic laboratory that can turn around blood, urine and sputum samples the same day. Most importantly, the adivasis don't feel out of place at the sub-centre.

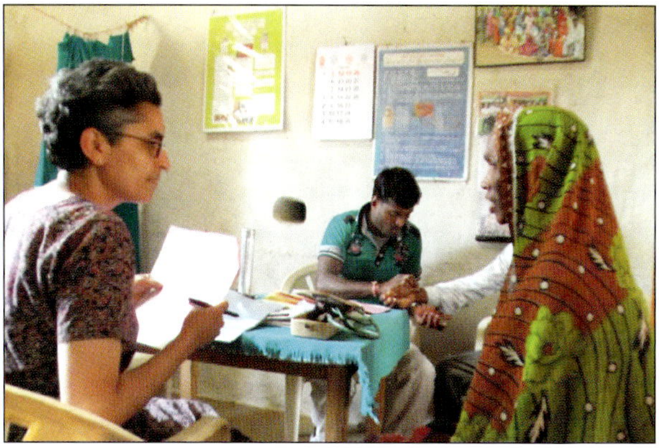

Rajkunwar like a large percentage of the people who come to JSS will not have to pay anything, but her care will be determined by her condition alone and nothing else. Others pay a very nominal fee. In 2010 JSS treated 470 cases of TB which increased to 587 in 2012.

If the message of JSS is not understood, the poor will continue to be deprived of rational healthcare while the rich will be sick of hospitals.

- Somnath Mukherji

Some More Examples of Appropriate Technology at JSS

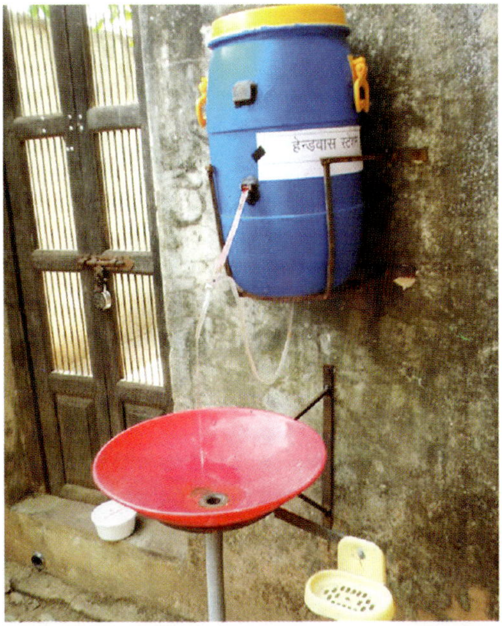

Hand washing station for village homes: The plastic pipe is fitted with an iron strip which when lifted is held by the magnet eliminating the need for a tap.

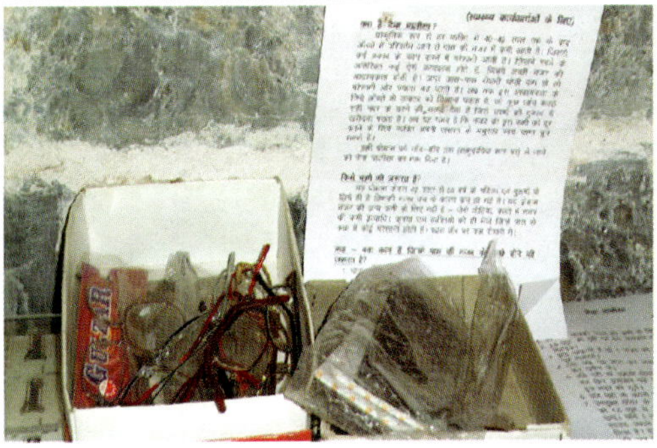

Naina Chalisa: A set of reading glasses over a range of power from which villagers can choose on their own without having to go to an ophthalmologist. This has been very popular with the people.

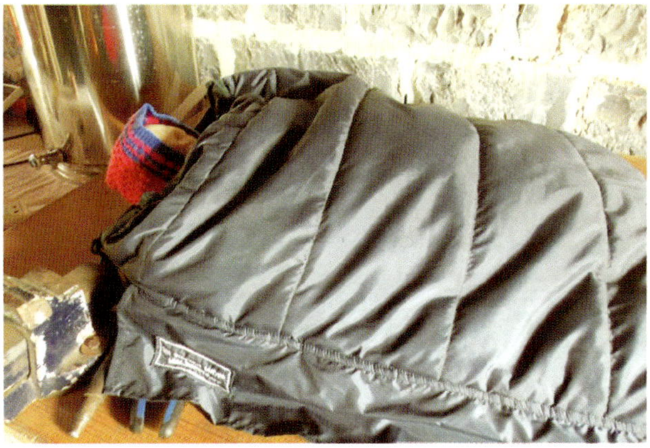

Baby sized sleeping bags: To save newborns from hypothermia in the mountain villages. The bag has a pocket where a big packet of palm oil can be heated in boiling water and inserted for additional heat.

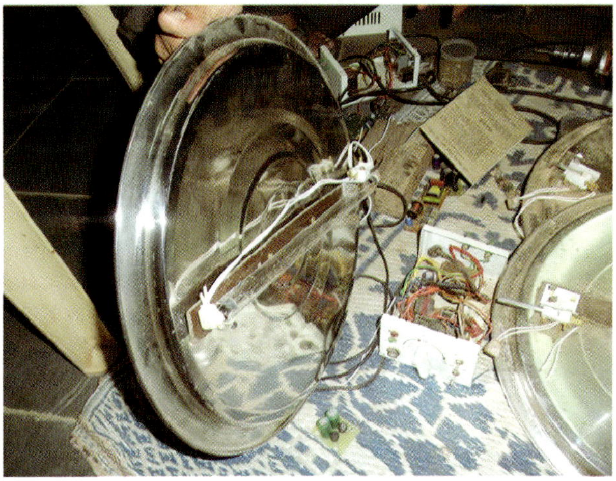

UV filter for drinking water: The lid for a 20 litre steel container is fitted with a UV lamp which can run either on 220V AC or 15V DC from solar power.

the 'health' deprived

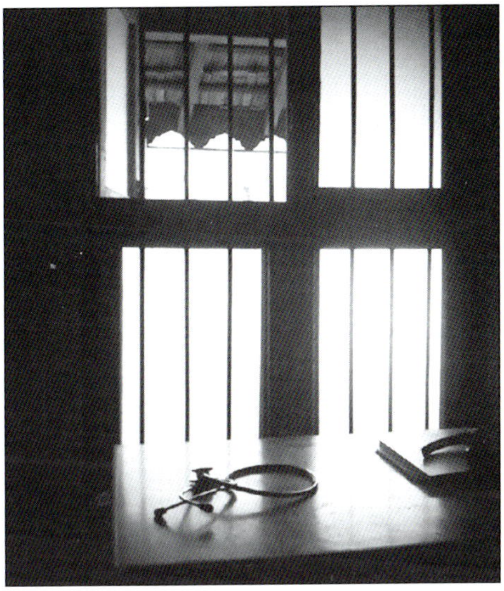

I was sitting in my room after lunch attempting to take a siesta one day, but failed. Took a random click on that afternoon, the stethoscope just a coincidence, but it stirred my conscious mind to think more philosophically, more deeply beyond a doctor. The window is the only thing through which you can see the outer world without knowing it. Our eyes are our windows through which you see but others cannot read you. But then I started to see through 'their' eyes, started to walk in 'their' shoes, started to empathise. 'They' are the Patients.

I started to put questions to myself and tried to get answers. But the search towards an answer generated more and more questions. I was confused. My mentor told me I was rightfully confused. This window showed me the crippling, futile efforts of mankind to attain this 'Health'. I wondered whether man in pursuing of Health or this extreme inequality was making 'Health' hungry of man.

W.H.O. says physical, social, mental, spiritual wellbeing defines 'Health'. I saw health dying due to poverty, hunger, inequality, inaccessibility, helplessness, unavailability, political lethargy and in so many ways. In other ways 'Health' is hungry of political willpower, education, accessibility, personnel, institution and empathy.

A child died of malnutrition; here Health was dying of this hunger. Every time I saw someone dying in an unjustifiable situation, I asked myself who is responsible?

While working at Jan Swasthya Sahyog (JSS) I came across so many such unjustifiable deaths, whether it was malaria, snake bite, gas gangrene, anaemia, tuberculosis or malnutrition. Making one of them responsible was like wearing black specs and saying the whole world is dark. The 'Cause of the Death' was just an excuse or an iceberg to mask the submerged injustice made by men causing the death of a fellow man unjustifiably. Wish we would genuinely have treated him as a fellow man.

I want to share some stories which are true and reflect the true nature of inequalities. I should dedicate this writing to these people, but a step to halt such losses further in the future would be more condolatory.

Cause of the Death : Postpartum Haemorrhage

It was a non-OPD day, still we saw patients almost like an OPD and mostly emergency cases. They brought her on a stretcher. I rushed to her, as I could clearly see her deep breaths from a distance. She was about 23 year old. Her gasps suggested a delay in coming to the hospital. Her pale face added more fear to the environment, as it was a signal for urgent blood transfusion. I was not able to feel her pulse and the heart had already stopped. Immediate resuscitative measures had to be taken, but all was in vain. She was declared dead within 30 minutes of her arrival.

Later we came to know that she was pregnant and had delivered a baby, but the bleeding was continuing. Only a young, unmarried girl was with her helping out. No trained Dai or any health worker or any PHC nearby. Her umbilical cord had not been clamped, also some injury happened during the delivery.

This all lead to a massive blood loss with loss of a life, and a loss of a mother.

We came to know that both husband and wife were working at a construction site for the last one or two years, in a place about 500 km from their native home. They were temporary migrants. She was 9 month pregnant but she needed to stay there to take care of her husband as he was not allowed to take leave. There was no one to take care of her.

Would you agree if I said the cause of death was postpartum haemorrhage? PPH was just one factor, but should we turn our eyes away from other factors which resulted in her 'unjustifiable death'? Why did someone have to leave their home in search of bread and butter? Why should an employer not bear the cost of his employee's disease? Isn't it a moral responsibility to provide an ambulance, a health worker in the work place? Why is a district/state not able to provide employment in someone's own place?

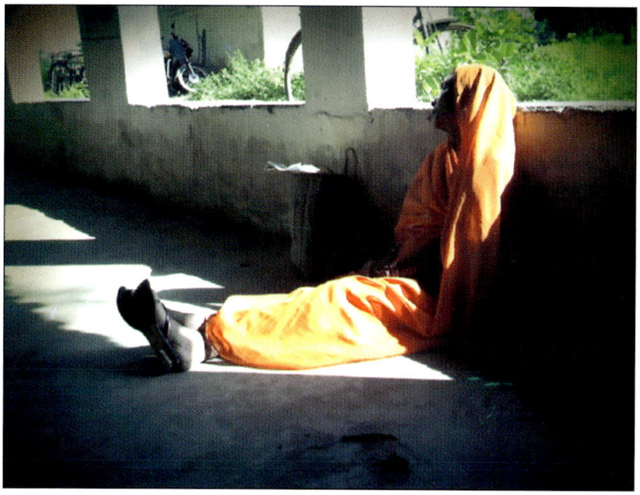

A patient who got tuberculosis while in Ladakh, another one who got silicosis when he was in Gujarat, both were thrown out of their job. They lost their working capacity and the employer had not given a penny. A woman suffered from acute psychosis because her husband, a driver and had to stay away frequently. A mother was unable to treat her child in time because her husband did not send any money this time.

PPH is a leading cause of post-delivery maternal mortality. It is disgraceful if we are losing mothers at the cost of development. There is a collapse of someone's family while doing construction for another. It's very unfortunate to feel the last pulse of a patient when you come to know that mortality was preventable. But it is more painful when death is premature.

We see workers, labourers, sweepers, drivers and vendors in all the cities. They work in cities to make hospitals, malls, colleges, roads available for us, they clean gutters and some are scavengers too. Most of us are unaware of the harsh reality linked with each of these people.

A young woman suffered from depression because she was unable to live with her two children, who were studying in a school outside her village. Her husband left her a few years back because she had TB. Depression was her companion now days. Antidepressants: we learnt to prescribe this, but did she really need this? We didn't know, but she knew, drugs could not bring her children back; the mere changing of a biochemical response is not going to change reality, 'the cause'. Often we are not interested to know the cause. Then what will work? Quality education at her village will definitely work, not drugs. This may prevent her children's educational migration. This will prevent a lot of havoc in millions of lives in our country.

Cause of the death: Malaria

I was in my 8th standard, when we heard that a classmate died of cerebral malaria. Death did not create any conspicuous worry among us; probably we had only heard of it, not seen any yet. Indeed while studying in medical college malaria was never appalling. But living more than a year now in Chhattisgarh; I get shivers as soon as I hear "there is a malaria patient". It shook me, from my head to toe when I saw a 4 year old girl dying of falciparum malaria.

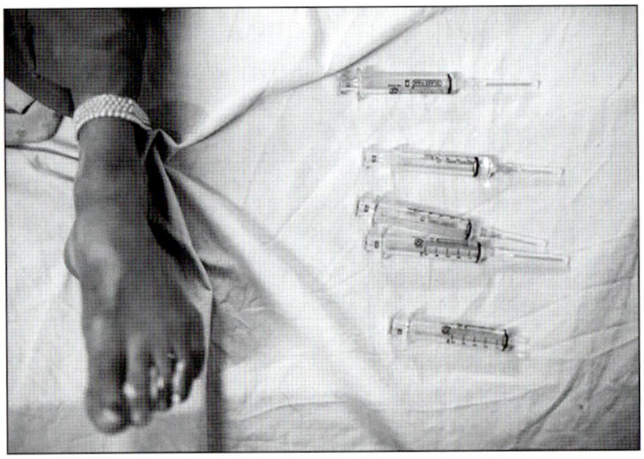

Plasmodium Vivax is the most common causative parasite which gives you malaria, but in Chhattisgarh it's the Plasmodium Falciparum. This parasite is more dangerous than Vivax. Resistance to chloroquine made it more lethal.

It was late January, and the four year old girl brought in by her parents, with the father holding her in his arms. We rushed to the casualty. She looked very dry like someone had sucked all the body's water out. Anaemia was looking at us through her pale skin. It was a seizure which compelled them to bring her to our hospital. She had seizures three hours earlier since when she was in a semi coma. Artesunate injection was immediately given, electrolyte imbalance assessed, and arrangements for blood transfusion made, treatment for the seizures given, as we tried to stabilise our patient. Vitals of the patient were stable for a while. After one hour she had another seizure, then again, another and, then another ...she was in status epilepticus. Fear replaced worry. At one time she went into respiratory arrest. I was witnessing the futility of modern medicine in the midst of uncertainties.

A few hours of tug of war to bring back life against death concluded in the victory of the latter. It was agonising to see a beautiful child dying. The father said she had had fever for four days, and they consulted a local quack. He diagnosed it as malaria but did not know whether it was Vivax or Falciparum. He might have given chloroquine as treatment. This was of no use as it was chloroquine resistant falciparum malaria. None of this would have helped except to bring her to the nearest PHC. The time wasted with the quack cost the parents their daughter.

This was not the answer to the question which haunted my mind since that child was admitted. Holding that quack responsible was like giving an answer to Yaksha's first question. There was a series of questions which needed to be answered. I did not get an answer to all the questions but it certainly generated unrest in me.

Why should I blame the quack when he was the sole health care provider in the village? The lack of knowledge could be blamed, but did he really not want to gain knowledge? Why was the government not certifying them as village heath workers and training them? Why were most rural hospitals not well equipped to handle cases like sever malaria? Almost 15-20% mortality is unavoidable even in the best ICU setup in case of severe falciparum malaria and cerebral malaria. This clearly signifies the importance of preventive initiatives. If India is unable to bear the cost of preventive measures then which India is ranked second among developing countries?

The recent death of a 22 year old photo journalist of Tehelka raised eyebrows of the media. Why then is the media more interested in bombarding us with the United States election news, while at the same time we were witnessing some unjustified deaths? Official documentation for malaria deaths is horrible. Figures are manipulated. If the patient died because of a complication of malaria, officially they don't record it as a death due to malaria.

Paul Farmer called such a death a 'Stupid Death' not because it was caused by a mere sting of a mosquito but a collective stupidity of policies, politics, health systems, inaccessibility, lack of doctors, lack of basic infrastructure and most importantly inequality.

Malaria is not just a disease, it used to be plague, but now a plague might be dengue, or cholera, and it may be malnutrition. These indicators of social injustice bestow the poor with prolonged suffering.

Questions should be raised against this prolonged suffering everywhere and with resonance. Single voices are buried and a synergistic effort is required. A solution is the need of the hour to prevent such stupid deaths because one day unknowingly these would engulf our so called civilised urban life too.

Cause of the death : Gas Gangrene

A 28 year old man came on a stretcher, a wound on his left leg smelling extremely foul; it was nauseating to even go past him. With just a cloth pulled over it, it was covered by maggots; hundreds of them. 'Gas gangrene' is one of the worst diseases a farmer may experience. This was an emergency, and a decision was taken to perform an above knee amputation. Surgery was done but the infection had already spread to other parts of the body. The patient went into shock and then respiratory failure. The dice was rolled in vain. The patient died.

'Cause of the Death' was Septicaemia.

It was not shattering...but the story began now.

He was a labourer, who worked for a rich man. He was doing his daily work as told by his master. That day they were filling a truck with some material in big sacks who his master wanted to sell in the local market. The truck was continuously being filled up, and unaware of the fact, that it was overloaded, when suddenly a sack fell on the man as he stood beside the truck. His leg was injured, probably fractured. There was much blood loss both internal and external. He fainted and was immediately taken to the nearest PHC. The doctor saw it and told him to go to the district hospital. He was kept there for two days but because of his bad condition they advised him to go to either Nagpur or Jabalpur medical college. Nagpur was 400 km and Jabalpur almost 250 km from his home. He could not afford to go to either, when someone told about the JSS hospital and he was rushed here.

JSS too was almost 240 km from his home and he had to sell his half acre land in just rupees 12000; arrange a vehicle for rupees 4000. But he died. His old parents left inconsolable.

Why did he have to suffer this; just because he was poor?

Why could a district hospital not manage a case of gas gangrene at least in the initial stages?

Why did a farmer have to sell his land for his health?

Why was there is no state transport in Chhattisgarh and Jharkhand?

Why are the health services different for village and cities?

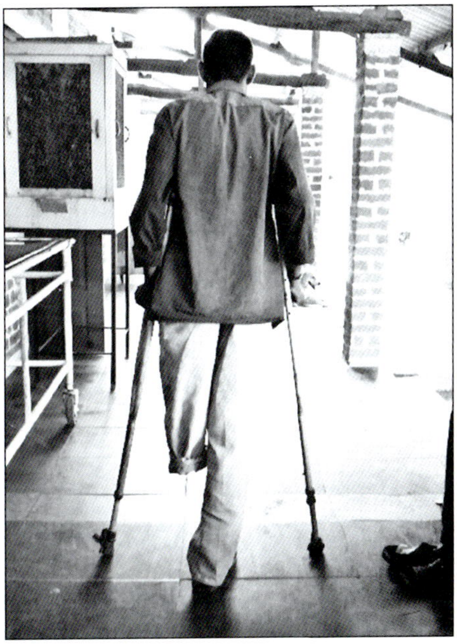

Why did local MLA's or MP's not go to government hospitals? Because they know these were ill-equipped and lacked personnel. But wasn't this their responsibility to make these facilities good? Instead poor facilities encouraged privatisation and increased inequality too. The day a MLA, MP, or District Collector chose to go to a government hospital an overnight change would be visible.

The question was still unanswerable...

And who owed the answer to his father?

Within a few days we had another patient, a young man with three children. He had minor prick on his limb while working in field. He presented almost fifteen days later. Gangrene was already set up to engulf his limb.

The reason behind his delay was different. It was the ploughing season and his 12 year old son could not do all of the field work in his absence. His wife had to look after a nine month old baby and a four year old girl. It was impossible to leave the work in the season as rain was unpredictable and he was not rich enough to have his own motor pump. He had to plough in that period only. He was in a dilemma: to choose between his own health and food for his family. Time passed and the small prick flared up into gangrene. The pain was unbearable; and it was pain alone that provoked people to think of a hospital. If all the diseases had not been painful; farmers, poor people, labourers would never be the visitors of hospitals.

The bacteria overwhelmed the body's defence. Every organ of the body was destroyed. He died after 4-5 hours.

His wife and baby were taken home by the hospital vehicle along with his body; there was no sign of life around. His son and four year old daughter were ploughing the field when his wife reached home with their dead father. The ambulance driver narrated this in pain. The mourning of the son and daughter looking at their dead father was the worst music ever played by destiny.

Pizza reaches our door within half hour, but there is no means of transportation in most of these villages. Does the speed of pizza delivery juxtapose development? Huge bridges have been made on the sea, but villages are kept separated from hospitals, with no bridges to cross forest rivers. Inequality is the root of the problem, and attitudes need to change to uproot this. Every citizen had to be treated equally.

Cause of the Death: Snake Bite

It was during the rainy season, and one Sunday morning around 6:45, I got a call from Yogesh sir. A doctor calling another doctor at this time fell mostly under 'emergency calls'. He had had a call from the JSS Bamhani clinic a short while earlier but being out of town, he called me. A woman had just arrived at Bamhani in severe respiratory distress (gasping) from a nearby village with a snake bite. Dr. Parag, Anil and I got ready to go to Bamhani with the emergency kit and a vehicle. It was an hour's drive to reach the check post to enter the tiger reserve into which Bamhani was situated. Then another 20 min of journey on a 'kaccha' road. This timing was crucial, and for a doctor, the 1 hour and 20 min was already too much for a patient in respiratory distress. Still we needed to take the chance to reach the patient.

Another natural obstacle awaited us in the form of a river. We crossed a more than 50 feet wide and 4 feet deep river which consumed another 15-20 min, but which was inevitable. A health worker was waiting with his bicycle across the river and we reached Bamhani just before 9 am. I examined the patient; there were no respiratory effort, not a single sign of life.

Her pupils were fully dilated and I realised we were late, much too late.

The patient had been bitten by a common krait (we came to know this on the basis of the timing of the bite and symptoms as told to us by the health worker) around 2 o'clock at night while sleeping. She was taken to some local 'baba'. He did some magic process on her claiming to take the venom out of her body. This detoxification process took nearly two hours. Within these two hours she was deteriorating and her parents had no choice but to take her to Bamhani as the baba's magic was not working. And the venom was already showing its effect of respiratory distress by the time she reached the clinic. There the health worker called immediately Yogesh sir who instructed her to give artificial respiration to the patient with an air bag and mask. But this was not sufficient to fulfil the patient's oxygen demand; she needed to be given oxygen and respiration by putting tube inside her throat. A village health worker could not be trained in this procedure as it was complicated, and even doctors needed to be trained well under supervision.

The reluctance of the parents and unavailability of even primary health care led a person's life to death. This was not the first time when I declared a patient 'dead', but this time there was some helplessness, pity and some anger in my feelings. After some formalities we left heavy heartedly for Ganiyari.

All of us were quiet, an unbearable quietness. Clouds of questions were churning in our brain and poking us to search for answers. We had not wasted any time to reach at Bamhani. Still we felt responsible. We talked about whom to hold responsible.

Was it the government's health care system that could not provide primary health care in a tiger reserve forest where snake bites were common? Was it the transport system that could not build a bridge just because it was a tiger reserve? Or was it the education system that failed to create awareness among tribals about snake bite and getting the right care? But here, even primary education did not reach. How would we teach them what to believe and what not to, in that forest? Once my sister asked me about modernisation of medical equipment and I told her the more the equipment was modern the more it was far from the reach of the poor. We had to try to make it appropriate and reachable to the poor. If we could not teach health workers to intubate, could we not develop instruments which simulated the work of intubation? Snake bite, scorpion bite, dog bite, wild boar bite, bear bite and various other encounters with wild animals are more common in village or tribal areas. It is always the poor who become victims and the treatments to these accidents are so expensive that he may die with that burden.

'Medical education and rural India'...my understanding at JSS

It's a paradox to use these words together. Young doctors are more and more moving or motivated to move or forced to move towards our so called 'civilized cities'. You would be considered a fool if you willingly went to villages. Only 26% of doctors served up to 73% of village population. I might not have been the right person to criticize the medical education system but these figures were not an illusion. Something was wrong.

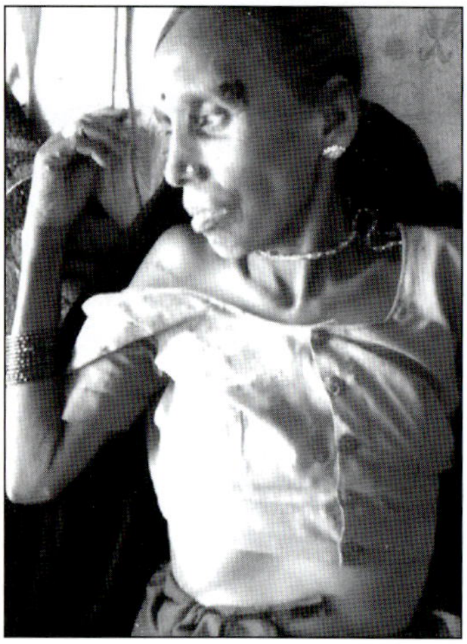

I finished my internship two years ago and got my MCI registration within 3-4 month of completion. Legally I was a doctor but socially and skillfully not. Every one of my batch was studying for the PG entrance. It's a dogma that if you do not do a PG (in any subject whether you like it or not) you are incomplete. I was not convinced. I was confused. I thought and decided to work for at least 2-3 years in a rural area. I wanted to explore various places and myself. I came to know about JSS and joined within 3 months of my internship. I did it quickly because I was suffocating in the four walls of medical education.

My real education was at JSS. Preventive and Social Medicine was a subject which we hated most in college. At JSS I actually realized what 'social' meant. To make aware and to implement the 'prevention' was more difficult than to read Harrison, or where tuberculosis was not just HRZE or DOTs, or PEM not just the lack of protein and energy or Malaria was not just giving Artesunate. Here I realized disease was the manifestation of social inequity and poverty.

Baba Amte used to say "In relationship with suffering". When I saw a 33 kg woman with TB, I was trying to imagine myself in her place but I could not even imagine it. I learnt the calorific value of various food materials at college but I learnt the significance of nutrition at JSS. A woman with TB was left by her husband along with three children, and there was no source of earning, what would you do? I asked myself this question and I was baffled. How could you learn this face of TB just by reading it 'social stigma'? There was a major difference between 'to be read' and 'to be seen'. Increase by 11 kg of weight after AKT was neither written in books nor taught in colleges. It told of how much the patient was starved of food. They don't teach Empathy and Approach towards a rural patient. You have to see the villages first.

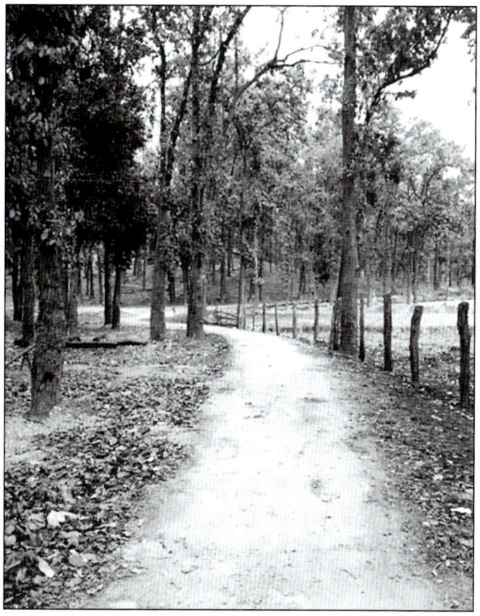

Investigations were one of the most abused parts of patient management. I never came across a thing like a rational investigation. We always used to advise a battery tests like – liver function test, renal function test but most of the time you did not need those investigations. I learnt that a significant amount of expenditure of the patient could be saved and also it stimulated us to improve our clinical skills.

Same with the medicines, we learn about generic medicines in colleges but while prescribing we used trade names. We had seen while in college, which MR (medical representative) was giving more money or gifts. We saw from residents to professors each one was seeking those gifts. Most of the time, they did not even think about the patient. I learned the importance of cost effectiveness and how important it was to cut the cost of treatment of a poor patient. This is why the approach was necessary.

One of my friends who was doing his PG, blamed rural people for not coming on time. I could have done the same thing if I had not experienced rural conditions. You never realized the woes of rural people sitting in a tertiary care hospital. A daily wage laborer cannot come on time without making arrangements of money for him and his family. A seven day stay at a tertiary hospital snatched so much from him. I saw this because I chose to witness it.

Many rural areas in India still lack primary health care. With no accessibility to hospitals, many die on the way. Many worsen on the way because of poor roads, poor vehicles or no ambulance. A few years back students used to prepare for PG from their internship, but now days it's from the second year of MBBS. You would be considered incompetent if you had not done PG. People would say "I will be settled once I get admission to MBBS" then during MBBS said "I will be settled after PG" and in PG some said "there is no point in doing plain PG, you have to do super specialty". I was confused, did we decide our skills or would our degrees decide our skills?

My perspective would not have been like this if I were doing PG now. I would not have understood this if would not come to JSS and to rural Chhattisgarh.

Some time I wonder is it just an illness which forces people to come to the doctor. Perhaps not, and being in their shoes and looking through their eyes I might get the answer. There was something beyond the illness, beyond the pain relief they needed. Probably, a word of togetherness, a word of consolation. They know that a doctor was a person who was able to hear so many sorrows so much pain throughout his lifetime. They hoped they had come to the right person. It was a responsibility to keep hope alive.
"It will be all right" these words may be sufficient for them.....I chose to be a doctor, I am happy to be a doctor.

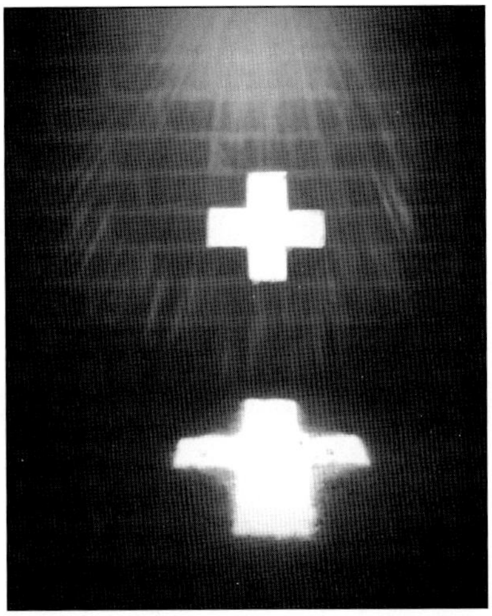

To tell someone that he should go to the villages and serve there is to force them. I liked to say "let's try". Being young I said "fasten your belts, lace your shoes and travel". You could not see the different colours of medicine unless you explore the 'Window', which I found. This window opened vast opportunities to learn and to develop one self. This window made your vision to see a 'person' not a 'patient'.

Abhijit Gadewar

Articles

health through the hunger lens

by Yogesh Jain with Jan Swasthya Sahyog

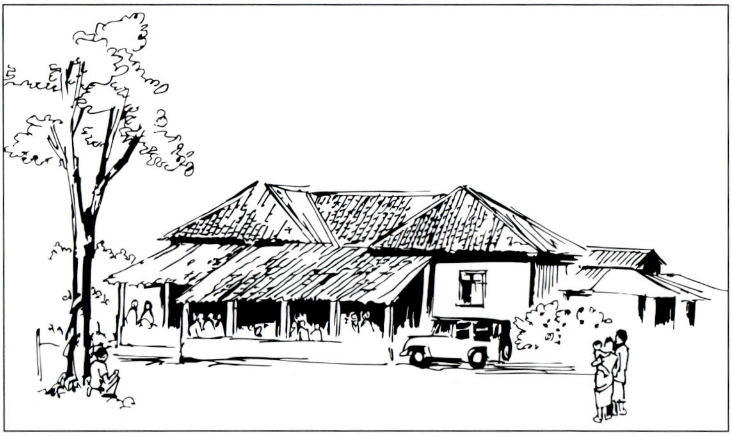

In tribal-dominated Chhattisgarh, where this writer works, men and women are at least 10 kg lighter than the reference Indian, and even the popular PDS rice scheme lasts a family only 11 days. The high burden of all diseases, from TB and malaria to cancer and heart disease, has clear links with the 'lifestyle' of poverty and hunger in this region.

On February 8, 2012, 36-year-old Dhansai Portey walked into our out-patient department. He was the image of a person literally consumed by tuberculosis. Though normal in height, he weighed just 35 kg. An x-ray of his chest revealed lungs that had turned almost white from the disease (normal is black). For the last six months or so, he had been experiencing several symptoms and had become too weak to pull a rickshaw to earn his living in Bilaspur, Chhattisgarh, in central India.

For me this was a familiar picture of deprivation and injustice, of which disease is only the embodiment. I have become immune to such medical situations which can only be described as 'violence'. The low body weight (at 36, Dhansai weighed as much as a 12-year-old child) led me to check for other causes of immune deficiency, such as HIV. Thankfully, these were negative. Dhansai told me that for the last six years he had been living with his wife and three children. Through the much-applauded public distribution system (PDS) in Chhattisgarh, he received 35 kg of rice a month, at Rs. 2 per kg. He ate almost nothing else. In fact, little remained of the Rs. 70-80 that he managed to earn from his rickshaw every day: Rs. 400 was spent on rent for his one-room tenement, and another Rs. 100 went on electricity every month.

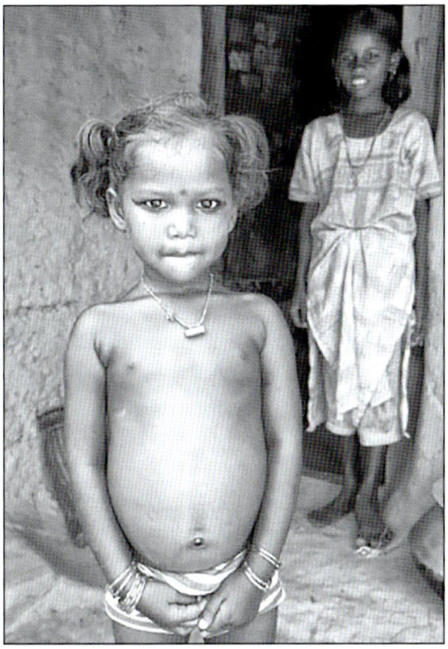

I thought about the drugs he should take; I worried whether he had acquired a resistance due to irrational anti-TB drug combinations prescribed by other doctors; I thought about the points that needed to be stressed during counselling; I wondered whether his weight loss was due to lack of food or because his symptoms had been ignored by the health system.

Records of his previous visit to Jan Swasthya Sahyog (JSS) seven months earlier showed his weight at 43 kg. He had come to look after his sister who was being treated for advanced tuberculosis requiring hospitalisation. Dhansai believed he had developed tuberculosis because he had been sleeping on the cold hospital floor. The physician who saw him then had prescribed analgesics for his bodyache and given him some iron tablets for his mild anaemia.

This long story taught me many things. One striking lesson was that we should have recognised that Dhansai was already at risk of developing tuberculosis when he came in with his sister last May. Though 8 kg heavier, he was already at much greater risk than someone like me, at 65 kg, who sees, along with others at JSS, over 500 new tuberculosis patients every year. Even in an organisation that is committed to understanding hunger as it relates to health, we did not appreciate Dhansai's greater risk of becoming a victim of what can only be called a 'disease of poverty or hunger'. Should something have been done when Dhansai first came to us at 43 kg?

Hunger

When I say that one-third of all men and about half of all women in India have weights or body masses less than Dhansai's 43 kg, it is not a mere nutrition statistic. Statistics confuse most of us, yet they are enormously significant. What the numbers tell me is that a large proportion of our people are at great risk of contracting illnesses like tuberculosis and worse. They are also less likely to survive these illnesses even if they do manage to receive the best treatment available. Those who survive may be left unable to work. Yet these facts do not impinge upon our consciousness, or even our conscience. Spurred on by Michelle Obama, American society, which recognises that the health costs of obesity due to overeating runs into billions of dollars, unleashes programmes to address the problem. We, on the other hand, occasionally distracted by the 'HUNGaMA' of statistics[1], continue to be blissfully smug and ignorant about the huge health costs of undernutrition, or its less sanitised synonym, hunger.

If the first question that occurred to me was: Should something have been done for Dhansai when he first came to JSS, the questions that followed were: What are 'good weights' for men and women? What about height? How does height and weight translate into an ability to earn, or into being healthy or unhealthy? How much food does a person require to remain healthy or to maintain a normal weight? What amount and type of food should the right to food entitlements and security and the right to good health translate to? And finally, when whole communities remain hungry what are the consequences on their health, at different points in life? Where do the present food entitlement programmes lead us? And is there hope for them?

I will explore some of these questions from the vantage point of the junction of health and hunger, situated as I am in a community health programme in an area where deprivation is entrenched; where, in fact, deprivation is actually promoted by the exploitation of rural areas, ineffective development programmes, and a public distribution system that has increasingly restricted its coverage. All of these lie within the rubric of structural violence.

If one gets enough to eat, the National Institute of Nutrition (NIN) recommends that, as a reference, a rural Indian adult man should weigh 60 kg and be 173 cm tall, and a woman should weigh 55 kg and be 161 cm tall[2]. These obviously are the ideal to which one must aspire. The mean heights of both men and women in India are lower than these references or standards by a little more than 10 cm. The National Family Health Survey does not publish data on weight alone, but it does give information on body mass index (BMI), a derived indicator representing weight for height, which is another measure of nutritional status. According to NFHS-3 data, going by the standards of BMI, as many as one-third of India's adults are undernourished, with a BMI of less than 18.5. There is also a clear pecking order in the social group, with scheduled tribes faring the worst, followed by scheduled castes, other backward castes, and the general category, in that order. There are also variations between states[3]. At JSS, among the people in tribal-dominated forest fringe villages, the median weights of men and women are 49 and 41.5 kg respectively, or at least 10 kg lighter than the reference Indian. And this has not changed in the last decade that we have worked here and collected such information.

Why are we so fixated on weights and heights? The reason is that these measures are robust indicators of food security. If you discount those who have certain psychiatric problems, no one would have a lower weight or height if he/she had access to adequate food. The proof of the pudding is in the eating. We can judge all processes like the efficacy of the PDS, the importance given to growing food crops, and the purchasing power of people by looking at body parameters like their weight and height. Besides, a person's height can also tell us whether adequate food was available during his/her childhood.

Why should we call undernutrition hunger? Let me give you a reason. Nutritionists say that to lose (as well as to gain) each kilo, the cost would be 7,000 calorie units. NIN and other bodies recommend 2,325 and 1,900 calories for the sedentary Indian man and woman respectively, and additional calories for physical work[4]. As mentioned above, Indian men and women weigh at least 10 kg less than what they would have weighed had they been eating well. Thus, the hunger cost of their nutrition is 70,000 calories. Even if we assume that an average Indian goes hungry by 500 calories every day, it would take at least 140 consecutive days to reach that state.

We can still choose to describe underweight and stunted people as 'malnourished' if we like. But I suggest the correct term would be 'hunger'.

How did food security get reduced to food 'entitlements'? That too, targeted at the officially poor? And that in turn into cereals alone? And that too into a magical figure of 35 kg, or, worse, 25? This is beyond my comprehension. One administrator in my own state of Chhattisgarh said it was his personal assumption -- not based on any research or guideline -- that an adult required 10 kg of cereals every month and a child 5 kg; thus, a family of five that had three children required 35 kg. Simple! The Food and Agriculture Organisation recommends that every person living on a predominantly, though not exclusively, cereal-based diet requires about 18 kg per month[5]. Our studies in Bilaspur, with an average family size of 5.5, aimed to look at how long PDS rice lasts. We learned that PDS grain (35 kg per family) lasts just 11 days. That leaves families to fend for themselves for the rest of the month, from the market or from their own produce. And the Food Security Bill is aiming for 25 kg per family!

Why only cereals? The Chhattisgarh government has piloted giving 2 kg of channa (gram) monthly to the officially poor in Bastar and Sarguja divisions; this may be extended to the rest of the state. It experimented with providing 1 kg of oil at a little less than the market rate, but that did not succeed. In Chhattisgarh, the JSS has recommended that the state implement a better PDS that would meet more than half people's calorie and protein intake[6]. We hope that the state will heed our plea.

Has the presence of a PDS ever shown an improvement in people's nutritional status, or in their food intake? I have not found any studies to show this, although some are still underway. It seems to me that at the very least, given that there are so many needs, the money saved due to the availability of subsidised foodgrain from the PDS allows people to buy other things, possibly other foods. With PDS food lasting just a few days, families are victims of spiralling food prices in the market.

Yet it is true that the public distribution system is quite popular, allowing the present government to come back for a second term. Efficient overseeing of this programme has plugged leakages, delays and non-delivery. It has weathered criticism from the middle class that people are less interested in agriculture due to easy availability of foodgrain for a majority of working people. Yet, it is inadequate. The people of Chhattisgarh have some of the poorest nutrition indicators in the country.

The consequences of food deprivation

How do we view the food situation from a health window? What we see are massive levels of morbidity which can be shown to be a consequence of deprivation, of which food deprivation is the most important one. In our clinics, we check the weights of everyone who attends any level of our health programme, and are astounded to find that the median weights of men and women are 42 kg in women and 49 kg in men. It may be argued that these are patients and therefore they have low weights. However, even among the healthy in the community, with 79% of them being adivasis, the median BMI is 19.1 among men and 18.4 in women, and the median heights are 160 cm and 151 cm respectively. These are in some ways not much worse than what is seen at the state or the country level. Given the stark association in our community between undernutrition on the one hand and high rates of disease and death on the other, we can easily imagine the situation across India for the deprived people of an entire country.

The first point that strikes us in our work is the massive numbers of people with sickness of all types. The prevalence rates of chronic illnesses like rheumatic heart disease, rheumatoid arthritis, cancers, asthma, low body weight, diabetes, hypertension and severe anaemia surprised us for some time, but now seem to make sense. The incidence rates of new illnesses like upper respiratory illnesses, pneumonias and soft tissue infections and tuberculosis are higher than we have seen in most literature on the health status of rural Indians, which itself is scarce. While the purists may question whether these huge numbers are directly attributable to hunger or food deprivation, or whether they should rather be associated with 'poverty', the weights and heights of people with these illnesses are compelling enough for us to attribute these diseases to food deprivation. At another level, we feel it is unnecessary to disentangle food deprivation from other forms of deprivation.

The second point is about the types of illnesses. If illnesses are biological 'embodiments' of deprivation, then we can really see the 'soul' of food deprivation through the illnesses. For example, we see a higher than expected incidence of maternal exhaustion during delivery, leading to higher caesarean rates for women with lower body weights. We also see a higher percentage of deaths in people with tuberculosis, among those with lower body weights.

Likewise, there are a massive number of hernias among underweight men.

We have wondered why we have malaria incidence and deaths peaking in November and December, months which are relatively cool and have lower mosquito biting rates (Figure 1).

Figure 1: Is malaria related to food availability or to nutrition?

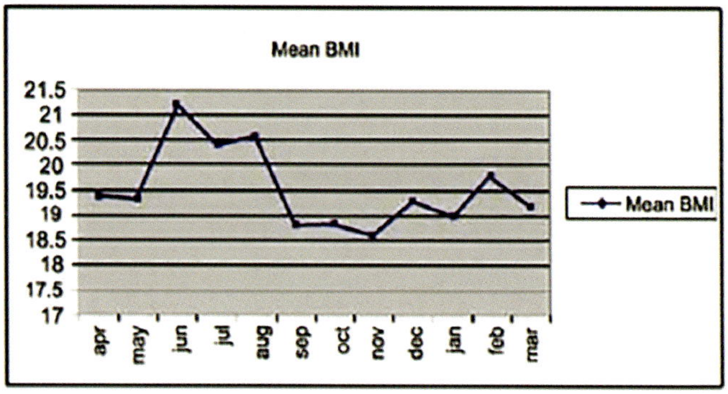

Figure 1-2: Seasonality of malaria 2002-2011, JSS Bilaspur

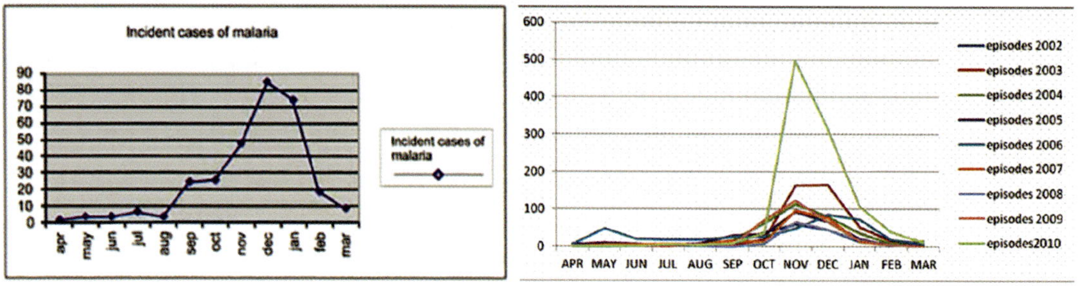

In most discussions on infectious diseases, the focus is on the agent -- the bacteria, virus or parasite -- the vector, and sometimes the environment. There is very little interest in the host, the person who suffers the illness. For example, in TB, one is obsessed with the bacteria and its spread through sputum, but not in people's weights which are so much more important. In malaria, the obsession is with resistance in the malarial parasite, or the mosquitoes, or water stagnation. There is very little about the determinants of the human being's vulnerability. One of the most important determinants is nutritional status.

In most of India, the major crop is sown pre-monsoon, in May-June, and harvested around November. Thus, food stocks for most people become available in December and then decrease over the year, even if there is a smaller, second crop. Food stocks are lowest just before the annual harvest in November. Indeed, when we check people's weights through the year, we find that weights are the lowest around harvest time. We suggest that the 'unseasonal' malaria outbreaks in central India are precipitated by the dip in nutrition in November and therefore an increased vulnerability in the host.

No one who works with malaria can deny the plausibility of this hypothesis. In fact, the association between hunger and malaria deaths has been elegantly argued in a study done almost a century ago in rural Punjab[7].

While tuberculosis, malaria, soft tissue infections, pneumonia with complications, and diarrhoeal deaths may be accepted as being due to the body's low immunity from hunger, which may have allowed these bugs to damage weak bodies, what surprised us is the pattern of what are called non-communicable diseases, or NCDs (Figure 2). The dominant discourse clamours for the recognition that NCDs are an emergency[8], and India is a diabetes capital.

The World Health Organisation has a uniform, single explanation for this problem -- the nutritional transition, or an improvement in people's nutrition, which gives rise to a new set of NCDs. But this discourse attributes NCDs to a sedentary lifestyle, an excessive intake of high-calorie refined foods with little of the fibre contained in fruit and vegetables, and tobacco use. Data from urban and peri-urban clinics and surveys links NCDs to increasing rates of obesity and higher weights. While this may be true in urban areas, the profile of

Figure 2: Community burden of illnesses in rural Bilaspur, JSS 2011

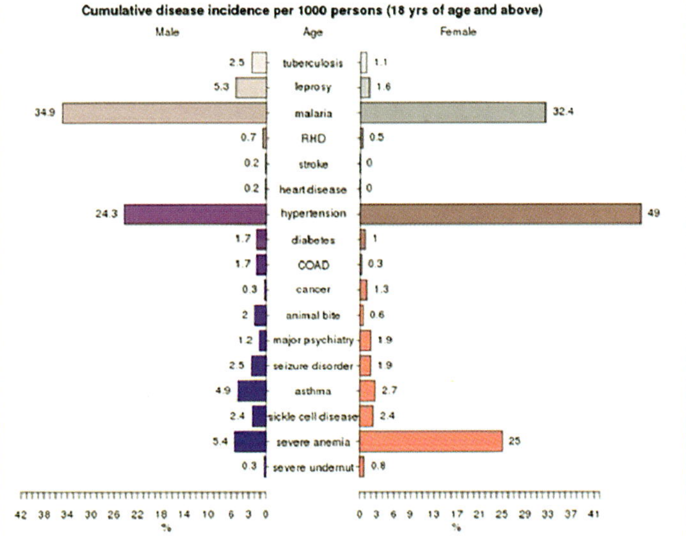

NCDs in rural areas has not been given due importance. In rural Bilaspur, we see a high prevalence of hypertension in the community; 16% of rural women more than 30 years old had hypertension and their weights or heights were not higher than in those without hypertension. In other words, their condition was not due to their nutrition. In 2011, we saw 400 new patients with cancers, 89 with rheumatic heart disease and 258 patients with diabetes (Figure 3). Similarly, 80% of people with diabetes seen here have low or normal weights, something that is the inverse of what is seen in urban areas. As a group of diseases, cancers are the second most prevalent morbidity at the JSS clinics, next only to tuberculosis. In fact, it would be appropriate to say that patients with diabetes or cancer or tuberculosis, in Ganiyari in Bilaspur, have more similarities to each other in terms of weight, dietary predicament, social and economic status than to people with the same biological ailment in a city like Delhi or Mumbai. We feel that NCDs in rural India are clearly linked to the same deprivation of food and other human needs as are tuberculosis and malaria; they are not linked to affluence. Illnesses are, in fact, reflections of local deprivation rather than mere biological events with universally common appearances.

Figure 3: Burden of major illnesses seen in the JSS community health programme, rural Bilaspur, January-December 2011

Illness	New patients seen
Tuberculosis	587
Leprosy	132
Hypertension	478
Rheumatic heart disease	89
Cancers	400
Condition requiring surgery	1,473
Sickle cell disease	99
Diabetes	258

There are some serious implications of neglecting the association between hunger and NCDs in mainstream discourse. If there is going to be a homogenous preventive clarion call for reducing NCDs by eating less, working or exercising more, and by stopping tobacco for both urban as well as rural people, for those who are overweight as well as those who have low weights, then there is a problem. If the 'lifestyle' of poverty and hunger that seems to be associated with these illnesses in rural central India is ignored and all NCDs globally are attributed to a sedentary lifestyle and excess consumption, then there is also a moral problem. In fact, by correctly highlighting the association between NCDs and deprivation, we can more strongly advocate another good and strong reason to ensure adequate and balanced food for all. The bluff of the WHO should be called.

Besides infectious diseases and NCDs, there are the core diseases of undernutrition, which deserve a third category. Rates of anaemia, including severe anaemia -- due to iron deficiency as well as malaria -- are frightfully high in both women and children, and are not much less in men[9]. While both mental and physical symptoms are attributed to even lower grades of anaemia for the rural person, it is the beginning of a vicious cycle of poor earning power, resulting in a reduced ability to purchase food, and so on. For a labourer, working with anaemia is like doing the job of a bull with the energy levels of a cow. Besides, it can't be stressed enough that anaemia poses the greatest risk of death and morbidity for women in labour because of a clearly increased chance of postpartum haemorrhage, which is the most important reason for maternal deaths in our country.

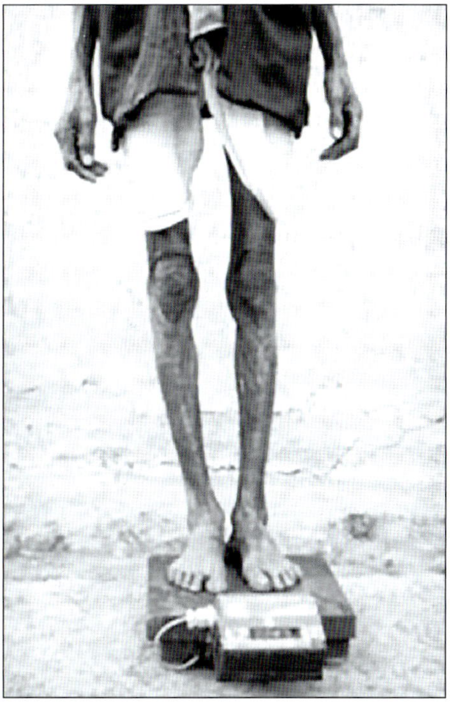

What about minerals other than iron? Most of them come from wholesome food that is associated with affluence. This includes foods that come from animal sources. Total body potassium falls in all patients with severe undernutrition, and this can lead to profound weakness. Similarly, calcium is a mineral that is more available in animal-based foods and its deficiency occurs due to deficiency of these foods plus the increased burden that women incur when they bear and suckle their babies, as calcium is extracted by the foetus as it grows, and then in breast milk. Its deficiency can cause severe painful spasms and weakness. Zinc too is a mineral of affluence and is often deficient in poor people's diets. While much is written in praise of this mineral, the best possibility of alleviating its deficiency comes from the consumption of more wholesome foods as well as increasing soil concentrations of the mineral.

And vitamins? We have a really confusing situation here. Certain minerals and vitamins are being promoted for the prevention of disease or to augment the effects of drug treatment. Micronutrient initiatives are posited almost as an alternative to the basic 'macronutrients' of calories and protein. We need to very carefully assess the health consequences of vitamin deficiency. In rural Bilaspur, we see high rates of night blindness among the poorest women during lactation and pregnancy. Vitamin A has reparative properties: it helps in the healing process, building tissue destroyed through infections. Deficiency of this vitamin can have important consequences in a situation where infections, even if they are minor, are so common. But it may be prudent to say that vitamin deficiency almost mirrors the deficiency of macronutrients, and thus ensuring food in a balanced way will surely be able to look after these deficiencies too. There do not seem to be compelling health reasons to have special vitamin deficiency treatment programmes.

The biggest wealth of poor people is their ability to labour. Thus, the biggest health consequence of poor nutrition that we see is in the ability to labour. This ability is clearly affected by lower weights and heights. This translates to poor earnings which, by reducing the purchasing power of people, results in a continuation of the vicious cycle. Given the fact that wages are given according to work output, according to prescribed rates, it would be interesting to see how the weights of people correlate with their work output and earnings at MGNREGS sites. It seems that people with hunger and poor weights are at a disadvantage compared to their peers who eat better and weigh more.

The unfairness of this is complete when one realises that all calculations of caloric requirement that may go into any food distribution systems are defined on the basis of a sedentary lifestyle. Who cares that people with heavy work schedules and who live off the land need almost double the amount of food compared to those who live off the pen or their minds!

Endnotes

1. The HUNGaMA Survey Report 2011. Available at www.naandi.org/CP/Hungama BKDec11LR.pdf

2. Nutrient Requirements and Recommended Dietary Allowances for Indians: A Report of the Expert Group of the Indian Council of Medical Research'. New Delhi: ICMR; 2009. pp 24-9

3. National Family Health Survey-3, 2005-2006. Chapter 10. 'Maternal and Child Nutrition. Nutrition and Anaemia'. p 304 4 ICMR, 2009. p 66

5. Indian Experience on Household Food and Nutrition Security: Nutritional Requirements in India. www.fao.org/docrep/x0172e/x0172e02.htm

6. Jan Swasthya Sahyog. 'An Enhanced PDS for Better Nutrition and Health of the People: Suggestions for Implementation in Chhattisgarh'. Recommendations submitted to the chief minister and chief secretary. 2011. March 18

7. Christopher S R. Malaria in the Punjab, Calcutta: Superintendent Government Printing. 1911

8. Narain J P, Garg R, Fric A. 'Non-communicable Diseases in the South East Asia Region: Burden, Strategies and Opportunities. National Journal of Medicine. India. 2011; 24: 280-7

9. NFHS-3. p 288

burden & pattern of illnesses among the tribal communities in central India : a report from a community health programme

Yogesh Jain, Raman Kataria, Sushil Patil, Suhas Kadam, Anju Kataria, Rachna Jain, Ravindra Kurbude & Sharayu Shinde

Jan Swasthya Sahyog, Village and Post Ganiyari, Bilaspur (Chhattisgarh), India

Tribals are the most marginalised social category in the country and there is little and scattered information on the actual burden and pattern of illnesses they suffer from. This study provides information on burden and pattern of diseases among tribals, and whether these can be linked to their nutritional status, especially in particularly vulnerable tribal groups (PVTG) seen at a community health programme being run in the tribal areas of Chhattisgarh and Madhya Pradesh States of India. This community based programme, known as Jan Swasthya Sahyog (JSS) has been serving people in over 2500 villages in rural central India. It was found that the tribals had significantly higher proportion of all tuberculosis, sputum positive tuberculosis, severe hypertension, illnesses that require major surgery as a primary therapeutic intervention and cancers than non tribals. The proportions of people with rheumatic heart disease, sickle cell disease and epilepsy were not significantly different between different social groups. Nutritional levels of tribals were poor. Tribals in central India suffer a disproportionate burden of both communicable and non communicable diseases amidst worrisome levels of undernutrition. There is a need for universal health coverage with preferential care for the tribals, especially those belonging to the PVTG. Further, the high level of undernutrition demands a more augmented and universal Public Distribution System.

Key words Burden of illnesses - Cancer - diabetes - non-communicable diseases - particularly vulnerable tribal groups (PVTG) - Tuberculosis - surgical needs - tribals - under nutrition

Introduction

While there is a broad consensus that tribals are among the poorest social groups in the country[1], and figures about high levels of undernutrition among tribal adults and children are available[2], a concomitant concern about the illnesses they suffer from is not so obvious[3,4].There is little and scattered information on the actual burden and patterns of the illnesses that afflict them[1,4,5-7]. The challenge of inaccessibility to health services and their health care seeking behaviour seem to dominate the discourse in tribal health[1,6]. Further, it is still believed that tribals suffer mainly from infections and selected non-communicable diseases such as hypertension while other illnesses like cancer, diabetes, mental illnesses, illnesses that require surgery and heart diseases are thought to be uncommon among them[8-12].

The context and the people

Jan Swasthya Sahyog (People's Health Support Group or JSS) is a group of health professionals running a community health programme with a three tiered structure that includes a referral hospital accessed by people from over 2500 villages drawn from seven districts of Bilaspur, Kawardha, Janjgir-Champa, and Korba of Chhattisgarh and Dindori, Anuppur and Shahdol of Eastern Madhya Pradesh (Fig. 1) for their major health care needs, three outreach clinics in forest fringe and forest village clusters serving about 150 villages and an intensive community programme served by two hamlet based village health workers each in 70 forest villages. in the intensive community programme 67 per cent of the people are tribals whereas 32 per cent patients who access the referral centre are tribals. The most common tribes in the area are the Gonds, Baigas, Kols, Kanwar, Oraons, Dhanuhar, Bhumias and Manjhis; 19 per cent of the total population in the intensive community programme and 2.4 per cent of those attending the referral centre belong to the particularly vulnerable tribal groups (PVTG) such as Baigas, Dhanuhars and Manjhis. In the community programme, 65.5 per cent families had a Below Poverty Line (BPL) card whereas 2.9 per cent had an Antyodyaya card. Twenty two per cent families were landless and the median land holding was 1.8 acres per household. At the referral centre, data from people attending one single outpatient clinic suggested that 77.5 per cent were living in kachcha houses, 14.8 per cent in semi-pucca houses and only 7.8 per cent were living in pucca houses. Fifty three per cent of the outpatients possessed a Rashtriya Swasthya Bima Yojana card, and almost 90.1 per cent had a food rations BPL card issued by the government of Chhattisgarh or Madhya Pradesh.

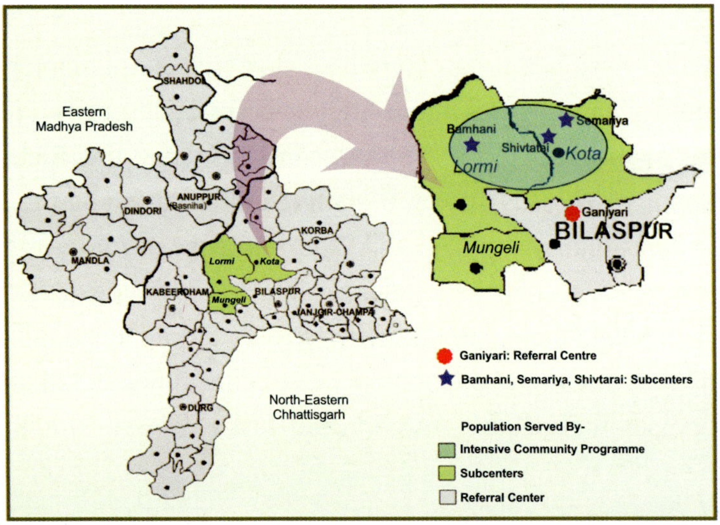

Fig. 1. Regions of Chhattisgarh and Madhya Pradesh States from where patients come to Jan Swasthya Sahyog (JSS) health centres.

This community health programme has been running for the last 15 years. The demographic, nutritional and disease related information on these tribal communities has been collected to understand the burden of illnesses we faced and tried to answer the following questions: (i) What are the burden and the spectrum of illnesses in a tribal population of this area when a reasonable effective health care service is provided?; (ii) Do tribals have a less complex pattern of illnesses than non-tribals?; (iii) Do tribals suffer from less or more proportion of common illnesses such as tuberculosis, diabetes, cancer and other illnesses than non tribals?; (iv) What is the nutritional status of the people who present with these illnesses, and does it differ between various people belonging to different social categories?; and (v) Do people belonging to the PVTGs have worse nutritional status or illness presentations than among non PVTGs?

The referral centre provides comprehensive primary, secondary and where necessary appropriate tertiary care for many illnesses; for example, obstetric emergencies, ultrasonography, CT/MRI and laboratory investigations for serology, microbiology, hormonal assays, blood transfusion where necessary, treating drug resistant and complicated tuberculosis, severe anaemia, severe falciparum malaria, sickle cell disease including crisis, offering common surgeries, surgical and chemotherapy based cancer care, group therapy to people with alcohol dependence and secondary level care for mental health problems.

We present here data on pattern of illnesses and undernutrition, collected and analysed for over a period of 14 years, but majority of the data are for four years, 2010 to 2013.

Anthropometric data as a measure of the nutritional status and data of several major illnesses as well as demographic information of all people were recorded electronically. Weights to the nearest 100 grams and heights or lengths (below 2 yr of age) to the nearest centimetre were recorded for all patients who attended the referral hospital and the sub-centres at each visit, and body mass index calculated.

Data were also collected for the serious manifestations of some illnesses in social categories. These manifestations included proportion of advanced forms of cancer cervix such as stages 2B, 3 and 4; proportion of sputum positive tuberculosis as proportion of all pulmonary tuberculosis; proportion of all extra-pulmonary tuberculosis as part of all patients with the disease; proportion of those illnesses that require major surgery; proportion of non-obese diabetes as proportion of all diabetes; and proportion of lepromatous or borderline lepromatous leprosy. The pattern of three indicative illnesses, tuberculosis, diabetes and cancers was studied. the overall health and nutritional status of the people belonging to the PVTG and other tribal groups was assessed.

In the JSS clinics, major illnesses such as tuberculosis, rheumatic heart disease (RHD), diabetes mellitus (DM), cancers, severe hypertension, illnesses that require surgery as their primary treatment and leprosy were seen in substantial numbers during 2010-2013 (Table I). The hospitalization rate for people who belonged to the community programme (n = 35,669) at the JSS health service was 14.6 per 1000 in 2012, which was similar to that of other urban areas in India[13]. All tuberculosis, pulmonary tuberculosis and cancers were disproportionately more among tribals than non tribals ($p < 0.001$), whereas diabetes and sputum positive tuberculosis as a proportion of all pulmonary tuberculosis was more common among the non tribals (Table I). Further, those illnesses that require major surgery

Table I. Patients seen at *Jan Swasthya Sahyog* (JSS) clinics, 2010-2013

Illness	All	Non-*adivasis*	Tribal excluding *Baigas*	*Baigas*	*P* value
OPD attendance	59039	40115	17560	1364	
All tuberculosis	1993	1070 (2.67)	812 (4.62)	111 (8.14)	<0.001
Pulmonary tuberculosis	1272 (of 1993)	587 (54.86)	601 (74.01)	84 (75.68)	<0.001
Sputum positive tuberculosis	894 (of 1272)	451 (76.83)	392 (55.92)	51 (60.71)	<0.001
Rheumatic heart disease	383	258 (0.64)	118 (0.68)	7 (0.51)	0.792
Diabetes	1061	825 (2.06)	224 (1.28)	12 (0.88)	<0.001
Severe hypertension (180 or diastolic 110mm Hg)	1153	734 (1.83)	396 (2.26)	23 (1.69)	0.002
Cancers	1635	1037 (2.59)	559 (3.18)	39 (2.86)	<0.001
Illnesses requiring major surgery	2192	1474 (3.67)	633 (3.60)	85 (6.23)	<0.0001
Leprosy	513	337 (0.84)	156 (0.89)	20 (1.47)	<0.05
Lepromatous leprosy	137	91 (27.0)	40 (25.64)	6 (30)	0.90

Values in parentheses represent percentages, *P* values according to Chi-square Test or Fisher's exact test.

for their treatment and leprosy were significantly more common among people belonging to the particularly vulnerable tribal groups than among the non tribals. Rheumatic heart disease was not observed to be differently distributed among the social categories.

In the intensive community programme, many communicable illnesses such as tuberculosis, malaria and leprosy and several non-communicable diseases such as cancers, epilepsy, sickle cell disease, diabetes mellitus and severe hypertension were observed. The prevalence of tuberculosis, cancer and leprosy was significantly higher among the tribals than among non tribals. The presence of epilepsy, and rheumatic heart disease was observed to be similar among tribals and non tribals (Table II). Further, the non tribals were observed to have a higher prevalence of those illnesses that require surgery for treatment (Table II). People belonging to the PVTG groups had a higher proportion of all tuberculosis, while they seem to have a lower prevalence of cancers, severe hypertension and diabetes than the others.

Comparison of different illnesses in the referral centre

Looking at the diagnostic category of all newly registered patients over one calendar month it was found that almost all illnesses such as cancers, infections (acute and chronic), non-communicable diseases, maternal and child health problems, nutrition deficiency diseases

Table II. Data from community health programme villages of JSS (2000-2013)					
Illness	Total cases	Non-tribal population	Tribal excluding PVTGs	PVTGs	*P* value
Total population of the villages		11771	17186	6712	
Tuberculosis	87	19 (0.16)	37 (0.22)	31 (0.46)	<0.001
Sputum positive tuberculosis	53 (out of 87)	14 (73.68)	25 (67.57)	14 (75.16)	0.083
Rheumatic heart disease	44	10/6534 (0.15)	24/10191 (0.24)	10/3074 (0.33)	0.227
Diabetes	50	20/5212 (0.38)	29/7580 (0.38)	1/3000 (0.03)	0.002
Severe hypertension	229	74 (0.63)	112 (0.64)	23 (0.34)	0.014
Illnesses requiring major surgery	336	136 (1.16)	156 (0.91)	44 (0.66)	0.002
Cancer	139	45/8274 (0.41)	71/12033 (0.59)	13/4763 (0.27)	0.032
Sickle cell disease	119	34/8274 (0.41)	54/14059 (0.38)	31/4763 (0.65)	0.05
Leprosy	62	13 (0.11)	44 (0.26)	5 (0.074)	0.001
Epilepsy	167	51/8274 (0.62)	84/12033 (0.7)	32/4763 (0.67)	0.281

Values in parentheses represent percentages. *P* values according to Chi-square Test or Fisher's exact test.

and those due to poor access such as neglected trauma, and those due to animal bites were seen (Fig. 2). When looked for numbers of selected communicable and non-communicable

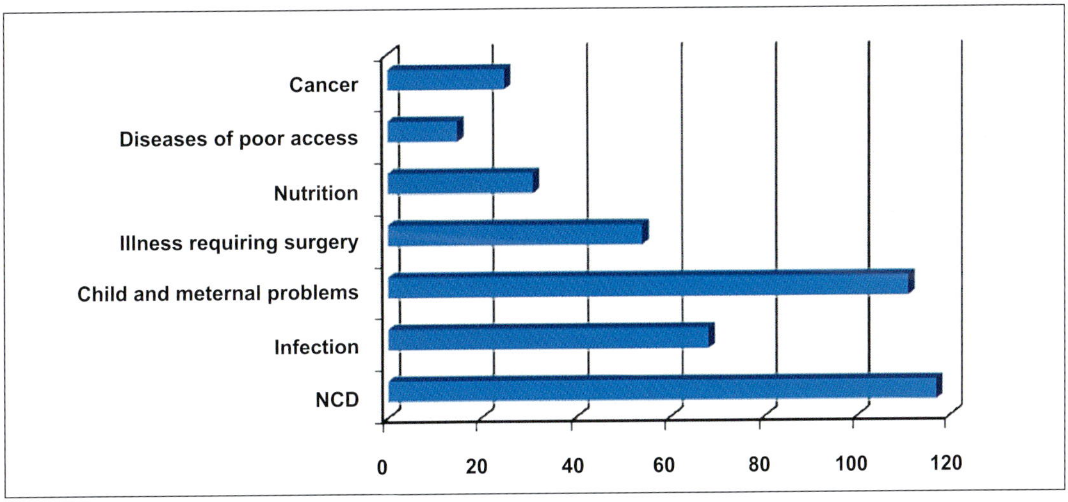

Fig. 2. Spectrum of illnesses for new patients over one calendar month (November 2010) in the referral centre. NCD, non-communicable diseases

diseases in one calendar year (2013) at the referral centre (Fig. 3), patients with severe hypertension, TB, cancer and DM were found in substantial numbers.

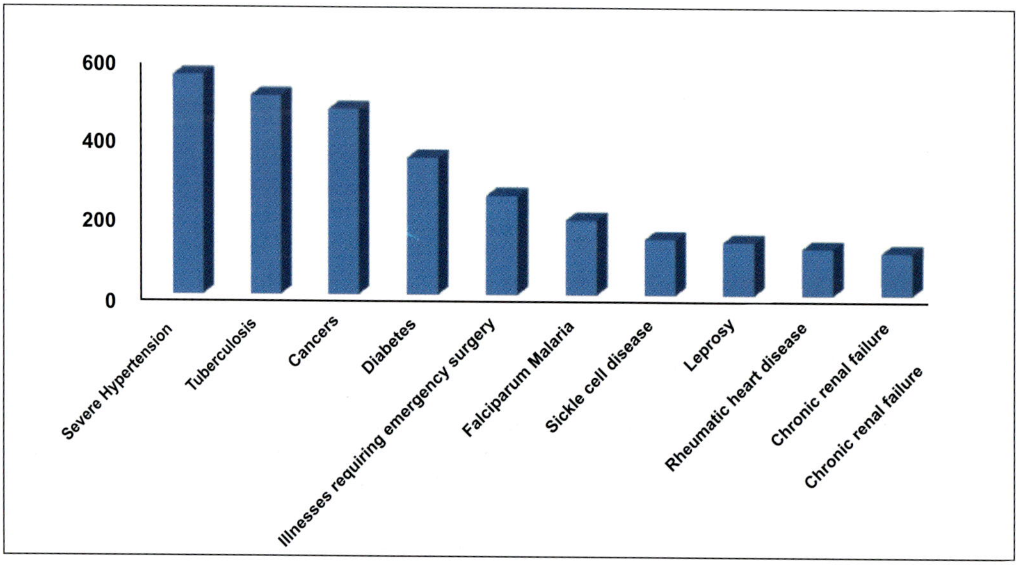

Fig. 3. number of new diagnosis of selected major illnesses in one year (2013).

Nutritional status of people

Anthropometric status of all new patients who attended the JSS referral centre during 2010-2013 showed a clear gradient of weight, height and body mass index across social groups, paralleling their socio-economic development (Table III).

The sex ratio of the patients seen for all illnesses suggested a clear preference for more women showing at the referral centre across all social groups. Over the last four years (2010-2013), 31,461 women attended the outpatient clinics compared to 27,578 men. Further, 47.9 per cent of people with body mass index (BMI) less than 16 kg/m2were tribals, but only 16.1 per cent of those with BMI more than 25 were tribals (Fig. 4). The proportion of tribals in the higher BMI categories appeared to have declined.

In the self-help groups in the community programme, the proportion of women with

Table III. Social group wise median weights, heights (cm), body mass index (bMI), gender disaggregated of patients seen at JSS referral centre OPD (2010-2013, n = 47,216 patients)

Social groups	Weight (kg) (n=47601)		Height (cm) (n=6336)		bMI (kg/m ^{2}) (n=6329)	
	Men (n= 21706)	Women (n= 25895)	Men (n= 2888)	Women (n= 3448)	Men (n= 2883)	Women (n= 3446)
PVTGs	46.3 (41.8-52.1)	40.55 (36-45.6)	160 (154-164)	151 (147-153)	17.55 (15.77-19.25)	17.68 (16.08-20.30)
Non PVTGs tribal	49.4 (44.6-54.6)	42.6 (38.1-47.7)	162 (158-166)	152 (148-155)	18.65 (16.93-20.40)	18.56 (16.90-20.69)
Scheduled Caste	50.9 (45.6-57.1)	44.2 (39.3-50.8)	163 (158-166)	151 (148-155)	19.38 (17.36-21.62)	19.46 (17.51-22.40)
ObCs	50.6 (45.5-56.6)	44.1 (39.5-50.1)	162 (158-166)	151 (148-155)	19.18 (17.51-21.53)	19.68 (17.66-22.07)
General	55 (48.3-63.8)	48.8 (42.3-58.4)	165 (161-169)	152 (149-156)	19.78 (17.84-22.63)	20.46 (18.38-23.67)

ObC, other backward classes; PVTGs, particularly vulnerable tribal groups.
Values in parentheses indicate 95% CI

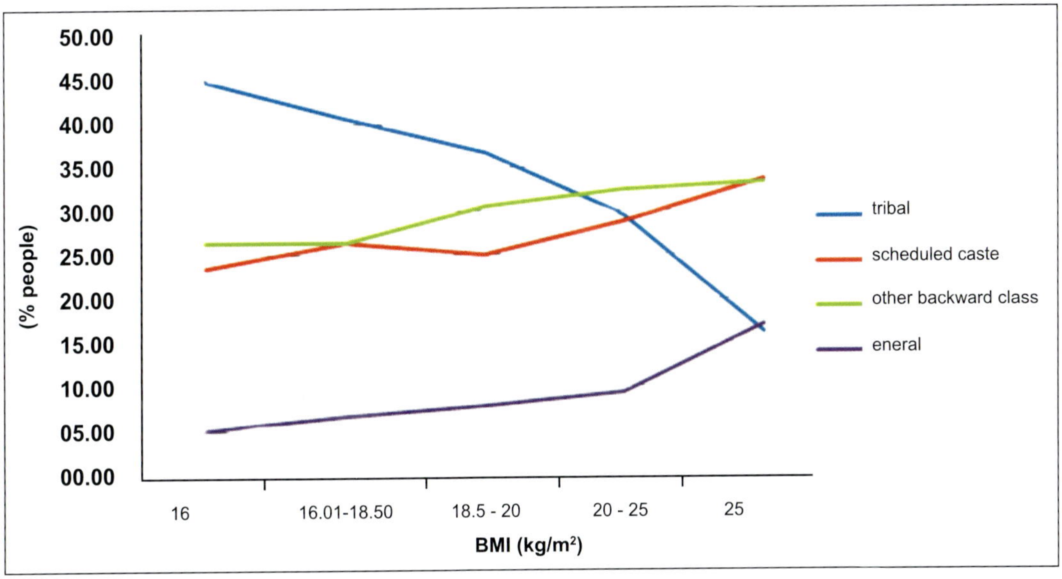

Fig. 4. Proportion of people (in %) in different BMI categories in each social category. STs, scheduled tribes; SCs, scheduled ceastes; OBC, other backward classes.

abnormally high waist-hip ratio was less in tribal women than in women of other social groups. The proportion of women with abnormally high waist-hip ratio (more than 0.9) was 32.5 per cent among OBCs and Schedule Castes, where as it was 23.4 per cent among tribal women.

Tuberculosis

The median weights and BMI of people with tuberculosis were 42.4 kg and 16.2 kg/m2 in men and 36.4 kg and 15.8 kg/m2 in women, respectively among 1517 adult patients seen over 2010 to 2013. More women (260 of 481, 54 %) than men (485 of 1036, 46.8%) had severe undernutrition (BMI $<$ 16 kg/m2) ($P = 0.008$). While people from several social categories such as tribal, Schedule Castes and OBCs had low median weights and BMI, no significant difference was observed between their anthropometric status. Median BMIs were not different between tribals and non tribals.

Not surprisingly, sputum positive tuberculosis was high as a proportion of all pulmonary tuberculosis in all groups of patients (894 of 1272; 70.2%), suggesting delayed presentation. Further, 443 of 685 tribals with pulmonary tuberculosis were sputum positive compared to 451 of 587 in the non tribals ($p < 0.001$) (Table I). There were 95 deaths (4.8%) in four years. Seventy two per cent of these deaths happened in those with BMI less than 16.

Diabetes mellitus

In the clinic, 1061 new patients presented with diabetes over the four years (2010 to 2013) (Table I). Overall, 75 per cent of them had a BMI <23, and 44.7 per cent had BMI <18.5 kg/m2. People from all social groups had diabetes, with tribals accounting for 22 per cent. The SC, ST and OBC accounted for 86.3 per cent of all diabetes patients, and as many as 90 per cent were living in rural areas. Among all, 29 per cent patients with DM presented before the age of 40 yr, and 59 per cent before the age of 50 yr. Median BMI of adult diabetes patients among tribals was lower than in other social groups according to the gender and the social category (Fig. 5). The proportion of patients with BMI <18.5 kg/m2 was high (70.69%) among tribals, compared to other groups (Dalits - 34.74%, OBCs - 43.62%, and general 23.68%). Sixteen per cent patients required insulin for treatment.

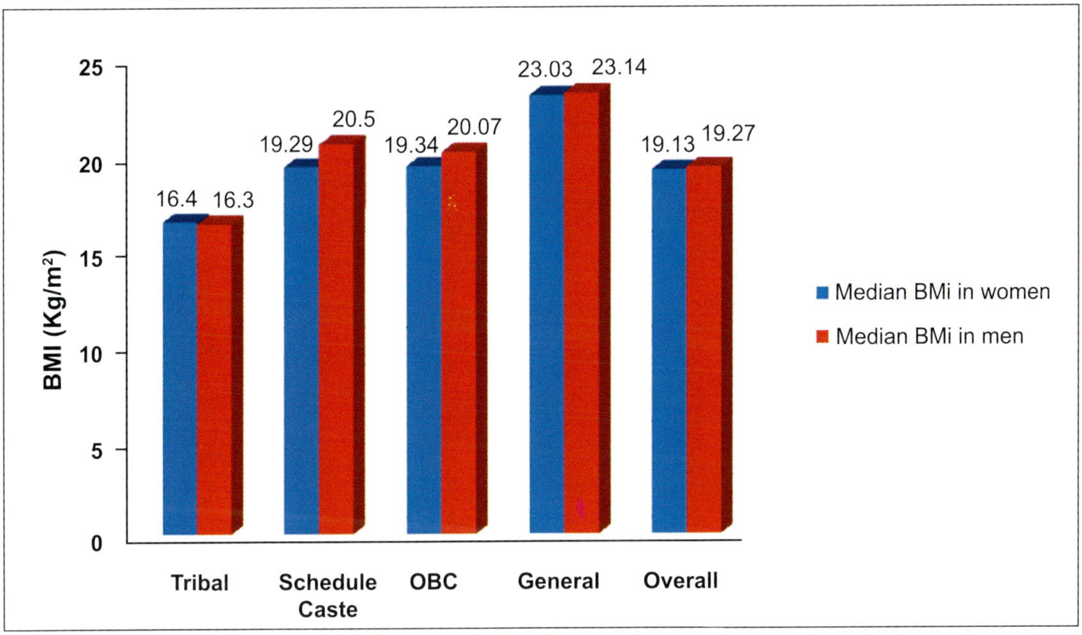

Fig. 5. Median BMI of all adults with diabetes according to the gender and the social category. OBC, other backward classes.

Cancer

Table IV. Types of cancers by gender at JSS referral centre (2009-2013)

Cancer types	Among men Number (%) of patients	Among women Number (%) of patients
Genitourinary (Cancer cervix for women)	63 (10.34)	601 (51.41)
Ovary	0 (0)	68 (5.82)
breast	0 (0)	154 (13.17)
Oral	177 (29.06)	94 (8.04)
Gastrointestinal	134 (22)	71 (6.07)
Others	235 (38.59)	181 (15.48)
Total	609 (100)	1169 (100)

At JSS, in five years (2009-2013) 1778 new patients were diagnosed with cancers. Women accounted for almost two thirds of the total cancer patients. Tribals accounted for 643 of these 1778 patients (36.1%). The proportion of women in each of the social groups varied between 60 to 70 percent (Table IV). The pattern of the cancers did not suggest any specific predilection for any type of cancer to occur in any specific social group.

Health of the particularly vulnerable tribal groups (PVTG)

In a quick evaluation of about 700 households drawn from 19 randomly selected Baiga PVTG hamlets during 2013-2014, it was found that 91 per cent of them were staying in kachcha houses, 34 per cent of them having wired electricity connection and erratic electricity supply and 10 per cent had toilet availability inside the homes. Further, while studying the nutrition status of the Baigas among the PVTGs, a worrisome situation of adult undernutrition in both men and women was observed. The median weights of men and women among 1200 consecutive adults Baiga PVTG were 47 and 40 kg, respectively. Compared with non Baiga PVTG women (median weights 45 kg) from the same villages, Baiga women were at least 5 kg lighter; 25 per cent of these apparently healthy Baiga PVTG women weighted 37 kg or lower. The median height of adult Baiga women was 150 cm and that of men was 160 cm. Using 3rd percentile of the National Centre for Health Statistics (NCHS) standards for height at 18 yr of age of 163 cm for men and 151 cm for women as a reference cut-off 10, 66.4 and 58.2 per cent of Baiga men and women, respectively were stunted, compared with 38.6 per cent of non Baiga women with stunted growth.

Table V shows that of the 1205 adult Baiga PVTG studied, about half (51.4%) had BMI <18.5 kg/m2 (47.7% men, 54.4% women). Of these, 10.8 per cent (7.2% men and 13.6 % women) had BMI <16 kg/m2. Only 1.3 per cent men and 1.8 per cent women had BMI >25 kg/m2.

This community health programme provides the estimates of disease burden largely reflecting passive case detection and is an underestimation of the true prevalence/incidence of most illnesses in the tribal community. An unequal high burden of illnesses was observed among tribals along with poor levels of nutrition.

There were several lacunae in the data such as completeness and small numbers in some illnesses. Further, data on maternal deaths were not collected. While there are studies documenting large numbers of people with hypertension and diabetes[9,14], the large numbers of tribals with rheumatic heart diseases, illnesses requiring surgical care, animal bites, chronic renal failure as well as large numbers and more complex presentations of major communicable diseases have not been documented before. With a relative risk of 4.49 for developing tuberculosis at a BMI 18.515 kg/m2[15] and a RR of 2 in the risk of death with BMI lower than 16[16], much higher burden as well as poorer outcomes would be expected in tribals due to their poorer nutritional status.

Falciparum malaria is one of the biggest illnesses being faced by tribals. Tribals constitute only 8.6 per cent of the population according to the census 2011 data but account for about 30 per cent of all cases of malaria and 50 per cent of malaria deaths[17,18].

Within the tribals, it was found that the health condition of PVTGs was much worse. The levels of undernutrition among the PVTGs were a cause of concern considering the fact that these were all normal adults working in the community. Compared to the national data of BMI in adults as seen in the National Family Health Survey-3 (NFHS-3)[19] which showed 35.6 per cent of women and 34.2 per cent of men in the age group of 15-49 yr were undernourished, among the Baigas 54.4 per cent men and 47.7 per cent women were at least 15 percentage points higher than them. As many as 13 per cent women and seven per cent men had severe undernutrition as suggested by a BMI < 16 kg/m2. The rates of undernutrition put half of all adult Baigas at five times higher risk of getting tuberculosis than if they had a normal nutritional status.

The Indian Council of Medical Research (ICMR) has recommended weights and heights of 60 kg and 173 cm for adult Indian men, and 55 kg and 162 cm for adult Indian women[20]. Only 1.3 per cent men and 1.8 per cent women among Baigas had a BMI > 25 kg/m2.

An obvious association between undernutrition and the burden of illnesses has emerged

Table V. body mass index (kg/m ^{2}) distribution among PVTG men and women

Category	Total adults	Per cent in all	No. (%) Men	No. (%) Women
bMI less than 18.5	620	51.4	251 (47.7)	369 (54.4)
• bMI less than 16	130	10.8	38 (7.2)	92 (13.6)
• bMI between 16.01 and 17	172	14.3	62 (11.8)	110 (16.2)
• bMI between 17.01 and 18.49	318	26.4	151 (28.7)	167 (24.6)
bMI between 18.50 and 24.99	566	47	269 (51.0)	297 (43.8)
bMI 25 and above	19	1.6	7 (1.3)	12 (1.8)
Total	1205	100	527 (100)	678 (100)

among these social groups. In illnesses like tuberculosis, the relative risk for undernutrition is well known, but similar associations for illnesses like diabetes, or hypertension or falciparum malaria are not so well known.

There is a need to have a more augmented and universal Public distribution system (PDS) that is not only looking at cereals, but also has a focus on promoting pulses and oilseeds cultivation by offering minimum support prices, by regaining highlands for cultivation and by offering cheap and good quality seeds.

We observed a high proportion of tuberculosis among the tribals, and within them among the PVTG. Among tribals there was a high proportion of those with tuberculosis and severe undernutrition (BMI < 16 kg/m2). This has been documented in the past[21,22].

There is a need to understand diabetes that we see among people in tribal areas. The median BMI of tribals with diabetes were 16.3 and 16.4 kg/m2, respectively for men and women and over 70 per cent had BMI less than 18.5. This is in contrast with the usual association between obesity and diabetes[22]. This high prevalence of undernutrition was in contrast to other clinic/hospital based reports from urban India which indicated the prevalence of low body weight in type 2 DM in only a 3.5-29 per cent[24]. It is possible that there are different phenotypes of adult onset diabetes. At JSS, the median age of onset among diabetes patients was found to be 37.5 yr in women and 45 yr in men of Baiga tribe, while it was 50 yr for both women and men with diabetes belonging to other social groups. This accelerated age of onset of diabetes in India has been noted in other studies[25,26] as well, but the reasons are unclear.

Given the spectrum of illnesses among tribals, universal health coverage is the only way forward as there is a heavy disease burden among the tribals.

Acknowledgment

Authors thank all the founding doctors- C Sathyamala, Anurag Bhargava, Biswaroop Chatterjee, Madhuri Chatterjee, Madhavi Bhargava, Pramod Upadhyay as well as Surabhi Sharma, Ramani Atkuri, Ravi D'Souza and other doctors who worked in this health programme as were as over 200 other health professionals who work and run this work.

References

1. Balgir R. Tribal health problems, disease burden and ameliorative challenges in tribal communities with special emphasis on tribes of Orissa; 2006. Available from: http://www.rmrct.org/files_rmrc_web/centre's_publications/NSTH_06/NSTH06_22.RS.Balgir.pdf, accessed on September 28, 2014.

2. Rao VG, Yadav R, Dolla CK, Kumar S, Bhondeley MK, Ukey 2. M. Undernutrition & childhood morbidities among tribal preschool children. Indian J Med Res. 2005;122 : 43-7.

3. Kshatriya G. Changing perspectives of tribal health in the 3. context of increasing lifestyle diseases in India. J Environ Soc Sci 2014; 1 : 1-7.

4. Das S. Childhood undernutrition: A comparative analysis of 4. Scheduled Tribes and others in the mid-Indian Tribal Region. Social Change 2008; 38 : 64-83.

5. Planning Commission of Government of India. 5. Report of the Working Group on Communicable Disease Burden for the 12th Five Year Plan. New Delhi: Planning Commission; 2011.

6. Planning Commission of Government of India. 6. Report of the Working Group on Non-Communicable Disease Burden for 12th Five Year Plan. New Delhi: Planning Commission; 2011.

7. Kasar PK, Toppo NA. Prevalence, awareness, treatment and 7. control of hypertension and diabetes among tribal population of central India : A cross-secttional study. IEA World Congr Epidemiol 2014; 1-2.

8. Tribhuwan RD. 8. Health, medicine, and nutrition of the tribals. New Delhi: Discovery Publishing House Pvt. Ltd.; 2004: p. 72.

9. Rizwan S, Kumar R, Singh AK, Kusuma YS, Yadav K, Pandav 9. CS. Prevalence of hypertension in Indian tribes: a systematic review and meta-analysis of observational studies. PLoS One 2014; 9(5) : e95896.

10. Muniyadi M, Singh N. Tribal health inequity: Challenges 10. remain. Tribal Heal Bull 2013; 17 : 8-14.

11. World Health Organization (WHO). In: 11. Global status report on noncommunicable diseases 2010: Burden: mortality, morbidity and risk factors. Geneva: WHO; 2010. p. 9-31.

12. Kerketta AS, Bulliyya G, Babu BV, Mohapatra SS, Nayak 12. RN. Health status of the elderly population among four primitive tribes of Orissa, India: a clinico-epidemiological study. Z Gerontol Geriatr 2009; 42 : 53-9.

13. Ranson M. Reduction of catastrophic health care expenditures 13. by a community-based health insurance scheme in Gujarat, India: current experiences and challenges. Bull World Health Organ 2002; 1 : 613-21.

14. Upadhyay RP, Misra P, Chellaiyan VG, Das TK, Adhikary 14. M, Chinnakali P, et al. Burden of diabetes mellitus and prediabetes in tribal population of India: a systematic review. Diabetes Res Clin Pract 2013; 102 : 1-7.

15. Cegielski JP, Arab L, Cornoni-Huntley J. Nutritional risk 15. factors for tuberculosis among adults in the United States, 1971-1992. Am J Epidemiol 2012; 176 : 409-22.

16. Bhargava A, Chatterjee M, Jain Y, Chatterjee B, Kataria A, 16. Bhargava M, et al. Nutritional status of adult patients with pulmonary tuberculosis in rural central India and its association with mortality. PLoS One 2013; 8 : e77979.

17. Sharma VP. Re-emergence of Malaria in India. 17. Indian J Med Res 1996; 103 : 26-45.

18. Singh N. Tribal malaria, an update on changing epideomiology. 18. available from: http://www.rmrct.org/files_rmrc_web/centre% 27s_publications/nsth_06/nsth06_6.n.singh.pdf, accessed on may 14, 2015.

19. International Institute for Population Sciences (IIPS). 19. National Family Health Survey 3. (NFHS-3), 2005-2006, India. Mumbai: IIPS; 2007.

20. Indian Council of Medical Research. 20. Nutrient requirements and recommended dietary allowances for Indians. Hyderabad: National Institute of Nutrition; 2010.

21. Yadav R, Rao VG, Bhat J, Gopi PG, Selvakumar N, Wares 21. DF. prevalence of pulmonary tuberculosis amongst the Baigas- a primitive tribe of Madhya Pradesh, Central India. Indian J Tuberc 2010; 3 : 114-6.

22. Chatterjee P, Baag P, Hossain A. 22. TB in tribal community in Uttar Dinajpur (West Bengal) in 2011. Available from: www.mfcindia.org/main/bgpapers/bgpapers2014/..../bgpap2014c.pdf., accessed on May 21, 2015.

23. Hossain P, Kawar B, El Nahas M. Obesity and diabetes in the 23. developing world--a growing challenge. N Engl J Med 2007; 356 : 213-5.

24. Das S. Low body weight type 2 diabetes mellitus. 24. Int J Diab Dev Countries 2003; 23 : 66-74.

25. Srivastava S. Early Onset of type 2 Diabetes in Pune. 25. Ethno Med 2013; 7 : 95-9.

26. Mohan V, Sandeep S, Deepa R, Shah B, Varghese C. 26. Epidemiology of type 2 diabetes: Indian scenario. Indian J Med Res 2007; 125 : 217-30.

Originally published in the Indian Journal of Medical Research (IJMR), May 2015.

letter from ganiyari

An Introduction

Ganiyari is a village in Chhattisgarh – nothing special, just another village in Central India. The health and social problems encountered in Ganiyari, like those in vast rural regions of India, include unchecked infections, widespread malnutrition, marginalization of certain groups, and poor public health systems.

Yet, Ganiyari, its problems, and the India it symbolizes, do not frequently affect the healthcare professional based in urban areas. By publishing a Letter from Ganiyari we hope to provide insights into healthcare issues of these areas to our readers through the experience of healthcare professionals who have lived and worked with the people of the region for over a decade.

The Jan Swasthya Sahyog (JSS, literally the People's Health Support Group) has been running a community health programme in the area for the past 15 years. It has focused on providing comprehensive healthcare to the people of the region, particularly tribals. Patients are drawn from a catchment area that spans seven districts and services are provided through a three tiered structure consisting of a referral hospital in Ganiyari, outreach clinics in forest areas and village health workers. JSS also provides nursing education and has recently started a postgraduate programme in family medicine.

The primary objective of all activities of JSS has been to address inequity in health while running a busy programme. JSS has tried to understand the causes of poor health and offer solutions through training, writing and other forms of advocacy. Some themes that have repeatedly emerged in the course of their work include neglected diseases, cost reduction without compromising quality and rationality, hunger–illness interaction, appropriate technology, tribal health, strengthening the public sector, generalist medical education, etc. We hope these issues will be relevant to a large group of healthcare professionals.

Tuberculosis and Undernutrition: A Tale of Twin Problems

Not surprisingly, tuberculosis (TB), as a classical illness of poverty, is one disease that we diagnose and manage in large numbers in our programme. Over the past 15 years, we have seen more than 500 new patients with TB every year who pose enormous technical, operational and financial challenges. We struggle to find solutions to these problems everyday.

The most striking feature in these patients is the extent of coexisting malnutrition. In an observational study over 6 years, the median body mass index (BMI) and body weight of patients with TB were 16 kg/m2 and 42.1 kg among men, and 15 kg/m2 and 34.1 kg among women, respectively, indicating that 80% of women and 67% of men had moderate-to-severe undernutrition (BMI < 17.0 kg/m2).[1] Six years later in 2014, there are no signs of improvement. At present, 52% of patients (57% of men, 48% of women) are stunted indicating chronic undernutrition. Only 3% of these patients have co-infection with HIV and another 8% have diabetes mellitus. These levels of undernutrition adversely affect the severity of the disease, make treatment difficult, and result in poorer short- and long-term outcomes.

Recently, a popular talk show[2] on television in India focused on issues related to TB care. By discussing issues such as the quality of drug regimens, problems of accessing diagnostic facilities, regulation of treatment providers, and vulnerability of healthcare providers, the show seemed to have conveyed that the biggest challenge is drug resistance. That certainly seems to be the case in urban Mumbai where among newly diagnosed patients the proportion of multi-drug resistant (MDR) TB is as high as 30% and it is 67% among those who have been treated before.[3] Treatment regimens for MDR-TB are known to be difficult to administer, expensive, often toxic, and only half the patients get cured.

A day after this programme was telecast, we reviewed the profile of admitted patients in our 7-bed TB ward. Five of them were tribals of which 3 belonged to a particularly vulnerable tribal group. They were 19–59 years of age, their body weight ranged from 24 to 41 kg and the BMIs were 10.3–15.1 kg/m2. All but one was sputum-positive, and one had empyema.

All were HIV-negative, while one of them had associated diabetes. The results from cultures of 3 patients showed that their bacteria were sensitive to isoniazid and rifampicin and we await results for the other 3. At Ganiyari, of the 717 positive sputum cultures of all consecutive 1151 patients with pulmonary TB over the past 42 months, 3% of isolates among new patients (n = 535) showed MDR-TB while it was 16.1% among those on retreatment (n = 186). These rates are much lower than those reported from Mumbai. Thus, drug resistance does not seem to be the most important issue among our patients in rural Chhattisgarh where coexisting undernutrition is an overwhelming concern.

BMI levels considered lethal,[4] i.e. < 13 kg/m2 among men and < 11 kg/m2 among women, were seen in 7% of patients. While these may represent an extreme end of starvation by selecting patients sick enough to require admission, half of our general patients, including those receiving outpatient treatment, had a BMI of < 16 kg/m2 at presentation. A BMI of < 16 kg/m2 makes for a precarious state for patients with TB. It not only doubles the risk of dying while on treatment, it results in much higher rates of sideeffects, poorer absorption of drugs, and poorer quality of life at the end of treatment.

With these life-threatening levels of weight and BMI in Ganiyari, the question 'Should we provide supplemental food to all patients with TB and undernutrition to improve their outcomes?' – a topic of intense, and often acrimonious debate – does not remain merely an academic question. The WHO guidelines on nutrition care for TB allow the implementation of food support. In view of the increased risk of mortality, the guidelines even include hospitalization of patients with severe undernutrition until a BMI of 18.5 kg/m2 is reached.[5] Yet, several experts quote the heterogeneity of demonstrated benefit of food supplementation in improving outcomes[6] as a reason for not including it in India's national policy. They perhaps overlook that none of the five trials in the Cochrane review managed to reach calorie intakes above the minimum recommended dietary allowances for an uninfected person! How can we then expect that these people would show significant weight gain? In at least two of these studies there was increased compliance with treatment as well as better weight gain,[7] yet this assertion of a 'lack of adequate evidence' is being used as evidence of the lack of benefit[8] with food! The result is that patients with TB in the Revised

National Tuberculosis Control Programme do not have any provision for food supplements regardless of their level of associated undernutrition. TB patients in India stopped getting supplementary food in 1962 after a major trial failed to show additional benefit on disease quiescence.[9]

This conundrum leads us to ask, while the main effort of research is to answer questions, is it not more important to ask the right questions first? We know that malnutrition and underweight increase all-cause mortality, regardless of whether or not one has TB. Here the clinical intervention would be nutritional therapy regardless of the aetiology of being underweight. So why does this question 'Should we offer food supplements to people with undernutrition and TB?' even arise? This is an example of the limits of induction.[10] We do not imply that we already know everything about this issue; there are important secondary questions which would benefit from more empirical studies. For example, what should nutritional therapy for TB patients consist of, or how is nutritional therapy best delivered in programme settings? This should be the focus of our enquiry and debate, not whether food is needed! In public policy, such demands for elusive evidence can often be a guise to avoid change and maintain status quo.

At Ganiyari, faced with the moral predicament of treating those adults who do not weigh even half as much as us, we have to work towards ensuring adequate food supplements for people with TB. People who are sick with TB and severe undernutrition deserve therapeutic nutrition support, as they would receive if they had severe undernutrition in any setting. Their need for calorie, proteins and micronutrients have to be higher than what is normally required. Their food packet could range from onsite or offsite daily rations, or even monthly rations. Besides cereal, dals and oil, in several programmes around the world the food packet has included beans, spray-dried milk, dried fish and eggs among other foods.[11,12] The support would also be dependent on the budget that the state allocates, as well as the problems of distribution of cooked food or those which spoil easily.

We are pleased to note that at the national level there now seems to be an acceptance towards adding supplemental nutrition in the care of TB, as was discussed in a recent meeting of the Central Tuberculosis Division, though the operational details are for the states to work out.

In Chhattisgarh, there is a much stronger motivation to add food supplements, and we hope that the programme would be rolled out soon. However, this is not the end of the story. There is a larger role for food, and that is in preventing TB. While we argue for food supplements for about 1.5 million people who develop TB annually in India, preventing TB in those 350 million Indians who have latent TB is possible only if they get adequate food. Undernutrition is a risk factor for the development of TB in at least half of the people[13] and thus ensuring adequate and balanced food for all makes sense so that, among its many benefits, fewer people get TB. Time will tell whether we will ever have a policy to ensure food adequacy for all, but the basis for such a decision is blowing in the wind.[14]

References

1. Bhargava A, Chatterjee M, Jain Y, Chatterjee B, Kataria A, Bhargava M, et al. Nutritional status of adult patients with pulmonary tuberculosis in rural central India and its association with mortality. PLoS ONE 2013;8:e77979.
2. Satyamev Jayate – Season 3 | Episode 4 | TB–The Ticking Time Bomb, Oct 2014. Available at https://www.youtube.com/watch?v=8G7VGXco4Vs (accessed on 15 Oct 2014).
3. D'souza D, Mistry N, Vira T, Dholakia Y, Hoffner S, Pasvol G, et al. High levels of multidrug resistant tuberculosis in new and treatment-failure patients from the Revised National Tuberculosis Control Programme in an urban metropolis (Mumbai) in Western India. BMC Public Health 2009;9:211.
4. Henry C. The biology of human starvation: Some new insights. Nutr Bull 2001;26: 205–11.
5. World Health Organization. Guidelines: Nutritional care and support for patients with tuberculosis. Geneva: WHO; 2013.
6. Sinclair D, Abba K, Grobler L, Sudarsanam TD. Nutritional supplements for people being treated for active tuberculosis. Cochrane Database Syst Rev 2011;11: CD006086.
7. Jahnavi G, Sudha CH. Randomised controlled trial of food supplements in patients with newly diagnosed tuberculosis and wasting. Singapore Med J 2010;51:957–62.
8. Available at http://rationalwiki.org/wiki/Absence_of_evidence (accessed on 15 Oct 2014).
9. Ramakrishnan CV, Rajendran K, Jacob PG, Fox W, Radhakrishna S. The role of diet in the treatment of pulmonary tuberculosis: An evaluation in a controlled chemotherapy study in home and sanatorium patients in South India. Bull World Health Organ 1961;25:339–59.

10. Available at http://en.wikipedia.org/wiki/Inductive_reasoning (accessed on 15 Oct 2014).

11. Sudarsanam TD, John J, Kang G, Mahendri V, Gerrior J, Franciosa M, et al. Pilot randomized trial of nutritional supplementation in patients with tuberculosis and HIV-tuberculosis coinfection receiving directly observed short-course chemotherapy for tuberculosis. Trop Med Int Health 2011;16:699–706.

12. PrayGod G, Range N, Faurholt-Jepsen D, Jeremiah K, Faurholt-Jepsen M, Aabye M, et al. The effect of energy protein supplementation on weight, body composition and handgrip strength among pulmonary tuberculosis HIV-co-infected patients: Randomised controlled trial in Mwanza, Tanzania. Br J Nutr 2011;107:263–71.

13. Bhargava A, Benedetti A, Oxlade O, Pai M, Menzies D. Undernutrition and the incidence of tuberculosis in India: National and subnational estimates of the population attributable fraction related to undernutrition. Natl Med J India 2014;27:132–7.

14. Swaminathan S, Padmapriyadarsini C. Undernutrition and tuberculosis: Strongly linked, but ignored. Natl Med J India 2014;27:129–31.

books on social medicine

1. **Revolutionary Doctors – Steve Brouwer**

   Revolutionary Doctors gives readers a first-hand account of Venezuela's innovative and inspiring program of community health care, designed to serve – and largely carried out by – the poor themselves.

2. **The Scalpel, The Sword – Sydney Gordon and Ted Allan**

   Originally published in the early 1950s, The Scalpel, the Sword celebrates the turbulent career of Dr. Norman Bethune (1890-1939), a brilliant surgeon, campaigner against private medicine, communist, and graphic artist. Bethune belonged to that international contingent of individuals who recognized the threat of fascism in the world and went out courageously to try to defeat it.

3. **Rakku's story – Sheila Zurbrigg**

   This book turns the usual approach to health analysis on its head. It begins by looking at continuing ill-health in India through the life of a labouring village woman, exploring the forces which keep her from adequately feeding and caring for her children and herself. It probes the source of ill-health, not by focusing on missing nutrients, drugs or skills, but by looking at the way disease and malnutrition are distributed in society - an approach which necessarily sheds light on the distribution of food and all resources, and thus also, the distribution of power. Inequalities within the existing healthcare system thus become a window on the structures and forces operating throughout society.

4. **Infections and inequalities – Paul Farmer**

   Paul Farmer has battled AIDS in rural Haiti and deadly strains of drug-resistant tuberculosis in the slums of Peru. A physician-anthropologist with more than fifteen years in the field, Farmer writes from the front lines of the war against these modern plagues and shows why, even more than those of history, they target the poor. This "peculiarly modern inequality" that permeates AIDS, TB, malaria, and typhoid in the modern world, and that feeds emerging (or re-emerging) infectious diseases such as Ebola and cholera, is laid bare in Farmer's harrowing stories of sickness and suffering.

5. **Mountains beyond Mountains – Tracy Kidder**

In Mountains Beyond Mountains, Pulitzer Prize – winning author Tracy Kidder tells the true story of a gifted man who loves the world and has set out to do all he can to cure it.

In medical school, Paul Farmer found his life's calling: to cure infectious diseases and to bring the lifesaving tools of modern medicine to those who need them most. Kidder's magnificent account takes us from Harvard to Haiti, Peru, Cuba, and Russia as Farmer changes minds and practices through his dedication to the philosophy that "the only real nation is humanity." At the heart of this book is the example of a life based on hope and on an understanding of the truth of the Haitian proverb "Beyond mountains there are mountains" – as you solve one problem, another problem presents itself, and so you go on and try to solve that one too.

6. **Infinite Vision: How Aravind Became the World's Greatest Business Case for Compassion – Pavithra K. Mehta (Author), Suchitra Shenoy**

When a crippling disease shattered his lifelong ambition, Dr. Venkataswamy (better known as Dr. V) chose an impossible new dream: to cure the world of blindness. The tiny clinic he founded in India defied conventional business logic and is now the largest provider of eye care on the planet. At Aravind, patients choose whether to pay or not. Millions are treated for free, yet the organization remains stunningly self-reliant. Serving everyone from penniless farmers to the president, it delivers world-class outcomes at a hundredth of what similar services cost providers in advanced nations. Its model is emulated by organizations everywhere from Rwanda to San Francisco.

7. **Where There is No Doctor: A Village Health Care Handbook – David Werner**

Perhaps the most widely used health care manual in the world. Useful for health workers, clinicians, and others involved in primary health care delivery and health promotion programs, with millions of copies in print in more than 75 languages, the manual provides practical, easily understood information on how to diagnose, treat, and prevent common diseases. Special attention is focused on nutrition, infection and disease prevention, and diagnostic techniques as primary ways to prevent and treat health problems.

8. **How the Other Half Dies – Susan George**

In, How the Other Half Dies (1976), Susan George uncompromisingly exposed the way in which capitalism destroys the lives of the poorest people on our planet. Her essential aim in the book is to explain world poverty not as a terrible but unavoidable phenomenon, but rather as something which flows from the logic of the system itself. More than this, George draws out the deliberate manner in which the inequalities of the system are maintained. She does this in a number of ways. She demolishes attempts by apologists for the system to explain away poverty as a thing unconnected with the normal workings of capitalism. She looks at the political and social mechanisms by which the wealthy elites of the poorer countries are brought into the fold of the West. George also argues that technological 'solutions' in and of themselves, imposed with no regard for local economies and cultures, bring misery to those who are pushed aside by such developments. Finally, she looks at the workings of the large 'agribusiness' corporations and the politics of food aid.

9. **Anatomy of an Illness – Norman Cousins**

The best-selling, groundbreaking classic by Norman Cousins on combating life-threatening illness through humor and patient participation in care.

Anatomy of an Illness was the first book by a patient that spoke to our current interest in taking charge of our own health. It started the revolution in patients working with their doctors and using humor to boost their bodies' capacity for healing. When Norman Cousins was diagnosed with a crippling and irreversible disease, he forged an unusual collaboration with his physician, and together they were able to beat the odds. The doctor's genius was in helping his patient to use his own powers: laughter, courage, and tenacity. The patient's talent was in mobilizing his body's own natural resources, proving what an effective healing tool the mind can be. This remarkable story of the triumph of the human spirit is truly inspirational reading.

10. **The Lost Art of Healing: Practicing Compassion in Medicine – Bernard Lown**

    The real crisis in medicine today is not about economics, insurance, or managed care – it's about the loss of the fundamental human relationship between doctor and patient. In this wise and passionate book, one of our most eminent physicians reacquaints us with a classic notion often overlooked in modern medicine: health care with a human face, in which the time-honored art of healing guides doctors in their approach to patient care and their use of medical technology.

11. **Towards a Critical Medical Practice Reflections on the Dilemmas of Medical Culture Today – Anand Zachariah, R. Srivatsan, Susie Tharu**

    High medical costs, the impersonality of technology-intensive specialty medicine and the difficulty in accessing curative primary care constitute a crisis for medicine in India. Towards a Critical Medical Practice is the outcome of a dialogue between a self-critical medicine and the new social sciences that offers original perspectives on the crisis.

12. **Taking Sides: The Choices Before the Health Worker – C. Satyamala, Nirmala Sundaram, Nalini Bhanot**

13. **Pathway to Light – Dr. Praksh Amte**

    An autobiography

14. Dr. Albert Schweitzer

A Biography (http://www.schweitzer.org/2012/en/work-and-life/biography-long)

15. Maila Aanchal – Phanishwar Nath Renu

Renu's Maila Anchal is one of the finest novels ever written in Hindi. The landscape of Bihar, the caste divide, Indian independence and changes in its aftermath, Maithali folklores and poems, the multiple love stories painted on a canvas with highly perceptive descriptions of village life make it one of the most important novels written in and about rural India.

The novel was first published in early 1950s, in the post Prem Chand era, at a time when young, independent India was trying to redefine its identity as a Nation. The novel is set in Bihar, and incorporates the regional contexts and references into its theme, making it into a perfect example of Anchalik Upanyaas (Regional Novel).

films on health

1. **Ek Doctor ki Maut**

   The film is based on a doctor who discovers a vaccine for leprosy; his superiors in the health ministry suppress him and transfer him to a remote village. Instead of him, two other doctors receive the credit for discovering the same vaccine.

   (Language: Hindi, Year: 1990, Medical theme: Medical research)

2. **Munnabhai M.B.B.S.**

   The film is based on a gangster (Bhai) called Munna who sets out to fulfil his father's dream of becoming a doctor. He tries to heal the patients with love and affection and humanity instead of treating them with traditional methods.

   (Language: Hindi, Year: 2003, Medical theme: Cancer, Humanity in medicine)

3. **Pather Panchali**

   Apu and his poor family live in a village where they try to make ends meet. The father leaves for the city to try and earn more money while his daughter dies of a fever which prompts the family to move.

   (Language: Bengali, Year: 1955, Medical Theme: Rural poverty and health)

4. **Gaman**

   The film depicts the day-to-day struggle of two individuals, who aim to attain a better life-style in the city of dreams, Mumbai.

   (Language: Hindi, Year: 1978, Medical Theme: Rural-Urban Migration)

5. **Dr. Kotniski Amar Kahani**

   The film is based on the life of Dr. Dwarkanath Kotnis who was sent to China during the Second World War to provide medical assistance to the troops fighting against the

Japanese invasion in Yan'an province. His main success was curing a virulent plague, but later he succumbed to the plague himself.

(Language: Hindi / English, Year: 1946, Medical Theme: Plague)

6. **Anand**

Anand, a cancer patient lives his life to the fullest. He fills everyone's life with happiness, which inspires his doctor, Bhaskar, to write a book on Anand's life.

(Language: Hindi, Year: 1971, Medical Theme: Cancer)

7. **Koshish**

Haricharan and Aarti, a hearing and speech impaired couple, give birth to a son and raise him well. Things change when Aarti dies and their young son falls in love with a hearing impaired girl.

(Language: Hindi, Year: 1972, Medical Theme: Hearing Disability)

8. **Black**

A stubborn teacher helps a deaf and blind girl Michelle, explore her potential as she takes on the challenge of becoming a college graduate.

(Language: Hindi, Year: 2005, Medical Theme: Hearing and vision disability)

9. **Anuradha**

Anuradha falls in love with an idealistic doctor (Dr. Nirmal) and wants to marry him against father's will. Dr. Nirmal asks her not follow the hardship of his life. She still marries him and soon after realizes the gravity of her choice of living in a village. After some years her father tries to persuade them to settle in the city but Dr. Nirmal rejects the offer because of his patients and Anuradha decides to remain with him.

(Language: Hindi, Year: 1960, Medical Theme: Travails of rural physician)

10. **Taare Zameen Par**

Day-dreamer Ishaan just can't seem to get anything right in his boarding school. Soon, an unconventional new art teacher, Ram Shankar Nikumbh, helps the dyslexic student discover his true identity.

(Language: Hindi, Year: 2007, Medical Theme: Dyslexia)

11. **Paa**

An unmarried, up and coming politician realises that he has a son. He also learns that the boy suffers from progeria, a rare genetic disorder that causes him to age rapidly and appear like an old man.

(Language: Hindi, year:2009, Medical Theme: Progeria disease)

12. **Sadma**

A man rescues from a brothel a grown up girl who behaves like a 6 year-old due to a brain injury. Weeks pass by as he cares and protects her from one and all. He takes the girl to the village's medical practitioner who cures her of the psychiatric ailment.

(Language: Hindi, year: 1983, Medical Theme: brain injury and regression of mentation)

13. **My Brother Nikhil**

Set in 1990's Goa, this is the story of a swimming champion who is forcibly kept in isolation because he has AIDS. While family and friends desert him, it is his sister and his boyfriend who stand by him.

(Language: Hindi, Year: 2005, Medical Theme: HIV-AIDS)

14. **Sparsh**

Anirudh, a blind man who successfully runs a school for the blind meets social worker, Kavita. The two fall in love but after they agree to get married, Anirudh starts having second thoughts.

(Language: Hindi, Year: 1980, Medical Theme: Blindness)

15. **My Name is Khan**

Rizwan Khan who has the disease called Asperger's syndrome, embarks on a journey to meet the President of the United States of America. Along the way he attempts to change people's perception about his religion.

(Language: Hindi, Year: 2010, Medical Theme: Asperger's syndrome)

16. **Woh Lamhe**

A possessive boyfriend dominates his girlfriend who is a famous actress. An aspiring director wants to cast her in his first film. The director is attracted to her and discovers her unstable world with schizophrenia.

(Language: Hindi, Year: 2006, Medical Theme: Schizophrenia)

17. **Devdas**

Devdas is in love with Paro since childhood. But when Devdas' family doesn't approve of their relationship, he leaves home and seeks refuge at a brothel, owned by Chandramukhi and starts drinking. Finally he dies due to alcoholism.

(Language: Hindi, Year: 2002, Medical Theme: Alcoholism and its Consequences)

18. **Apana Asmaan**

A couple imposes their dreams on their mildly autistic child only to later feel distraught at its consequences.

(Language: Hindi, Year: 2007, Medical Theme: Autism)

19. **Lajja**

The journeys of four different women who are all victims of male chauvinism are brought together due to common circumstances. However, they refuse to get abused and decide to fight for their rights.

(Language: Hindi, Year: 2001, Medical Theme: Women's issues)

20. **Ganashatru**

Dr Ashok Gupta faces opposition from his elder brother after he finds a huge amount of bacteria in the holy water of a temple that is the cause of death for many locals.

(Language: Bengali/English, Year: 1989, Medical Theme: Epidemics)

The microbe is nothing, the terrain, everything.

– Louis Pasteur

Medical statistics will be our standard of measurement: we will weigh life for life and see where the dead lie thicker, among the workers or among the privileged.

– Rudolf Virchow

Maps of Inequity

These maps of inequity have been created with help of a cartogram software tool Scapetoad. Scapetoad uses Gastner-Newman algorithm, which is a diffusion based method for producing density equalizing maps by modifying the area polygons according to statistical parameters. These distortion maps are more impactful in visualising relative inequalities and ill-distributions of a variable, as compared to the traditional heat-maps. By including these maps in this public health book we hope to stimulate and channelize human efforts towards solving the grave issues described herein.

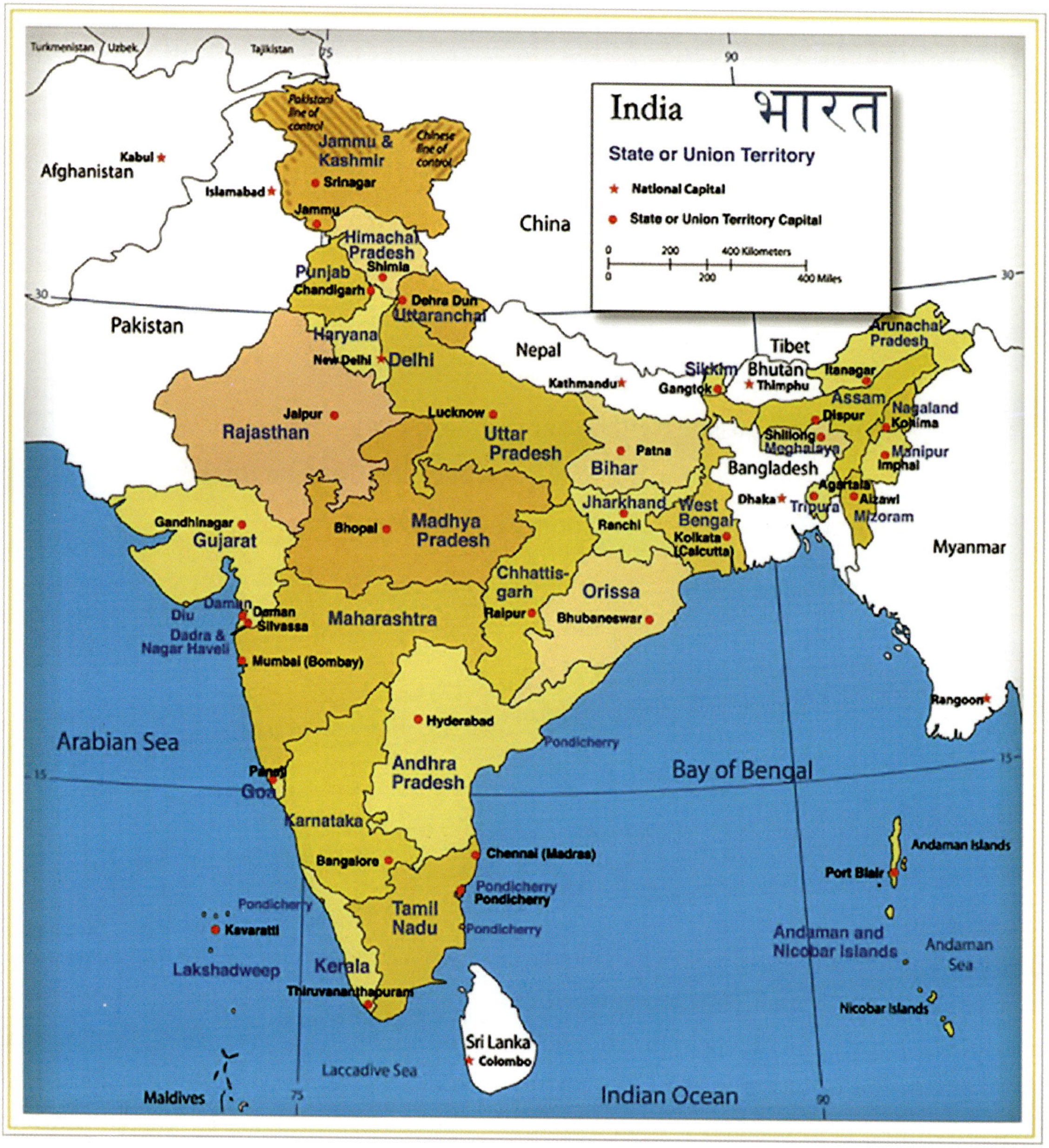
India
भारत
State or Union Territory
National Capital
State or Union Territory Capital
0
200
400 Kilometers
0
200
400 Miles
Turkmenistan
Uzbek.
Tajikistan
Afghanistan
Kabul
Islamabad
Pakistan
China
Nepal
Kathmandu
Tibet
Bhutan
Thimphu
Bangladesh
Dhaka
Myanmar
Rangoon
Sri Lanka
Colombo
Maldives
Pakistani line of control
Chinese line of control
Jammu & Kashmir
Srinagar
Jammu
Himachal Pradesh
Shimla
Punjab
Chandigarh
Dehra Dun
Uttaranchal
Haryana
New Delhi
Delhi
Rajasthan
Jaipur
Uttar Pradesh
Lucknow
Bihar
Patna
Sikkim
Gangtok
Arunachal Pradesh
Itanagar
Assam
Dispur
Nagaland
Kohima
Meghalaya
Shillong
Manipur
Imphal
Tripura
Agartala
Mizoram
Aizawl
Jharkhand
Ranchi
West Bengal
Kolkata (Calcutta)
Gujarat
Gandhinagar
Madhya Pradesh
Bhopal
Chhattisgarh
Raipur
Orissa
Bhubaneswar
Diu
Daman
Dadra & Nagar Haveli
Silvassa
Mumbai (Bombay)
Maharashtra
Hyderabad
Andhra Pradesh
Pondicherry
Panaji
Goa
Karnataka
Bangalore
Chennai (Madras)
Tamil Nadu
Kerala
Thiruvananthapuram
Kavaratti
Lakshadweep
Arabian Sea
Bay of Bengal
Laccadive Sea
Indian Ocean
Andaman Islands
Port Blair
Andaman and Nicobar Islands
Andaman Sea
Nicobar Islands
75
90
30
15

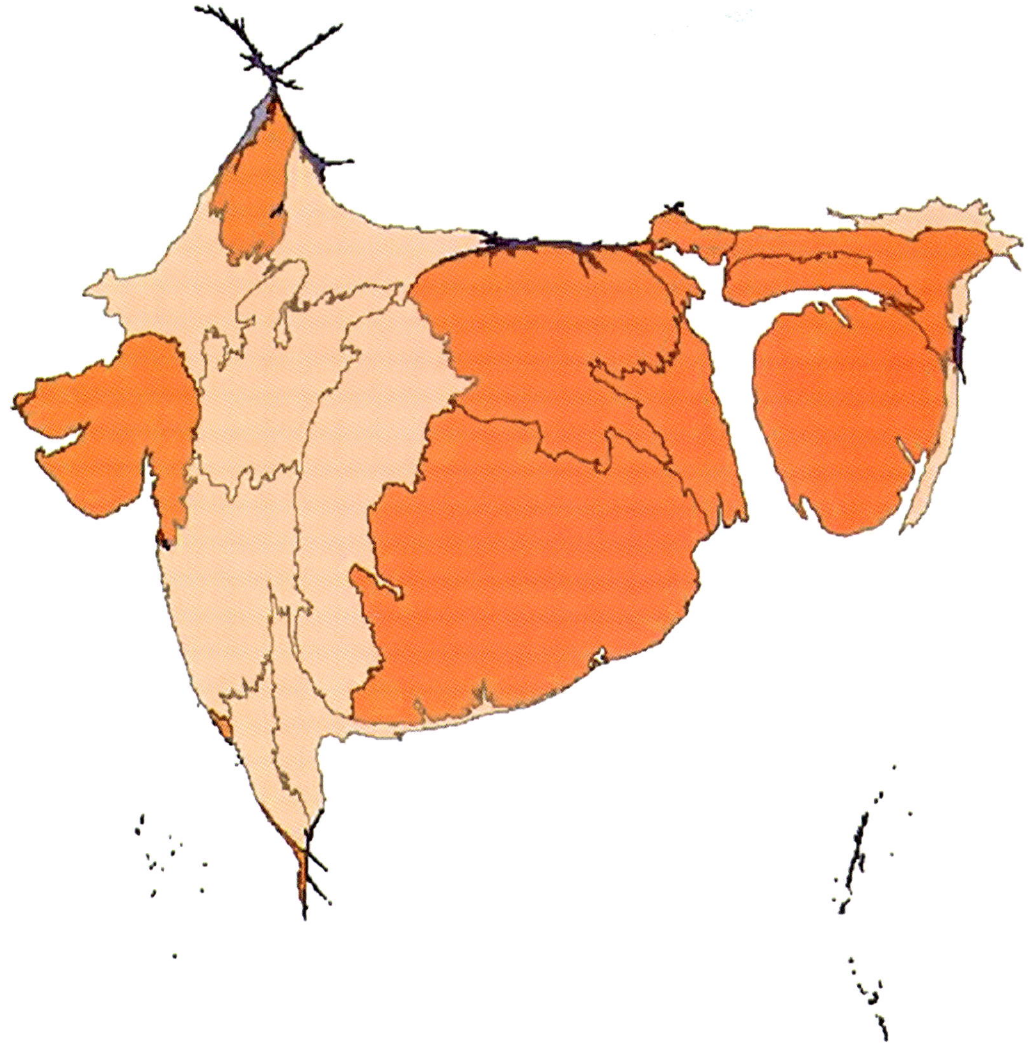

Malaria is caused by Plasmodium parasite which is transmitted by the Anopheles mosquito but we humans determine its frequency and lethality, by our mode of development and the way we handle water resources, and by the way we organise our treatment and control programmes. Officially India lost 535 people to malaria in 2014, though the Million Death Study estimated it to be 1,50,000 to 2,25,000 annually. Himalayan states are immune to it while the worst hit states are Tripura, Odisha, Chhattisgarh and West Bengal.

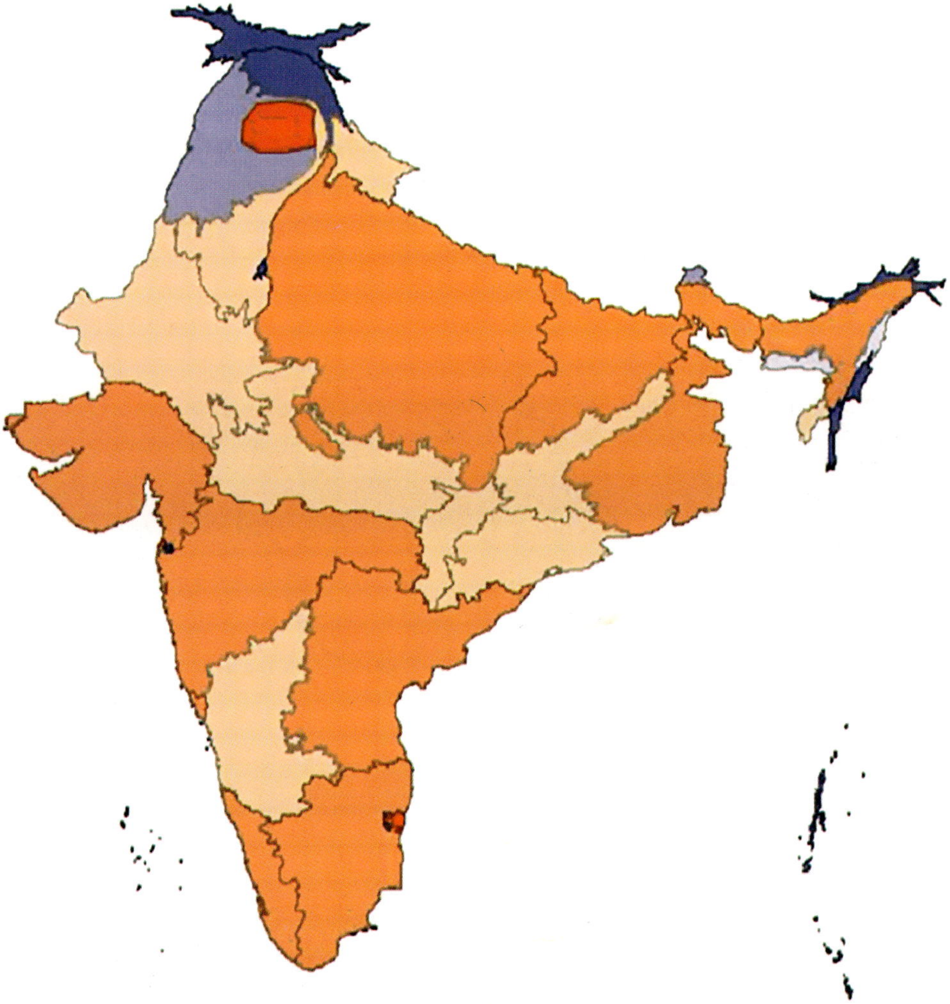

Shown here, is the relative distribution of smear positive TB cases in 2013, while total smear positive cases diagnosed in 2013 in the country were 9,28,190. Not only is tuberculosis caused by poverty and consequent food and income deprivation, the disease itself is capable of worsening the poverty status of affected people. This infectious disease shares strong associations with malnutrition and HIV. One person with untreated infectious TB can pass the illness on to 10-15 people annually therefore, countries with limited access to healthcare are worst affected. Indian society is also known to have social stigma surrounding TB affecting employment and marriages, forcing people into a spiral of poverty.

deaths due to acute diarrhoeal disease (2013)

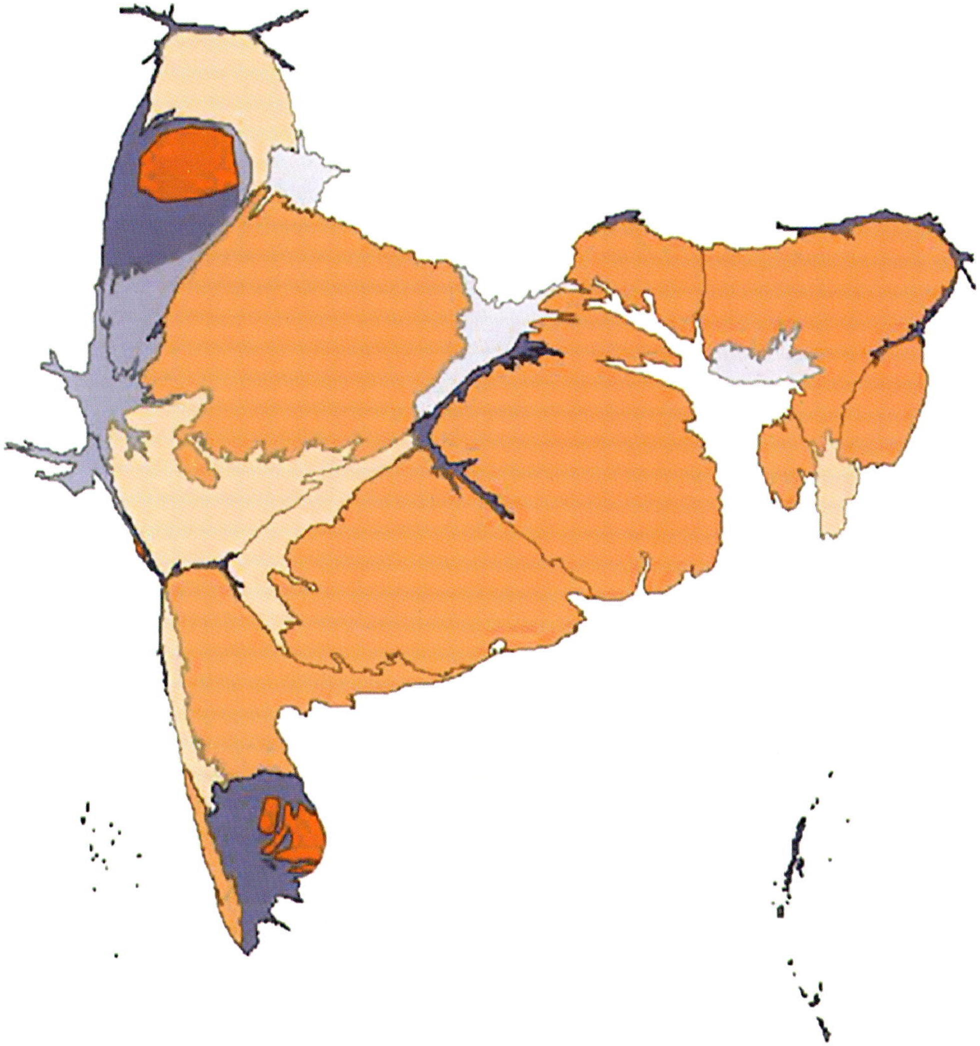

In poor countries, diarrhoea is a leading cause of morbidity. It is still a major killer of children under five. Inadequate sanitation, poor hygiene practices, contaminated food and malnutrition affect the spread and severity of diarrhoea. Emphasis on oral rehydration therapy and improved access to healthcare are necessary for control of morbidity and mortality.

HIV prevalence (2013)

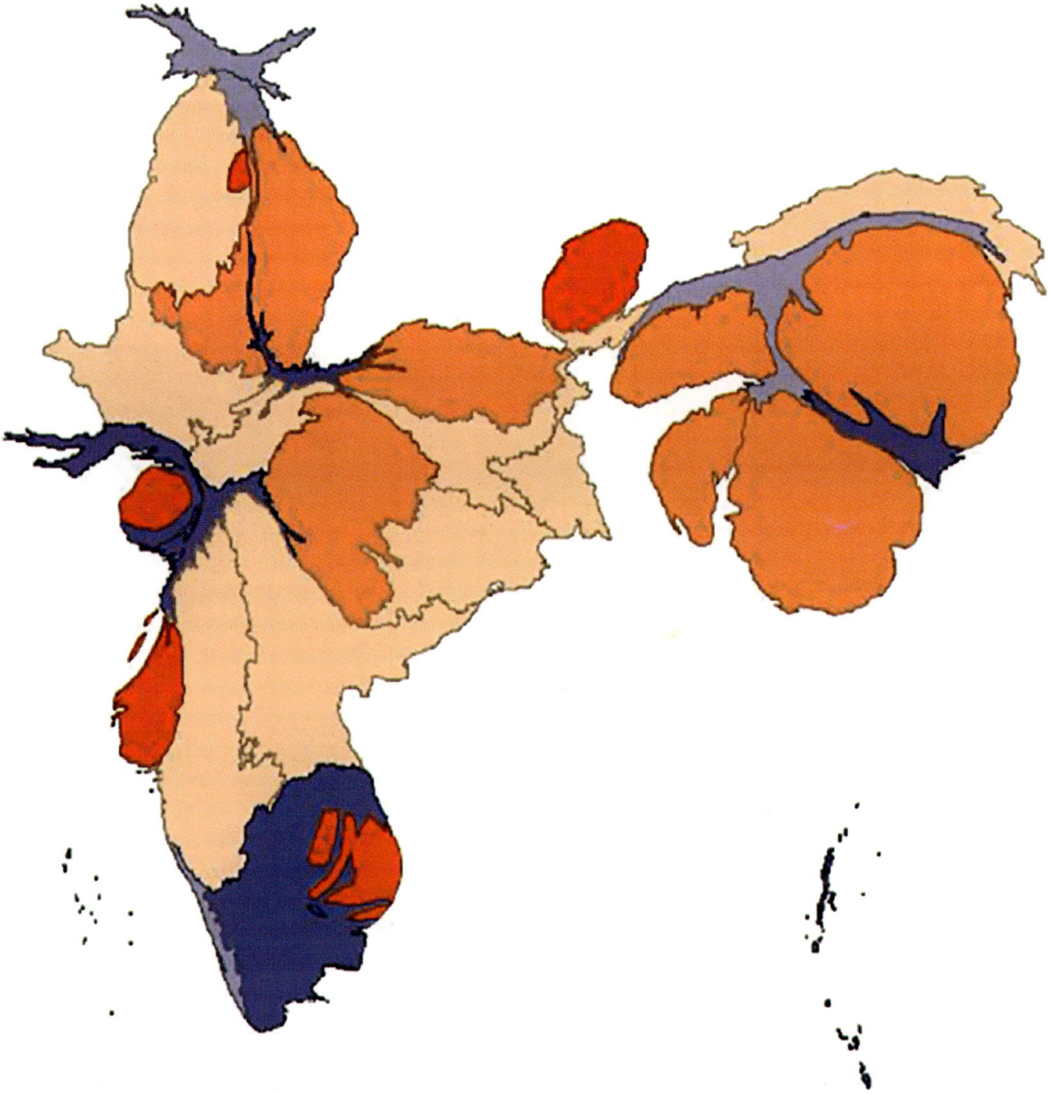

India has the third largest HIV epidemic in the world with 2.1 million people living with HIV while the country prevalence is 0.35%. There was a 38% decline in AIDS-related deaths between 2005 and 2013. Despite, this 51% of HIV deaths in Asia are in India. North East states, Andhra Pradesh and Chhattisgarh are worst affected.

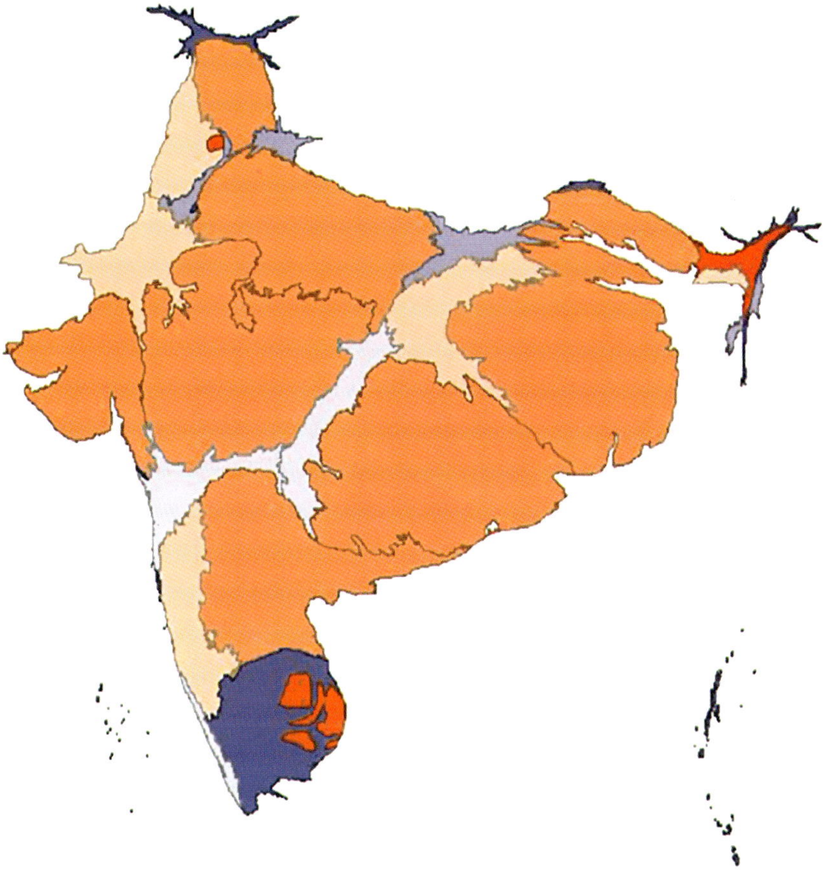

India is estimated to have the highest snakebite mortality in the world. The Centre for Global Health Research gives an estimate of 46,000 annual deaths by snakebite in the country whereas the Government of India's Central Bureau of Health Intelligence reported only 1,350 deaths each year for the period 2004 to 2009. The Million Death Study states "Snakebite remains an underestimated cause of accidental death in modern India. Community education, appropriate training of medical staff and better distribution of antivenom, especially to the 13 states with the highest prevalence, could reduce snakebite deaths in India." There are 13 known species that are poisonous and of these four, namely common cobra (Najanaja), Russell's viper (Dabiolarusselii), saw-scaled viper (Echiscarinatus) and common krait (Bungaruscaeruleus) are highly venomous and believed to be responsible for most of the poisonous bites in India.

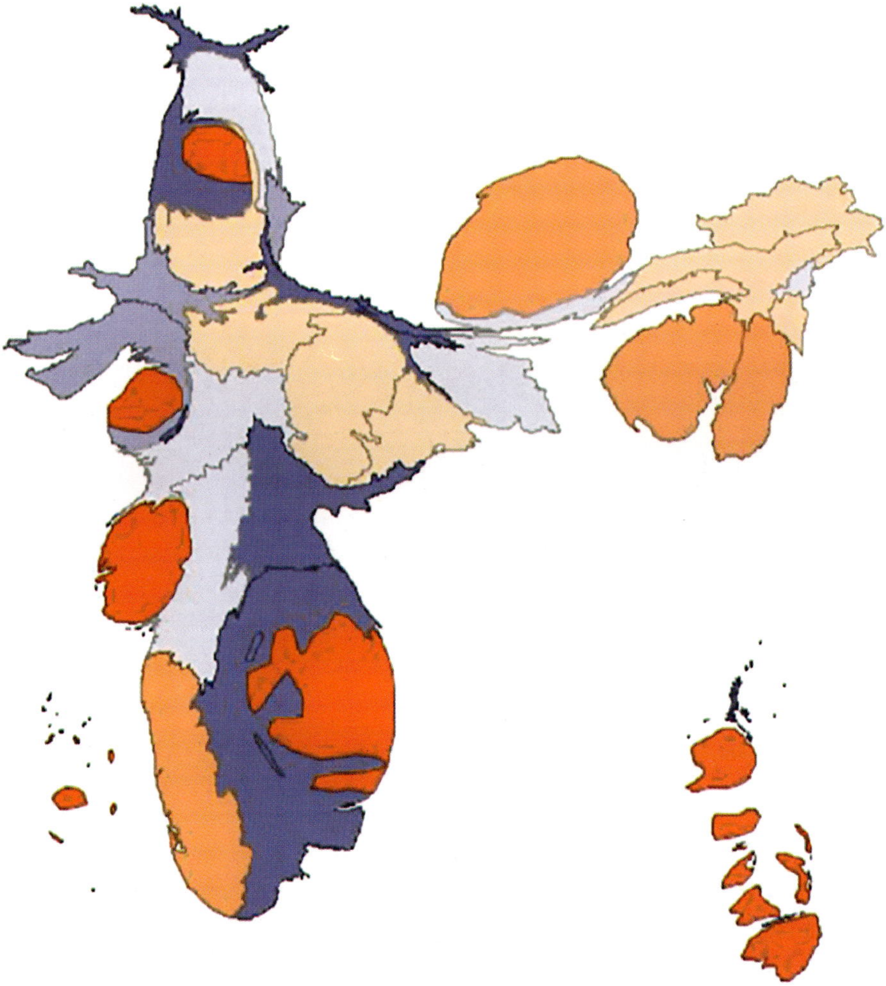

According to the W.H.O., India accounts for the highest number of suicides in the world. In year 2014, 1,31,666 people committed suicide in India. The all India rate of suicides was 10.6 during the year 2014 according to NCRB's ADSI-2014. Rate of suicides is defined as the number of suicides per one lakh population. Puducherry reported the highest rate of suicide (40.4) followed by Sikkim (38.4), A & N Islands (28.9), Telangana (26.5), Kerala (23.9) and Tamil Nadu (23.4). Our own data (JSS Community Programme) showed a suicide rate of 43 in the programme villages. 'Other Family Problems' and 'Illness' were the major causes of suicides among the specified causes, accounting for 21.7% and 18.0% respectively of total suicides.

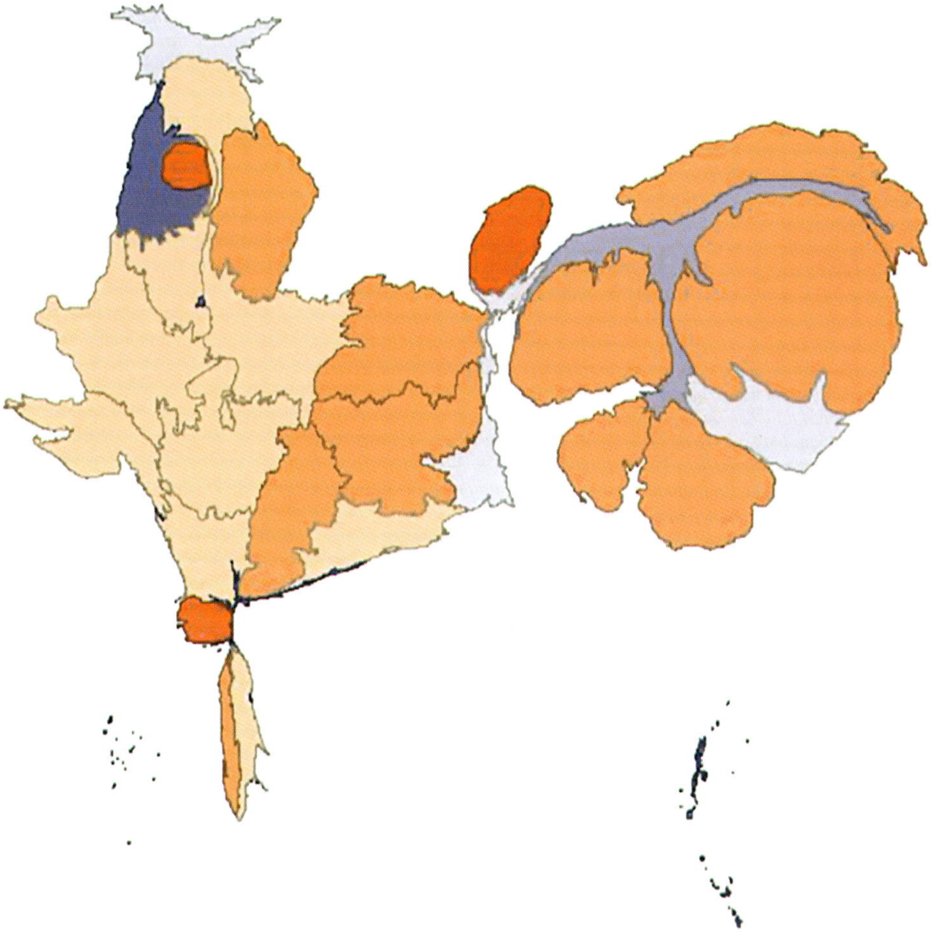

Caesarean section (CS or C-section) is a surgical intervention which is carried out to ensure the safety of mother and child when vaginal delivery is not possible (emergency CS) or when the doctors consider that the danger to the mother and baby would be greater with a vaginal delivery (planned CS). Proportion of CS to total births is considered as one of the important indicators of emergency obstetric care (World Health Organization, 2009). A figure below 5% implies that a substantial proportion of women do not have access to surgical obstetric care; on the other hand a rate higher than 15% indicates over utilization of the procedure for other than life saving reasons (WHO, 1985; WHO, 1993). States performing low on C–section rates are Rajasthan, Madhya Pradesh, Arunachal Pradesh, Meghalaya, Bihar, Jharkhand, Chhattisgarh, Uttar Pradesh, Manipur, Mizoram, Assam, Tripura, Odisha, Gujarat and Maharashtra.

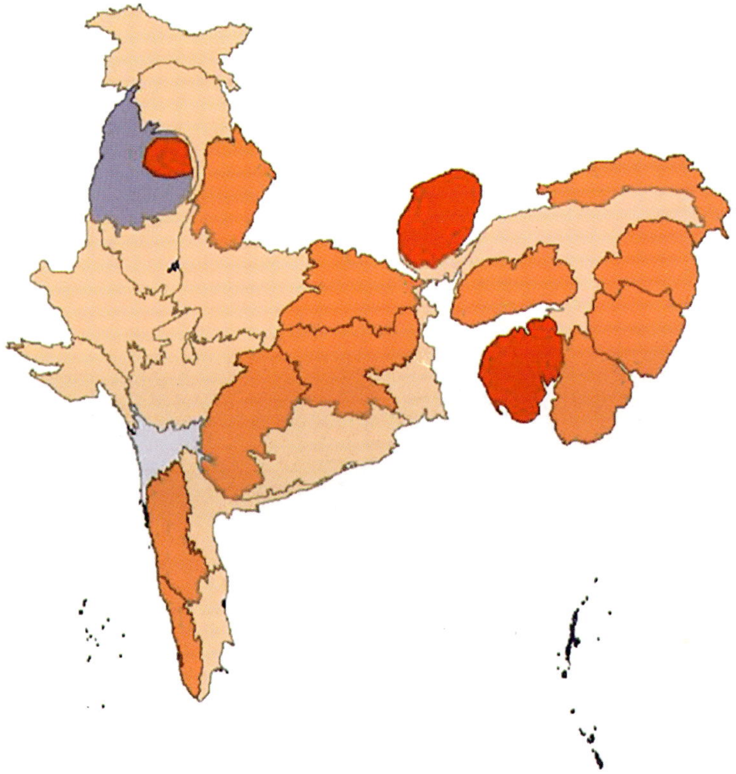

Maternal mortality ratio is the number of women who die from pregnancy-related causes while pregnant or within 42 days of pregnancy termination per 100,000 live births. The major causes of maternal mortality are postpartum bleeding, complications from unsafe abortion, hypertensive disorders of pregnancy, postpartum infections, obstructed labour and pre-existing comorbidities. Moreover, for every maternal death, there are approximately thirty times as many cases of pregnancy related illness or disability. For example, obstetric fistula (an opening between the bladder and the vagina) is usually the result of obstructed labour, can have tragic consequences for women as seen in the vesico-vaginal fistula narrative. Most of these deaths and morbidities can be prevented with good obstetric care which should be every mother's right.

MMR of India is 167 per 100,000 live births (2011-2013), and estimated to be at 140 in 2015, against the Millennium Development Goal (MDG) of 109. While Kerala at 61, Maharashtra at 68 and Tamil Nadu at 79 have shown what is possible, we must also look at and question Madhya Pradesh where MMR is 221, Rajasthan- 244, Chhattisgarh-244, Uttar Pradesh-285 and Assam at abysmal low of 300. According to recently announced sustainable development goals (SDG) India's MMR target for 2030 is to lower down maternal mortality to 70 per lakh live births.

(Source of map data: SRS 2011-13; CRS 2012 for Delhi; Annual health survey 2012-13 for Uttarakhand, Jharkhand and Chhattisgarh. Due to the unavailability of data, Union territories and Goa are not included.)

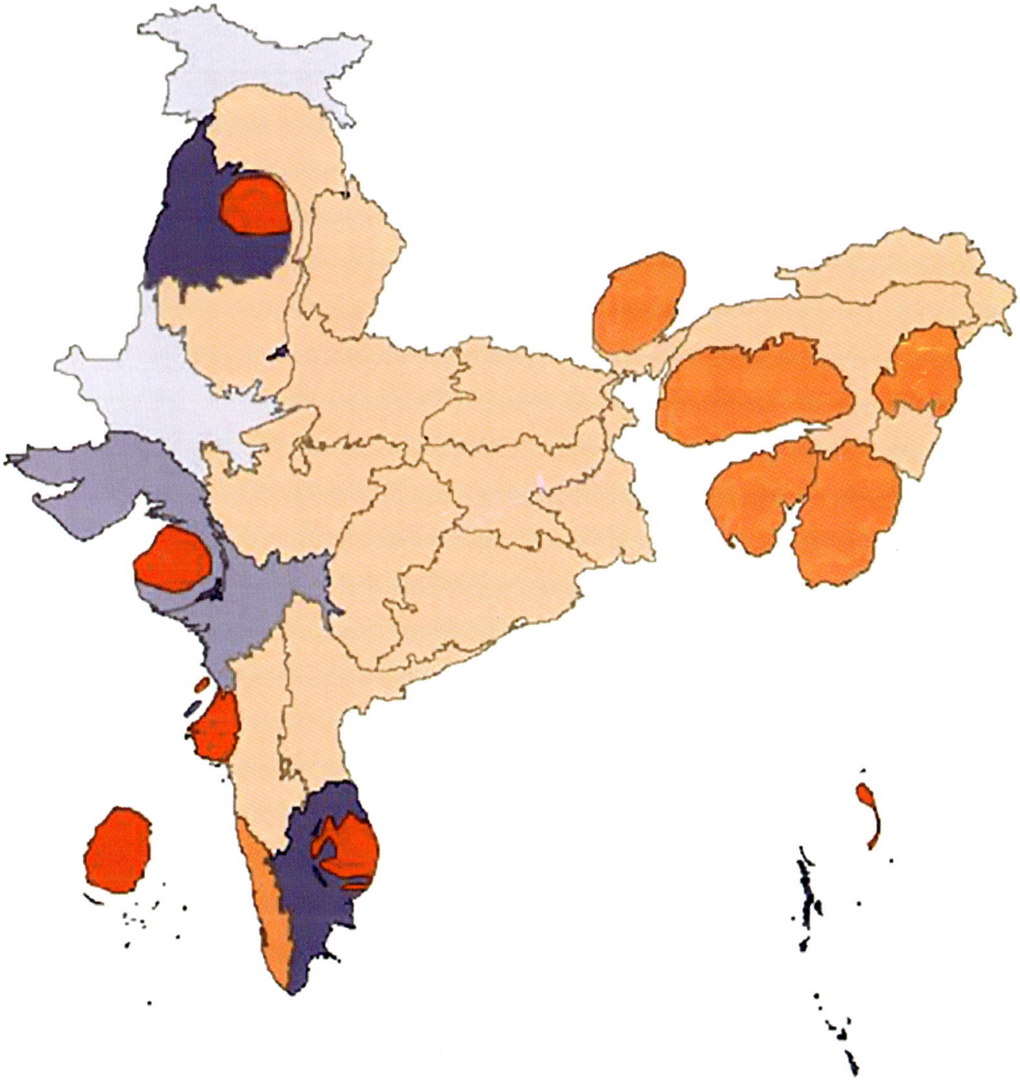

IMR is defined as number of deaths of children under one year of age per 1000 live births. The leading causes of infant mortality are birth asphyxia, pneumonia, pre-term birth complications, neonatal infection, diarrhoea, malaria, measles and malnutrition. India had MDG target of 27 to be achieved in 2015, which she could not.

population per government allopathic doctor (2013)

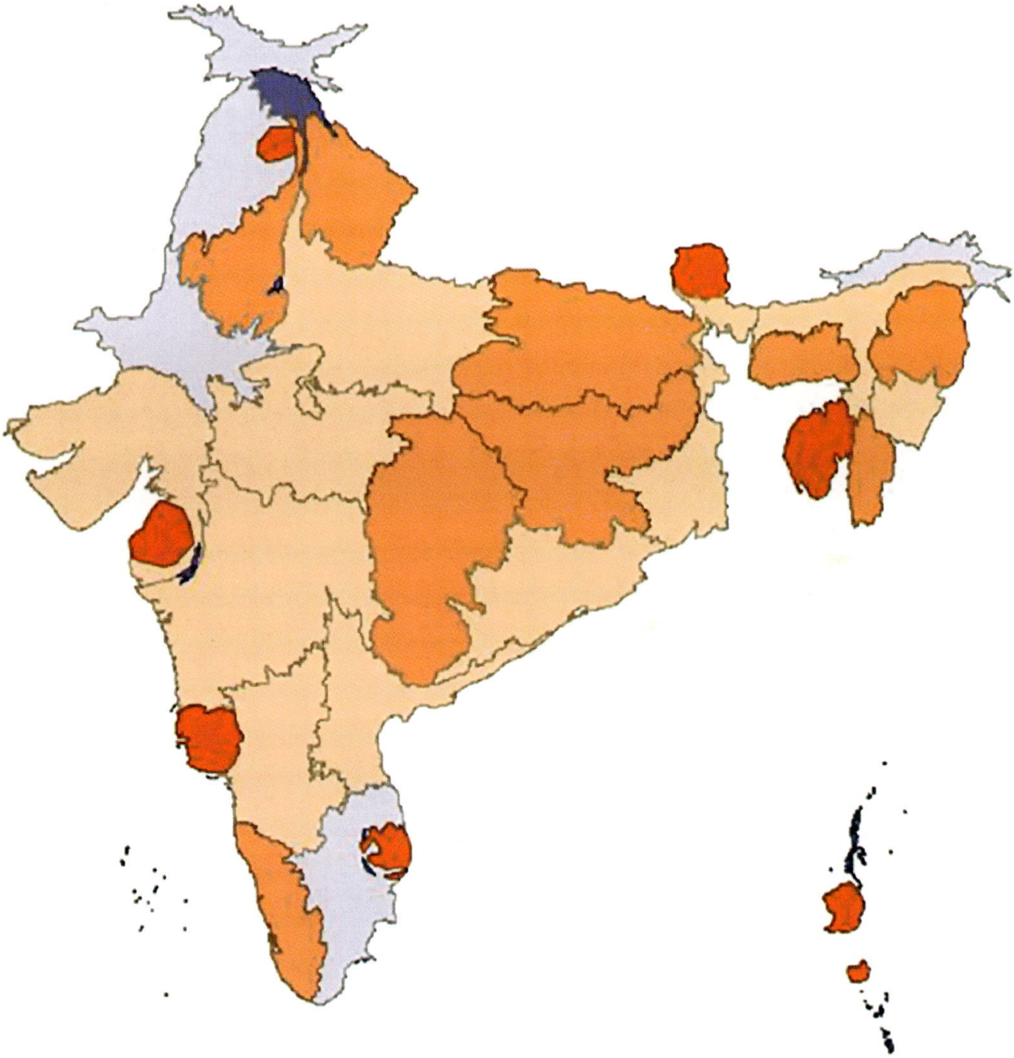

The doctor-patient ratio or physician per 1,000 population are good indicators of human resource in healthcare. But for the poor who are mostly reliant on the government for their health needs, "population per government allopathic doctor" seems to be a more reliable parameter. According to CBHI data, India has 11,455 population per allopathic doctor. The worst performing states according to this parameter are Maharashtra (28102), Chhattisgarh (24,711), Uttar Pradesh (21,122) and Bihar (20,207).

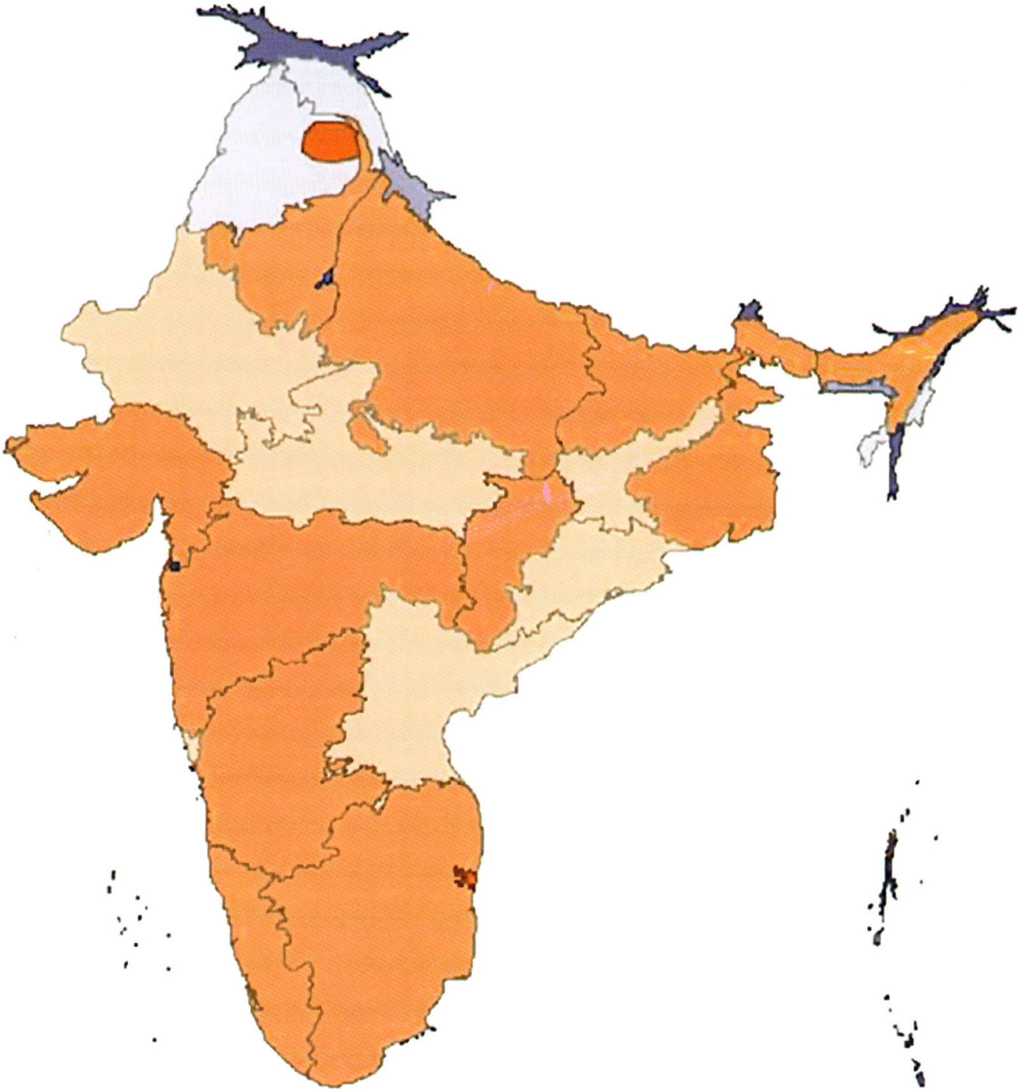

During 2014, a total of 4,50,898 cases of 'Road Accidents' were reported which rendered 4,77,731 persons injured and 1,41,526 deaths . 51 cases of road accidents took place every one hour during 2014, wherein 16 persons were killed. The major causes of road accidents are over speeding and careless driving.

the people

That man I remember well, and at least two centuries
have passed since I last saw him;
he traveled neither on horseback nor in a carriage,
always on foot
he undid
the distances,
carrying neither sword nor weapon
but nets on his shoulder,
ax or hammer or spade;
he never fought with another of his kind –
his struggle was with water or with earth,
with the wheat, for it to become bread,
with the towering tree, for it to yield wood,
with walls, to open doors in them,
with sand, to form it into walls,
and with the sea, to make it bear fruit.

I knew him and he goes on haunting me.

The carriages splintered into pieces,
war destroyed doorways and walls,
the city was a fistful of ashes,
all the dresses shivered into dust,
and for me he persists,
he survives in the sand,

when everything previously
seemed durable except him.

In the comings and goings of families,
sometimes he was my father or my relative
or almost was, or, if not, perhaps
the other one who never came back home
because water or earth swallowed him,
a machine or a tree killed him,
or he was that funeral carpenter
who walked behind the coffin, dry-eyed,
someone who never had a name
except as wood or metal have names,
and on whom others looked from above,
not noticing the ant,
only the anthill;
so that when his feet no longer moved
because, poor and tired, he had died,
they never saw what they were not used to seeing –
already other feet walked in his footsteps.

– Pablo Neruda

keywords

Accessibility

Accessibility refers to the ability of a given patient to obtain health care. There are several features that make a health care system accessible. First, adequate health care services must exist within a given geographic range. Second, people must be able to afford the costs of obtaining health care, including fees for services as well as the costs of transport and lost work time. Third, people must not face unduly high barriers to entry to the health care system that might include lack of information about an institution, dismissive treatment by the health center staff, or a fear of harmful procedures.

Addiction

Addiction refers to a condition in which a person compulsively consumes substances due to a physical or psychological dependence. The substances (or other stimuli such as gambling or sex) must be rewarding and reinforcing. The substances provide short-term rewards but long-term negative consequences such as the destruction of relationships, health problems, wasted money, and lost livelihoods. Addictive substances include alcohol, tobacco, cannabis or ganja, nicotine, and other illegal drugs. Addictive tendencies are both inherited and conditioned by social and personal factors such as chronic or acute stressors like poverty and undernutrition as found in our population. As a simultaneously physiological and psychological condition, addiction requires both medical and psychosocial treatment modalities.

Adivasi [Scheduled Tribe]

Adivasi directly translated means original inhabitant. It is used to refer to India's tribal groups. These groups are also referred to as scheduled tribes (STs) because they are listed in a schedule, or list, designated by Article 338 of India's 1950 Constitution. Scheduled Tribes consist of 8.6% of India's total population. Chhattisgarh has a large adivasi population, making up about 32% of the state's total population of around 28 million. Despite reservations in education and government jobs and special social welfare provisions, adivasis are one of the most deprived social groups in India. Adivasis fare the worst on any number of health and development indicators, starting with nutrition. In our area where adivasis make up the dominant social group, men and women are at least 10 kg lighter than the reference Indian. There are some sub-categories within the broader category of STs. For example, some tribal groups are labeled as particularly vulnerable tribal groups (PVTGs). In our area, Baigas fall into this category.

Anaemia

Anaemia refers to a condition in which there are a decreased number of red blood cells in the blood, causing the blood to have lowered oxygen. Symptoms include fatigue, weakness, dizziness, heart palpitations, shortness of breath, headaches, spoon shaped nails, and pica (a craving for unusual substances such as dirt, sand, chalk, or ice). Anaemia predisposes patients to a variety of negative health and social outcomes including fatigue, cognitive impairments in children, susceptibility to infection, and lost work time in adults. Most but not all anaemia is caused by prolonged iron deficiency in the diet. In this area, the diet includes meat only rarely and a limited amount of leafy green vegetables or citrus fruits. It primarily depends on rice and therefore iron consumption is very low. Anaemia is extremely common in India with over half the Indian population anaemic. It is even more common in women with some estimates finding anaemia in over 70% of premenopausal women in India. Iron deficiency anaemia is a good example of the gendered aspect of health inequity: due to menstruation women have much higher rates of iron-deficiency anaemia and also bear its burden in increased rates of maternal mortality, since anaemia predisposes women to postpartum haemorrhage. Iron deficiency anaemia can be treated with supplementation through iron pills and blood transfusions in severe cases. It is especially important to for all pregnant women to take iron pills regularly as part of a robust antenatal care program.

Baiga

In our context in central Chhattisgarh, Baiga has two meanings. First, Baiga refers to an *adivasi* or Scheduled Tribe group living in our area. Baigas are one of the most deprived social groups in this region. Traditionally they have depended on *bewar* (slash and burn or swidden agriculture) and the collection of forest products. Often they live physically apart from other social groups. Some commentators believe that the Baiga tribal groups should be provided the benefits of mainstream development that will bring them into settled agriculture and standard education systems. Others think that Baigas should be provided with culturally appropriate medical care and education but be allowed to preserve their lifeways to the extent they choose. Baiga in common parlance also refers to a traditional healer whom other social groups call on to provide magical or *jhadaphuk* healing rituals in times of distress.

Blood bank

An accessible and functional health care institution requires quick access to reserve blood supplies, or a blood bank. Blood is required in a variety of situations including for treating postpartum haemorrhage and acute crises of sickle cell anaemia and in many surgeries. However, rural India faces a critical shortage of blood supplies due to government regulations about blood banking. Currently a hospital like JSS can store blood so that it is available quickly but it cannot serve as a blood collection facility. Outside of the JSS system, 45% of patients have to purchase blood in the private market rather than receive voluntary blood donations. Many patients have erroneous notions about the impact of blood donation. Many think that blood takes a long time to regenerate and blood donation will result in the need to take time off from work and rest to recover.

Body Mass Index

Body Mass Index is an index of the relationship between weight and height. It is calculated by dividing the body mass (in kgs) by the square of height (in centimeters). BMI is an important indicator of health and a low BMI makes people vulnerable to a wide variety of diseases from tuberculosis to hypertension to malaria. The National Institute of Nutrition recommends that a rural Indian male of 173 cm height should weigh 60 kg and have a Body Mass Index of 20. A rural Indian female should of 161 cm height should weigh 55 kg with a Body Mass Index of 21. A BMI of less than 18.5 is considered undernourished. Up to one third of India's population falls into this category. A BMI of less than 16 is considered severely undernourished and it greatly increases the chance of death. The BMI of a population can be used as an indicator of its food security. In our region of rural Chhattisgarh, the low BMIs of the population indicate the low level of food security. The patients who are seen at our clinic and community health centers have median BMIs between 17.6 and 18.5.

Cancer

Cancer is an often life-threatening disease in which cells abnormally divide and spread. Cancers are a major health threat among all populations, no less in our rural population in central Chhattisgarh. Risk factors for cancer in rural India are similar to urban India and include lifestyle habits like tobacco smoking or chewing, genital infections that predispose to cancers, and genetic predispositions. They also include factors specific to rural India such as occupational exposures to kitchen smoke or chemicals in factories and mines. Most health care centers accessible to rural Indians lack cancer treatment facilities whether for surgery, radiotherapy, or chemotherapy. A policy of screening and education would assist in identifying cancers earlier, which would result in fewer cancer deaths and less pain. The government has undertaken the commendable steps of warning the public about the risks of tobacco smoking through messages on cigarette boxes and media campaigns but other common cancers have not received the same public attention. Most patients present with later stage cancers due to the distance and cost involved in traveling to seek treatment as well as lack of awareness. There is a gendered dimension to cancer as well. Women often fail to seek treatment for cervical cancer because symptoms like discharge are perceived to be normal. Women have very low awareness about breast cancer and the need to seek prompt treatment. According to the most recent figures, the top five types of cancers among men and women in India are breast, oral, cervical, colon and rectum, and stomach. The top five deadliest in India are stomach, liver, esophageal, tracheal, bronchus and lung, and breast.

Caste

Caste is a term used to describe the hierarchical division of Indian society based on religious-occupational categories. India is made up of thousands of highly specific caste-occupational categories that are local rather than pan-Indian in nature. Caste is important in determining appropriate marriage partners, mobilizing credit and capital, and gaining and using political power. The most oppressed castes in India are labeled “Scheduled Castes” or SCs. This refers to those castes listed in "schedules" of the Constitution. SCs are entitled to reservations in state employ and education and other ameliorative measures. Despite these ameliorative measures, SCs continue to face a great deal of structural oppression and violence. SCs also have poorer health outcomes on a variety of measures due to the lack of accessibility of health care. Caste often but not always maps onto class status. In common parlance, the English word caste usually maps onto the Hindi term *jaati*.

Class

Class is both a descriptor of income status as well as a sociological category of analysis for understanding life chances. In Indian health care, class influences a wide variety of health conditions. Financial capabilities determine the chances of life itself. In an acute situation, greater wealth allows the patient to obtain a higher standard of care in better-equipped facilities. Members of wealthier classes have access to inherited resources and privilege and, with these, the opportunity to influence political directions. Those with fewer financial resources are less likely to receive preventive and promotive health care, less likely to be able to seek prompt treatment, and more likely to face financial ruin due to health care costs that often represent a trivial portion of a wealthier patient's budget.

Diabetes

Diabetes is a metabolic disease in which there is too much glucose in the blood. Type 1 diabetes results from the failure of the pancreas to produce insulin. It is genetic and often presents in childhood or young adulthood. Type 2, which is by far the more common type, results from the pancreas producing insufficient insulin and the failure of the body's cells to respond to the insulin. A third type, gestational diabetes, occurs in women during pregnancy. Commonly thought of as a disease of the wealthy who over-consume sugars and carbohydrates, diabetes is a neglected disease among poor and rural Indians. It affects at least 34 million rural Indians and 28 million urban Indians, though many cases in low resource settings go undiagnosed. In poor and rural India, diabetes is most often a product of the limited availability and accessibility of any food besides cheap carbohydrates, especially rice. The rice heavy diet results in poor glycemic control in this population. This has led us at JSS to term diabetes among the undernourished as "thin diabetes." Diabetes severely limits livelihoods and health outcomes. It results in neuropathy, retinopathy, nephropathy, and complicated infections. The costs of measuring sugars and purchasing insulin are often prohibitive and patients lack the means to properly refrigerate insulin. In common parlance the disease is known as "sugar ki bimari" or sugar illness.

Epilepsy

Epilepsy is a brain condition or disorder in which abnormal neuronal activity causes recurrent seizures. A single seizure is not sufficient to diagnose epilepsy; rather the clinical definition of epilepsy requires two or more unprovoked seizures that lack another explanation. Epilepsy has a variety of causes including low oxygen during birth, head injuries, infections, tumors, and genetic conditions. A common preventable cause in India is neurocysticercosis, a parasitic infection by *Taenia solium,* a tapeworm found in pigs and transmitted through food and water. However, the cause of epilepsy is often unknown. Though pharmaceutical treatment is relatively straightforward and effective in the majority of cases, epilepsy goes undiagnosed in part due to a lack of knowledge among frontline health care workers and a severe shortage of neurologists. In India at least 12 million people have epilepsy. Left untreated, epilepsy can have a range of severe consequences including social stigma, loss of livelihoods, broken bones, burns (especially common in rural India where people cook over open flame), drowning, brain damage, cognitive decline, and death. With appropriate management, many people with epilepsy lead normal lives. Some cultures have viewed people with epilepsy as spiritual savants or seers. On the other hand, in some parts of India people with epilepsy are seen to be as cursed with black magic or witchcraft.

Forest

For much of India's history, the area that makes up modern Chhattisgarh state was part of the Great Central Indian Forest. In the past 150 years, Chhattisgarh's rich forest resources have been seriously depleted by commercial forestry to supply wood for railroads and ships (in the colonial period) and, more recently, to clear land for settled agriculture. Currently, forest land comprises 44% of Chhattisgarh's land. One important forest in our area is the Achanakmar Tiger Reserve. The JSS Bamhani clinic is sited in the core zone of the Tiger Reserve. The 2006 Forest Rights Act (FRA 2006) recognized India's *adivasi* communities' rights to forest land and produce. The Act provides the tribes with title rights over forest land and produce, rights to non-timber forest products, and rights to influence development activities, among others. While the FRA delineates the lofty goal of remedying "historical injustices" to the forest-dwellers, in central Chhattisgarh the Act has been violated a number of times. In our area in 2009, six villages were relocated before their claims to land under the FRA had been settled, in the name of designating the Achanakmar Reserve a Tiger Reserve under Project Tiger. When families lose their traditional farmlands to such conservationist projects without adequate compensation, they also lose a crucial source of income and food.

Food Insecurity

Food insecurity at the household level refers to the persistent shortage of nourishing and sufficient food. Although India has, on paper, an extensive public distribution system for rations like rice and salt and oil, numerous gaps in this system prevent its full efficacy. Families designated as Below Poverty Line are entitled to 35 kg of rice per month. Currently 44.61% of rural Chhattisgarhis are living below the poverty line of Rs. 738 per month. In our rural region the number of our patients with BPL cards is around 90%. Even when citizens receive the full amount of rations they are due, the quantities fall short of the amount necessary to feed a family, often only feeding a family for 11 days out of a month. Many times citizens do not receive their full share due to "leakages" or the supply of inferior goods. Even if the public distribution system worked perfectly, at current levels it would not sufficiently meet any family's food needs let alone provide for adequate nutrition. The public distribution system centers on cheap calories provided by rice rather than a diversity of vegetables, pulses, and complex carbohydrates. The emphasis on rice (or wheat in other regions in India) represents the victory of agricultural monoculture at the expense of nutritional diversity. The prevalence of simple carbohydrates in the Indian diet is not solely or even mostly an expression of cultural factors; it is also a political condition. Such simple carbohydrates perversely predispose those who can least afford it to greater risk for diabetes among other conditions. The opening of the Indian economy and its rising GDP has not heralded a concomitant rise in the nutritional status of its population.

Gender

Gender refers to the social constructions of biological differences between men and women. While sex differences are a biological fact, gender allows us to examine how those differences are perceived and managed in a variety of social settings. Gender is a crucial category of analysis for understanding health and society because gender disparities influence a wide variety of health outcomes. To give just one example, due to the biological fact of menstruation coupled with the social condition of patriarchy that limits women's nutritional intake more than men's, women in rural India have far higher rates of iron deficiency than men.

Generic medicines

Generic medicines are those whose patents are not exclusively owned by the drug company that developed them. Drugs that are still in patent are often prohibitively priced especially for rare diseases for which there is only a small market. Patients can be priced out of treatment simply because they have a rare condition. In contrast, the formulas behind generic drugs are not patented, allowing any number of players to manufacture them. In Indian patent law, patents on new forms of medicine are prohibited unless the new form represents a substantial advance. This prevents drug companies from repeatedly renewing their exclusive patent rights on the basis of minute changes to their drugs. A number of drug manufacturers have taken advantage of India's patent laws to produce low cost drugs sold within India and across the developing world. One such organization is *Locost*, a non-profit trust dedicated to making essential drugs. Physicians should be attentive to drug costs when they make prescribing decisions. Affordable and available drugs are an essential part of health care equity.

Gond

The Gonds are the largest Scheduled Tribe group in our region of central Chhattisgarh. In contrast to the Baigas, many have adopted the lifeways of settled agriculture and have adopted some Hindu practices. Nonetheless they have retained egalitarian tribal social structures: they do not practice caste in terms of rules of purity and pollution around food and human contact.

Health Care Equity

Health care equity is the principle that all people have access to high quality health care based on their needs. An equitable health care system should provide high quality, accessible health care to all. Health equity should be distinguished from health equality. Complete health equality is impossible to obtain because different people and population groups have different chances of developing various conditions. Different people and population groups begin in different social locations and circumstances that then determine medical outcomes, and an equitable health care system caters to those differing needs.

Health Insurance

Health insurance is a form of risk management in which an entity like a government or corporation agrees to cover health costs of a large group of people so as to limit individual health costs. Insurance is a necessity to make health care accessible. Universal health insurance is one important component of health care equity. Countries with universal health insurance tend to have better health outcomes. Currently, the Indian health insurance market is divided between relatively expensive private insurance schemes that are beyond the reach of poor rural Indians and government-sponsored schemes. One government scheme, the Rashtriya Swasthya Bima Yojana (RSBY) is aimed at workers in the unorganized sector (the vast majority of Indian workers). It provides a "Smart Card" with a credit of Rs. 30,000 for families living Below the Poverty Line (BPL). The money can be used to cover medical costs as well as transportation costs. However, there are some limits to this plan's benefits. First, the benefit is limited to cases where the patient is hospitalized. This leaves the millions of rural Indians suffering from chronic illnesses or acute illnesses or injuries not requiring hospital admission without adequate coverage. In so doing it continues the misguided policy of pushing health care resources toward treatment of crises rather than preventive and promotive health. Second, many families have yet to be enrolled. Third, the RSBY is planned for a nuclear family of five: two parents and three children. In the many cases where families do not fit this pattern, the scheme falls short of the mark. Fourth, beyond a Rs. 100 transportation charge per hospitalization, families do not receive any support for the material and in-kind costs they will surely face during hospitalization, such as food charges for the family members who take care of the patient, transport costs above Rs. 100, and lost work time. Fifth, the RSBY scheme does nothing to make insurance a public good; rather, it pays private and state-run insurance companies who are not accountable to voters or taxpayers. This will also eventually lead to increasing premiums on the part of the private insurers, driving up health care costs. Sixth, the scheme leaves out those who are just above the poverty line but whose livelihoods may be demolished by an unexpected health care expense.

Hypertension

Hypertension or high blood pressure is the most common diagnosis among our patient population in central Chhattisgarh. Often hypertension goes undetected since it commonly does not result in any symptoms. This has led JSS to implement an active screening program. Hypertension, like diabetes, is commonly conceived of as a disease of affluence since obesity and low physical activity are risk factors. However, in our patient population these are not problems. Here as in much of rural India factors such as overconsumption of salt, tobacco use, stress, and genetic factors predispose patients to hypertension. Salt is commonly used to improve the taste of food, especially rice, that otherwise lacks variety. Acute and chronic stress due to deprivation and poverty also surely contribute. Hypertension can lead to heart attacks, strokes, aneurysms, heart failure, and cognitive decline.

Injections

Injection, *suji,* or *bottle lagana* refers to the common practice of turning to unlicensed medical practitioners, and often licensed practitioners, to receive injections or saline IV drips for a variety of complaints from cough to fever to pain to generalized weakness. This practice reflects patients' desire for prompt and accessible medical treatment since these injections are widely available with little wait time in small towns and even from roaming unlicensed doctors in villages. However, this practice can have a number of negative effects. First, it often delays more comprehensive treatment in serious situations. Second, the injections themselves can cause damage. They are often given at the wrong site and might damage important nerves and cause paralysis. Sometimes the site of the injection can become infected. Third, usually these injections are an inappropriate treatment, meaning that the patient's time and money goes to waste.

Malaria

Malaria is an infection of plasmodium parasites transmitted by the Anopheles mosquito. There are several types of plasmodium parasites; *Plasmodium falciparum*, present in our area of central Chhattisgarh, can cause death within 24 hours if left untreated. Clinically, malaria is characterized by high fevers, chills, headache, and, often, an enlarged spleen. In our experience, malaria is as much a political problem as a medical problem. Outcomes of malaria infection are substantially influenced by the accessibility of health care and the health levels of the patient population including factors such as anaemia and undernutrition rates. The reporting of malaria deaths is a political issue as well: many malaria cases are not diagnosed in government health institutions and thus not reported in official figures, leading to an underestimation of the malaria problem in high-burden states which are, not coincidentally, also the poorest states in India. JSS has dramatically reduced malaria rates in its catchment area through persistent surveying efforts, wide reaching bed net distribution, patient education, and training of Village Health Workers to test for and treat malaria quickly. Malaria in pregnancy predisposes mother and baby to a range of harmful outcomes including miscarriage, premature delivery, low birth weight, and maternal and neonatal death. For this reason, JSS tests each pregnant woman in its antenatal care system for malaria.

Mental illness

Mental illness refers to a variety of illness that are caused by both physiological and social factors. Such illnesses present in the same or greater proportions in rural settings as in urban settings. Some of the most common mental illnesses in our population include depression, anxiety, bipolar disorder, schizophrenia, and psychosis. In most of India, practitioners refer to the World Health Organization's *International Statistical Classification of Diseases and Related Health Problems* (ICD-10) to diagnose and classify mental illnesses. It is akin to the *Diagnostic and Statistical Manual of Mental Disorders* (DSM) used in America. In rural populations where health care is difficult to access, the primary modality of treatment for mental illness is pharmaceutical rather than psychosocial. Even then, many patients face challenges in obtaining regular medication due to medicine costs as well as travel costs and lost labour time. Patients are often unfamiliar with the allopathic model especially as it relates to the less visible mental illnesses and are therefore more likely to delay allopathic treatment and rely on folk practices until the symptoms become unbearable, including suicide attempts. *Bandhna* or the practice of tying up patients who pose risks to themselves or family members or who wander outside of the home due to their mental illness is also widespread as families face the challenges of managing their daily livelihoods alongside the need to manage a sick and disruptive patient. The acute stresses of poverty such as unemployment or low wages and under nutrition must also be considered as risk factors for and contributors to mental illness.

Postpartum Haemorrhage (PPH)

postpartum haemorrhage is one of the most common problems in pregnancy and is the leading cause of maternal mortality worldwide and in India. postpartum haemorrhage is defined as the loss of more than 500 ml or 1000 ml of blood in the mother after the delivery of a baby. It can result in anaemia, hypovolaemia (decreased blood volume) and haemorrhagic shock. It is most often caused by the retention of the placenta or membranes in the uterus or uterine atony wherein weakness of the uterine muscles prevents the compression necessary to reduce blood flow. In a population with high rates of anaemia as in much of rural India, mothers are at greater risk of harm and death from PPH. Active rather than expectant management in the third stage of labour has been proven to reduce cases of postpartum haemorrhage. postpartum haemorrhage can be prevented through administration of oxycotin or mioprostol. Manual uterine compression is also a simple technique that we at JSS have taught to our Trained Birth Attendants and Village Health Workers to stop postpartum bleeding. Since even highly trained caregivers consistently underestimate blood loss, low resource settings require an inexpensive and simple method for measuring blood loss. In about 10% of cases postpartum haemorrhage is caused by tears in the cervix that can cause the woman to rapidly bleed to death and must be repaired by suturing. The lack of adequate blood supplies for transfusion contributes to the mortality rate from PPH. While India's

Maternal Mortality Ratio (defined as maternal deaths per 100,000 live births) has declined over the past twenty years, Chhattisgarh state's ratio remains much above the national average. The India-wide ratio is, according to the most recent data, around 167 deaths per 100,000 live births. Chhattisgarh has a far higher ratio with 221 maternal deaths per 100,000 live births.

Sickle Cell Anaemia

Sickle cell anaemia is a hereditary form of anaemia in which red blood cells take a sickle shape rather than the round form healthy round blood cells. Due to their sickled shape, the red blood cells block circulation, leading to a variety of outcomes such as severe anaemia, severe joint pain crises, cardiac emergencies, strokes, and organ damage. Sickle cannot be cured but its effects can be managed through appropriate medical treatment. The drug hydroxyurea can prevent red blood cells from sickling and reduce the chances of an acute crisis. Blood transfusions when available can also help. Sickle cell disease is inherited in an autosomal recessive pattern. In other words, it is a genetic disease that occurs when both parents carry the gene. When both parents carry the gene, there is a one in four chance that the child will have sickle cell disease. Sickled cells seem to have been an evolutionary adaptation to malaria since they protect against malaria. A person with sickle cell trait will not develop severe life threatening malaria and thus the genes for the disease got selected for among populations resident in malariaous zones. While the number of sickle carriers may be an objective constant in a population, the burdens of acute sickle crises, acute chest syndrome, infection, countless missed days of school and work, depression, and death are the product of both medical and social forces which, with the requisite political will, could be substantially reduced. The disease and the sickle trait are very common in our area of Central India. In India, unfairly it seems, the disease is found among tribal group and those lower castes labeled by the state as the scheduled castes (SCs) and other backwards classes (OBCs). In our present location in central Chhattisgarh, the rate is estimated to be between 10 and 15%. The swathe of central India ranging from Maharashtra to Odisha has a high proportion of tribal residents and has been labeled "the sickle cell belt."

Tuberculosis

Tuberculosis is an infection caused by mycobacterium tuberculosis. Though most commonly thought of as a disease of the lungs, tuberculosis can manifest in any part of the body such as the spine, brain, stomach, the skin, the lymph nodes, and the joints. Multiple sputum cultures are usually required to diagnose the disease in suspected pulmonary TB but even then the tests can give false negatives. About one third of the world's population carries latent TB. Among healthy populations only about 10% ever come down with active TB. However, in our deprived and malnourished region, latent cases are far more likely to become active due to weakened immune systems. TB is difficult to treat because it requires a six month long course of multiple drugs. The length and complexity of treatment often leads patients to default. In cases of treatment failures, patients are at a higher risk for drug resistant TB. TB is a good example of a biosocial disease because the progression from latent to active TB and prognoses are determined by nutritional status, HIV status, and other social factors. Among 1517 adults with TB seen from 2010 to 2013, males with TB had a median BMI of 16.2 and women had a median BMI had 15.8 BMI. Among the 95 deaths in this sample, 72% were in patients with BMIs less than 16, stark evidence of the ruinous effect of low nutritional status on TB outcomes.

Undernutrition

Undernutrition refers to the inadequate consumption of one or more major nutrients, often but not always due to food insecurity. Severe undernutrition is defined as a body mass index lower than 16. Undernutrition can cause a number of health problems including anaemia, fatigue, vision problems, cognitive impairments, depression, skeletal deformities, uneven gait, and difficulty in healing from infection. Childhood malnutrition results in lifelong low weight and height and can also cause permanent cognitive impairments. Malnutrition opens the door to the opportunistic attacks of tuberculosis. The connection between malnutrition and tuberculosis has lead JSS to advocate for the prescription of nutritional supplementation (food) to TB patients. While this is an important part of treating active TB cases, it does little to prevent TB in the first place in the current conditions of food insecurity and undernutrition. Most social scientists now agree that famines and food deprivation are the result not of shortages of food overall but the maldistrubtion of food.

Unlicensed medical provider/Jholachhap

An unlicensed medical provider is someone who sees and treats patients without a formal medical license. Unlicensed medical providers can take a variety of forms and often provide frontline medical care in areas where licensed medical providers are unwilling to settle and practice. Unlicensed medical providers lack the requisite training to provide high quality medical care and make mistakes that may put lives at risk. Also, unlicensed medical practitioners may provide unnecessary treatments to patients that amount to a waste of money for the patient. One alternative name for unlicensed medical practitioner is *jholachhap*, or one who moves around carrying a *jhola,* the bag full of medical supplies carried by many of these roaming practitioners. The prevalence and influence of the unlicensed medical practitioners is a reflection of the shortage of accessible medical practitioners especially in rural areas and reflects peoples' need and desire for accessible health care.

acknowledgement

Jan Swasthya Sahyog gratefully acknowledges the Tata Trusts for their generous and continuous support that allowed us to share these stories from Ganiyari and to produce this Atlas of Rural Health. We would also like to thank the Tata Trust for their support of the services we have been able to provide to the people of Chhattisgarh.

TATA TRUSTS

SIR DORABJI TATA TRUST • SIR RATAN TATA TRUST • JAMSETJI TATA TRUST • N.R. TATA TRUST • J.R.D. TATA TRUST

end note

Many people have contributed to the making of this book over a number of years. They shared stories, brought us photos, spoke of the people they met. All these accounts were slowly gathered and are presented here in the form of this Atlas.

This has been a collective and collaborative effort with what at times seemed impossible deadlines particularly for those working at the busy Jan Swasthya Sahyog clinics. We would like to thank all the doctors who have worked here, past and present, nurses and health field coordinators.

We would particularly like to mention Jonathan Fine, Priyank Jain, Timothy Laux, Sri Shamasundar, Brett Lewis, Somnath Mukherjee, Prashant Gogia, Ajay Verma, Anupam Kanodia, Ashwini Mahajan, Vivek Muthuramalingam, Victor Patterson and Abhijit Gadewar – who wrote narratives, commentaries and blogs and Rebecca Grapevine for the keywords and index.

Tom Pietrasik, Vivek Muthuramalingam and numerous amateur photographers, thank you for your photos that speak, at times more than any number of words could.

Also many thanks to Rukminee Guha Thakurta for all her inputs and advice on making a book and Yasmeen Tayebbhai for designing the book cover at such short notice. Grateful thanks are due to Moyna Mazumdar, for her expert editing of the narratives and many useful comments, also at short notice.

Thanks also to Vrinda Manocha and especially Priya Jain, for their help in editing and putting together this book. But for their final heave, this Atlas might never have been made.

index

C

D

E

F

G

H

I

J

K

L

M

N

O

P

R

S

T

Z

My Notes

My Notes